The Pneumonias

Monroe Karetzky Burke A. Cunha
Robert D. Brandstetter

The Pneumonias

Foreword by John B. West

With 55 illustrations

Springer-Verlag
New York Berlin Heidelberg London Paris
Tokyo Hong Kong Barcelona Budapest

Monroe Karetzky, MD
Director, Pulmonary and Critical Care
Assistant Director of Medicine
Newark Beth Israel Hospital
Newark, NJ 07112
USA

Burke A. Cunha, MD
Chief, Infectious Disease Division
Vice Chairman, Department of Medicine
Winthrop-University Hospital
Mineola, NY 11501
USA

Robert D. Brandstetter, MD
Associate Director of Medicine
Chief, Critical Care Division
New Rochelle Hospital Medical Center
New Rochelle, NY 10802
USA

Library of Congress Cataloging-in-Publication Data
Karetzky, Monroe.
The pneumonias/Monroe Karetzky, Burke A. Cunha, Robert D. Brandstetter.
p. cm.
Includes bibliographical references and index.
ISBN 0-387-97945-X.—ISBN 3-540-97945-X
1. Pneumonia. I. Cunha, Burke A. II. Brandstetter, Robert D. III. Title.
[DNLM: 1. Pneumonia. 2. Respiratory Tract Infections—diagnosis. WC 202 K18p]
RC771.K37 1993
616.2'41—dc20
DNLM/DLC
for Library of Congress 92-49615

Printed on acid-free paper.

Production managed by Dimitry L. Loseff; manufacturing supervised by Jacqui Ashri.
Typeset by Best-set Typesetter Ltd., Hong Kong.
Printed and bound by Edwards Brothers, Inc., Ann Arbor, MI.
Printed in the United States of America.

9 8 7 6 5 4 3 2 1

ISBN 0-387-97945-X Springer-Verlag New York Berlin Heidelberg
ISBN 3-540-97945-X Springer-Verlag Berlin Heidelberg New York

Dedications

The text is dedicated to all clinicians and scientists who have enhanced our understanding of the etiology, recognition and management of pneumonias.

M.K.

For Marie, Zachary, and Cheston—Thank you for your constant love, support, and encouragement. You mean everything to me.

B.A.C.

To God, my wife Deanne, children, family, colleagues, friends, and especially Dr. Martin Weiner, who have kept me alive with love and therapy to complete this book.

R.D.B.

Foreword

It is a pleasure to contribute a brief foreword to this new, comprehensive text on the pneumonias. The 1980s saw an explosion of knowledge in pulmonary science, and there is every reason to expect it to continue through the end of the century. As a result, it is becoming increasingly difficult to keep up with all the important advances, even in a restricted area of interest. For this reason, books such as the present one that collate the latest findings on an important clinical topic in a convenient, readable form provide a valuable service.

This book is a salutary reminder that there is life beyond molecular and cell biology. Important though these disciplines are, some of us regret the lemming-like rush into these fashionable fields at the expense of more traditional pulmonary science. One result of this rush has been an increasingly large number of residents and fellows who are unable to interpret the results of blood gas assays or who are completely at sea when presented with a patient who requires mechanical ventilation. The present perception that research funding is available only in molecular and cell biology has produced some unfortunate distortion of training programs. I pity the poor medical student in some of our most prestigious medical schools who is taught by a molecular biologist or neurophysiologist how the lung works.

I wish the book well. The pneumonias have been with us since the beginning of medicine and look well able to survive into the twenty-first century. Indeed, with a little help from the human immunodeficiency virus, they seem to be more enterprising than ever. But then, the pneumonias have never been respecters of persons and traditionally have invaded the very young to the very old. If patients ultimately benefit from the knowledge presented here, the book will have served its purpose.

John B. West, M.D., Ph.D., DSc
La Jolla, California

Preface

There are few texts devoted to lower respiratory tract infections, and those available approach pneumonia principally from an infectious or pulmonary disease perspective. *The Pneumonias* is the first and only multidisciplinarian book to address the scientific and clinical aspects of pneumonia. It is an integrated presentation of the pathophysiology and clinical basics of pneumonia, treating lower respiratory tract infections as a generic pathologic process. It attempts to strike a balance in the practice of science and the art of medicine. The book, however, does not suggest eliminating the need for consultants' services; indeed it focuses on the diagnostic and therapeutic indications for seeking their assistance. In some cases, it even encourages early consultation when their expertise would be most opportune at that time in the illness. The goal of this book is to enhance interaction between specialist and generalist, thereby ensuring a more favorable outcome for the patient.

The book is divided into chapters organized in chronologic order, so each topic provides a basis for the succeeding chapter. We have also written each chapter, however, so the incorporated material is independent from that in other chapters in the book. This approach is accomplished by discussing infectious pneumonias as clinical syndromes rather than as individual infections caused by specific organisms. We have also avoided the inclusion of exotic etiologic agents, which can readily be reviewed in standard texts.

We believe we have included a wealth of useful information concerning assessment of infectious lung diseases not available in this format elsewhere. For example, there are chapters on clues to the etiology of pneumonia and pulmonary disorders mimicking lung infection, and pitfalls to avoid when diagnosing infectious pneumonia. Finally we have included a novel chapter on hospital-discharge strategies for physicians managing patients with pneumonia. This book should be of practical use to all individuals treating patients with pneumonia.

Robert D. Brandstetter, M.D.
Burke A. Cunha, M.D.
Monroe S. Karetzky, M.D.

Acknowledgments

It is with respect and admiration that I have had the pleasure of working with Eleanor Mangieri and Lucille Mellaci.

R.D.B.

Much thanks to the staff of Springer–Verlag for sticking with the three of us to the completion of this text.

M.K.
B.A.C.
R.D.B.

Contents

Contributors

Robert D. Brandstetter, M.D., F.C.C.P., Associate Director of Medicine, Chief, Critical Care Division, New Rochelle Hospital Medical Center; Professor of Clinical Medicine, New York Medical College

Burke A. Cunha, M.D., F.A.C.P., Chief, Infectious Disease Division, Vice Chairman, Department of Medicine, Winthrop-University Hospital, Mineola, New York; Associate Professor of Medicine, State University of New York at Stony Brook

Leonard D. Epifano, M.D., Director, Pulmonary Function Laboratory & Respiratory Laboratory, New Rochelle Hospital Medical Center

Monroe Karetzky, M.D., F.C.C.P., Director of Pulmonary & Critical Care Division, Assistant Director of Medicine, Newark Beth Israel Medical Center, Newark, New Jersey; Associate Professor of Medicine, Associate Director; Division of Pulmonary Medicine, Associate Director; Division of Critical Care Medicine, UMDNJ-New Jersey Medical School

Andrew Pugliese, M.D., Infectious Disease Fellow, Winthrop-University Hospital, Mineola, New York

1 Historical Aspects of Pneumonia

LEONARD D. EPIFANO and ROBERT D. BRANDSTETTER

The search for knowledge and understanding of respiration and pulmonary diseases dates back to ancient times, in particular to the Greeks. Led by Hippocrates (circa 460–360 BC), the first systematic method for analyzing individual diseases was developed.[1] Hippocrates' approach to establishing the diagnosis of pneumonia was translated from the original description by Francis Adams of Great Britain in 1859 as follows[2]:

> Peripneumonia and pleuritic affections, are to be thus observed: If the fever be acute, and if there be pains on either side, or in both, and if expiration be attended with pain, if cough be present, and the sputa expectorated be of a blond or livid color, or likewise thin, frothy, and florid, or having any other character different from the common . . .

which implies in sequence that the clinical diagnosis of peripneumonia is established. His description of the findings characteristic of recovery from the disease is as follows.[2]

> When pneumonia is at its height, the case is beyond remedy if he be not purged and it is bad if he has dyspnoea, and the urine is thin and acrid and if sweat comes out about the neck and head, for such sweats are bad as proceeding from the suffocation, rales, and the violence of the disease which is obtaining the upper hand, unless there be a copious evacuation of thick urine, and the sputa be concocted [sputa are concocted when they resemble pus]; when either of these come on spontaneously, that will carry off the disease.

Claudius Galen was born in Pergamos, Greece in 130 AD and died in the city of his birth in 199 AD.[3] He contributed little to the clinical concepts related to pneumonia, but his work in anatomy and physiology established permanent recognition for him in medical history.[1] Although Galen lacked Hippocrates' objectivity and exactitude when describing medical phenomena, he was looked on as the greatest Greek physician after Hippocrates. His major contribution to the understanding of pneumonia was the anatomic demonstration of the difference between pleurisy and pneumonia.[3]

Aretaeus (130–199 AD), a Cappadocian, left a significant legacy of medical information, but unfortunately there has been little documentation detailing his activities. It is believed that he lived during the second century AD and that he was a contemporary of Galen. He practiced medicine in Cappadocia, a mountainous area in Asia Minor and did his medical writings in Greek. As a clinician, Aretaeus is ranked next to Hippocrates in regard to his presentation of the characteristics of a large number of diseases, including pneumonia, diabetes, tetanus, elephantiasis, diphtheria, epilepsy, and mental disorders. Amazingly, he was the first to describe decussation of the pyramidal tracts within the central nervous system.[3]

Aretaeus, in a description of the physical findings of acute pneumonia, made the observation that if the pleura becomes involved with infection pain related to respiration appears.[2]

> This is what we call Peripneumonia, being an inflammation of the lungs, with acute fever, when they are attended with heaviness of the chest, freedom from pain, provided the lungs alone are inflamed, but if any of the membranes by which it is connected with the chest, be inflamed, pain is also present.

Aretaeus' observation represented a pioneer effort in the understanding of the difference in the nerve supply to the lung compared to the pleura.

After the deaths of Galen and Aretaeus, a movement surfaced that discouraged all forms of scientific advancement. This attitude became so pervasive that it often gave rise to acts of violence, typified by the burning of a library at Alexandria by a fanatical group of Christians in 391 AD. Progress in European medicine was then to remain dormant for almost 14 centuries.[1]

Fortunately, the hiatus in the advancement of medical knowledge within the Greco-Roman world was filled by a group of Arabic-speaking physicians who lived in Syria, Persia, and later Spain. Of this group, Rhazes (860–932 AD) was the most famous and respected.[3] His quote with respect to the optimal approach to achieving a cure in various illnesses in essence is a restatement of the Roman dictum *primum non nocere* and is as follows[4]:

> In treating a patient, let your first thought be to strengthen his natural vitality. If you strengthen that, you remove ever so many ills without more ado. If you weaken it, however, by the remedies that you use, you always work harm.

Rhazes' management of serious diseases of the lungs and trachea was far ahead of his time. He recommended tracheotomy in situations where severe difficulty breathing existed and even described the technical surgical approach to it.[4]

Following the era of Arabic dominance in medicine, European influence resurfaced with the death of the Medieval Period and the advent of the Renaissance Period. The philosophy of the Middle Ages was slowly but inexorably replaced by acceptance of individual contributions not only in the field of medicine but in all other areas where progress could be achieved only through enlightenment, objectivity, and abandonment of superstition.

The predominant emphasis during this period was on morphology. It was the era of anatomists, who, by elucidating the structure and function of organ systems, paved the way for the eventual effective management of diseases of these organ systems. Interestingly, the major contributions to anatomy during this period was through the efforts of a large group of artists, whose masterful works have survived to the present day: Luca Signorelli, Michael Angelo, Raphael, Verocchio, and his student Leonardo Da Vinci (1452–1519).[1]

Leonardo Da Vinci's efforts were probably the most notable of the group; and through sketches of dissected subjects he left the medical world a legacy of accurate representations of the entirety of human anatomy. His major efforts were directed toward the musculature, but accurate drawings of the heart, lungs, and blood vessels provided a foundation for future anatomists. After Leonardo, Andreas Vesalius (1514–1564) took the reins of anatomic study and with a great deal of dynamic effort succeeded in converting the image of anatomy from a dull, uninteresting subject to a viable, absorbing science. Vesalius eventually achieved a reputation as the most dominant figure in European medicine following Galen and preceding William Harvey (1578–1657).[1]

William Harvey's place in medical history was secured by his description of the cardiovascular circulation, and the Italian anatomist Marcello Malpighi (1628–1694) ensured his own position by demonstrating the pulmonary circulation, including the capillary anastomosis between pulmonary arteries and veins.[1] After the anatomists provided the world of medicine a tangible understanding of the morphology of the lungs, there appeared on the horizon a group of clinicians who capitalized on their descriptions. These men concentrated their efforts on formulating a systematized collection of data that would provide clinical insight into confirming the diagnosis of pneumonia at the bedside. Utilizing the five senses to the fullest advantage, they established the principles of physical diagnosis; in this light, they could be viewed as the first medical detectives.

The first of these gifted individuals was Leopold Auenbrugger, an Austrian (1722–1809) who owed his discovery of percussion to the fact that his father was an innkeeper who kept a large number of wine casks. As a young man Leopold's duty was to check periodically the wine level in his father's casks. He subsequently applied this experience to the discovery of percussion. Auenbrugger imaginatively wrote in connection with the eventual medical applications of percussion that: "Casks, as long as they are empty are resonant everywhere, but when filled lose this resonance in proportion as the volume of air they contain is diminished." Auenbrugger's text, *New Invention by Means of Percussing the Human*

Chest as a Sign of Detecting Obscure Diseases in the Interior of the Chest, was published in 1761 and has endured as one of the great classics of medicine.[2]

In Garrison's *History of Medicine*, Auenbrugger's approach to percussion is described as follows.

> Our author's first proposition is that the chest of a healthy subject when struck, sounds like a cloth-covered drum. He then proceeds to outline his special method of eliciting information by striking the chest gently with the points of the fingers brought together (stretched out straight and forward flexed), the patient holding his breath; a muffled sound or one of higher pitch than usual indicates the presumable site of a diseased condition. He ascertained the sounds produced by tapping over fluids injected into the chest of a cadaver, localized pectoral fremitus, and carried his finding over into bedside practice including treatment by thoracentesis.

These efforts by Auenbrugger were largely criticized and voided by his contemporaries, and they remained unaccepted until Corvisart began to employ them in 1808, one year before Auenbrugger's death. Out of respect for Auenbrugger's contributions and because he truly believed in their accuracy and authenticity, Corvisart adhered strictly to his predecessor's methods. Corvisart quoted, "It is he and the beautiful invention which of right belongs to him that I wish to recall to life."[3]

Rene Theophile-Hyancinthe Laennec (1781–1826) made a large number of contributions to medicine, the most significant of which was his invention of the stethoscope in 1816. It was followed by his classic, *Traite Auscultation Mediate*, which was published in 1819.[2] Maurice Letulle, who lived during the midnineteenth century and who collaborated with Jules Dejerine in work on Friedreich's disease, is credited with stating that, 'Every physician throughout the world, who auscultates any part whatsoever of a human being, is by this act alone a disciple of Laennec!"[2] This comment in essence immortalized Laennec throughout all future ages of medicine.

Laennec's stethoscope evolved from a roll of paper to a rod of wood and finally to a cylinder of wood 1 foot long. During his writing of the *Traite*, Laennec was in poor health and sensed his imminent death. He wrote before his death, "I know that I risked my life, but the book I am going to publish will be, I hope useful enough sooner or later to be of more value than the life of a man." Ironically, Laennec died in 1826 of tuberculosis, shortly after publication of the second edition of *Traite*. Laennec's major contribution to pulmonary medicine was his accurate description of the physical findings of pneumonia and other pulmonary diseases.[2] Indeed the level of exactitude he achieved in his work on auscultation was never surpassed, and the terminology he organized and created has remained for the most part until the present day. He described the crepitus rattle[2] as a pathognomonic sign of the first stage of pneumonia. In sequence, he then observed the gradual disappearance of the rattle as hepatization takes place.[2]

In his treatise on the diseases of the chest and on mediate auscultation, he wrote, "I regard it [the crepitus rattle] as the most practically useful of all the stethoscopic signs, inasmuch as it points out in its very earliest state one of the most severe and most common diseases, and thereby enables the physician to apply his means with much more chance of success than he could have done even a few hours later."[2]

Laennec's insight and genius are clearly demonstrable in his description of the physical findings elicited during evolution of the pneumonitic process, and he carefully provided documented descriptions of the percussive and auscultatory findings during the phases of hepatization, suppuration, and resolution.[2]

In his treatise he further quoted in sequence.[2]

> When the inflammation has reached the degree of hepatization, we no longer perceive in the affected part, either the crepitus rattle or the respiratory sound; and the absence of the phenomena is frequently the only sign we have of hepatization having taken place. Bronchophonism exists near the roots of the lungs, or in the upper lobes, in which places the bronchial tubes are largest. When the pneumonia is central, bronchophonism either does not exist at all, or is very obscure; it becomes more and more manifest as the inflammation approaches the surface of the lungs. By means of this sign, I have frequently been able to indicate, previously to opening the chest, the precise point where a central peripulmonary had reached the exterior of the organ. This is easily accounted for by the fact that a hepatized lung is a better conductor of sound than a healthy one,—bronchophonism being nothing more than the resonance of the voice within the bronchia of the inflamed part. A pleuritic effusion, if posterior to the hepatization, renders bronchophonism stronger by compressing and condensing the superficial parts of the lungs not yet affected by the inflammation.

With a great degree of exactitude, Laennec was able to distinguish precisely the auscultatory differences between bronchophony and pectoriloquy: "When the hepatization is near the surface, and involves within it bronchial tubes of a considerable size, as when it has its seat at the roots or in the top of the lungs, bronchophonism becomes then almost like pectoriloquism."[2]

Laennec was well aware of the diagnostic clues provided by percussion of the lungs.[2]

> These are the physical signs of hepatization, which is always further accompanied by a dull sound on percussion, over the affected parts, except in the case where the pneumonia is central. In this case, and especially if the hepatization occupies the centre of the left inferior lobe and the lower part of the right side be naturally imperfectly sonorous, as commonly happens, percussion will frequently furnish us with no useful result or will at most lead us to suspect the affection of the left lower lobe.

Laennec was also aware of the potentially equivocal findings on auscultation of the right lower lobe because of the anatomic position of the liver, and he recognized the limitations of percussion for substantiating the diagnosis of pneumonia by physical findings.[2]

> [I]f the hepatization occupies the right inferior lobe, percussion will only then enable us to recognize its presence where we had previously ascertained the natural sonorousness of this part; since there are many persons in whom the right side of the chest, as high as the fourth or fifth rib, is naturally destitute of sound. In almost all cases, when the points hepatized are of small extent, percussion gives us no assistance.

Concerning the auscultatory findings associated with suppuration, Laennec wrote,[2]

> The infiltration of pus within the pulmonary tissue furnishes no new sign as long as the pus remains concrete. When this begins to soften, we perceive in the bronchia a more or less distinct mucous rattle occasioned either by the introduction of the pus into them or by the more copious mucous secretion which then takes place, sympathetic of the suppurative process going on within the pulmonary substance.

Finally, concerning the auscultatory findings on resolution of pneumonia, Laennec made the following observations.[2]

> When resolution takes place before hepatization has supervened, the crepitus rattle becomes daily less perceptible while the natural sound of respiration becomes gradually more distinct, and at last is alone heard. When hepatization has taken place, its resolution is invariably announced by the return of the crepitus rattle. I have never seen this sign wanting in any case which I have been able to examine daily. I commonly denominate it—the renewed crepitus rattle (rhonchus crepitans redux). M. Andral has noticed it in most of his examples of pneumonia cured [an anecdotal communication by one of Laennec's contemporaries]. To the crepitus rattle is gradually joined the natural sound of respiration which becomes daily more distinct and at last exists alone. The crepitus rattle equally announces the resolution of the pneumonia when it has arrived at the stage of suppuration, but in this case, it is usually preceded by a mucous or submucous rattle, indicating the softening of a part of the pus. In this case, the natural sound of respiration returns much more slowly than in the preceding instances. At the expiration of a few days, or even sometimes of a few hours, the crepitus rattle becomes subcrepitus, indicating the supervention of oedema which usually attends the resolution of this stage of peripneumony. The same thing is observed when oedema accompanies the resolution of the other two stages of the inflammation. When the disease has extended to the greater part of the lungs, the extreme points and the parts most recently attacked are usually those in which resolution commences, the contrary, however is sometimes the case.

Josef Skoda (1805–1881) of Pilsen, Bohemia carried on the efforts of both Auenbrugger and Laennec by expanding observations and adding refinement to percussion and auscultation.[2] Skoda was one of the most revered members of the Vienna school of physicians and was famous for his diagnostic capabilities.[2] His ability to unravel and clarify difficult problems in medical diagnosis was recognized throughout Europe, and he astonished his peers with the acuity and accuracy of his conclusions at the bedside. He paid particular attention and concentrated his efforts on diseases of the chest, writing extensively on the physical findings elicited during the course of a wide variety of pulmonary diseases including pneumonia. His treatise on percussion and auscultation (*Abhandlung uber Perkussion und Auskultation*) was published in 1839 and remains one of the great contributions to the understanding and application of physical diagnosis.[2] In this work, Skokda "classifies the different sounds in the chest by categories, ranged according to musical pitch and tonality and alternating from full to hollow, clear to dull, tympanitic to muffled, and high to deep."[3] Much of its contents and principles remain in use in medical school curricula today. Skoda was the first to discover that hyperresonance or an increased tympanitic sound is present above any portion of the lung that was decreased in volume, either by an accumulation of pleural fluid or atelectasis. He also discerned that the percussion sound in patients with otherwise normal lungs is distinctly more resonant in individuals with thin chest walls compared to those with chests of greater girth.[2] The term *skodaic resonance*, representing the drum-like sound heard with pneumonia and pericardial effusion, remains a tribute to the man and is used today as accepted medical terminology.[3]

Following the expert and ingenious observations of these men who provided medicine with the means to diagnose pneumonia and all of its associated complications effectively, there appeared the pioneers who studied the causative factors involved in the appearance of this disease. Some of these individuals obviously made their appearances concurrently with their colleagues who contributed so much to the physical findings observed in pneumonia.

The founders of this new world of investigation and identification of the invisible creatures who were responsible for pneumonia were Louis Pasteur and Robert Koch. The former was also the pioneer of modern preventive inoculation against disease, and Koch developed the correct theory of the existence of specific infectious diseases.

Louis Pasteur (1822–1895), initially a fisherman, finally developed an interest in chemistry and embarked on his true destiny while a student at Bescancon. Pasteur obtained his degree at the Ecole Normale at Paris in 1847.[3] Pasteur's contributions to infectious disease stemmed from his basic work in identifying and associating microorganisms with myriad disease processes, in both animals and humans. He was the first to recognize the differences between aerobic and anaerobic bacteria, and the terms aerobism and anaerobism are credited to him. The ability of microorganisms to convert oxygen to carbon dioxide (1861) was discovered by Pasteur. His work paved the way to the eventual discrediting of the erroneous principle of spontaneous generation that had prevailed for centuries.

Pasteur's achievement in the application of vaccines to successfully immunize infected animals and humans represents one of the monumental discoveries in the history of medicine. The effectiveness achieved by the vaccination process was based on Pasteur's demonstration of the principle that the pathogenic properties of microorganisms could be attenuated or increased by successive passages through the bodies of appropriate animals. In other words, the origin or extinction of any infectious disease could be due to variations in external conditions that might either strengthen or weaken the causative agent.[3] This concept provided major enlightenment to the medical world, not only of that time but to the present day. It represented application of Darwin's theories of natural selection and survival of the fittest to a new world of organisms, invisible to the naked eye but capable of destroying the visible creatures of the world, including humans, if not effectively controlled. Because of Pasteur's disinterest in bacteriologic morphology, he has received a much lesser degree of recognition for his discovery of the staphylococcal organism (*Staphylococcus pyogenes*) found in boils and for the streptococcus responsible for puerperal sepsis (*Streptococcus pyogenes*). Pasteur's genius was not limited to medical achievements alone, as he was also responsible for the instruction and inspirational motivation of a large coterie of investigational giants who subsequently made monumental contributions to the world of medicine that have remained significant to the present day. Pasteur's followers included Metchnikoff, Roux, Yersin, Calmette, Chantemesse, Chamberland, and Pottevin.[3]

Robert Koch (1843–1910) was born in Klausthal, Hannover and obtained his medical degree at Göttingen in 1866. Predominantly known for his three postulates, Koch also contributed a vast compendium of bacteriologic information to medical science. Koch initially embarked on a career in private practice after service in the Franco-Prussian War but soon became bored and sought greater stimulation by providing private microscopic studies and analysis.

He launched his career in bacteriology in 1876 with an extensive study of the life history of the anthrax bacillus. Koch was able to grow the anthrax organism in pure culture over a period of several generations and showed that the bacillus was capable of producing the disease in various animals. His findings were strongly refuted by many of the medical investigators of his day but were subsequently confirmed by Pasteur. Koch's work in establishing a means for identifying bacteria by the use of fixing, drying, and staining them with various dyes represented the initial milestone in achieving an understanding of all infectious disease followed by the eventual discovery of appropriate forms of therapy.[3] In 1882 Koch's greatest achievement, discovery of the tubercle bacillus, ensured him a permanent place in medical history. The discovery was accomplished by special culture and staining methods, and the publication included a statement of the first of "Koch's postulates" establishing the pathogenic character of a given microorganism. He was appointed professor of bacteriology in 1885 at the University of Berlin, where like Pasteur he was sought out by pupils from all corners of the medical world. Among these men who were later destined to become renown in their own right were Gaffky, Loffler, Pfeiffer, Welch, and Kitasato.[3]

Pneumonia of the Preantibiotic Era

Bubonic Plague

Because of the enormous impact bubonic plaque has had on the world's population, and because of the even greater lethality of the pneumonic complications of plague, this great decimator of humankind through the ages should have some mention in any review on the history of pneumonia.

Bubonic plague is a highly epidemic disease that has claimed millions of lives. There have been three recorded outbreaks of the plague in human history. The first started during the sixth century AD, the second during the fourteenth century, and the third just prior to and through World War II. The bacterium responsible for bubonic plague is *Yersinia* (formerly *Pasteurella*) *pestis*. The organism thrives in the rodent population, particularly rats, and is transmitted to humans by the rat flea (*Xenopsylla cheopis*). The human body flea (*Pulex irritans*) is a poor transmitter of the disease, and so it is rare to see the disease passed from one human to another. Consequently, maintenance of the chain-like continuity of any epidemic depends on a large population of infected rats. Infected humans have such low levels of the plague organism in their bloodstreams that they do not represent a serious contagion factor when afflicted with the disease. However, should the patient develop the pneumonic form of the plague, the disease can be readily transmitted from human to human via droplets contained in every breath or cough. The pneumonic form of the plague follows a highly accelerated course, and death may occur within a matter of hours.[5]

Influenza

Although sporadic outbreaks of bubonic plague occurred from the fourth to the twentieth century, the major toll on human life was inflicted by the "black death" that claimed close to 43 million European lives during the fourteenth century.[5] Six centuries later, influenza became the plague of modern times.

The history of influenza has not been clearly understood because of poor documentation and the overlap of influenza symptoms with so many other diseases. There have been many entities described in the medical literature that either bore a resemblance to influenza or indeed may have represented true influenza but were too nonspecific to categorize accurately. Medical historians generally accept the sixteenth century accounts of influenza as the most accurate. Isolated accounts of influenza epidemics date back as far as the twelfth century AD and subsequently during the thirteenth to eighteenth centuries, predominantly in Europe. The world's first accepted pandemic of influenza was recorded in 1580.[5]

This failure to focus attention on the disease is probably related to its usual innocuousness associated with a low death rate. Certainly, influenza was not looked on with the same dread as was the devastating bubonic plague. It was not until the pandemic of 1918–1920 that the medical world became aware of the lethal capabilities of this disease. The 1918 outbreak gained as much respect as the plague in terms of its ability to kill because of the frequency of pneumonia with which it was associated and the subsequent high mortality rates. The progress of the pneumonia was accelerated, and death usually occurred within 48 hours. All efforts to treat the pneumonia and its secondary complications were futile. The premortem descriptions of victims were as horrible as the previous descriptions of the plague and created enormous fear of the disease throughout the world. Patients were described as "turning blue" and their bodies "the color of slate" by eyewitnesses who survived.[5]

The available statistics, including both incidence and mortality, are not accepted as accurate because of the worldwide disorder related to the ravages of World War I. The situation was further clouded by the fact that influenza was not a reportable disease in many countries, and mortality as a result of pneumonia was often listed under an independent category. Conservative estimates, however, serve to indicate the truly devastating consequences of this pandemic. The worldwide death toll was estimated conservatively at 22 million. India was hardest hit, with a death rate of 4% population and a total death rate with a low estimate of 12 million.[5]

The impact of both the bubonic plague and the influenza pandemic of 1918–1920 certainly left humankind with a healthy respect for the great killer that pneumonia could be in the appropriate setting and conditions. Despite the many creative investigators who labored long hours to identify the bacteria that cause of pneumonia and to uncover and describe physical findings that aid in diagnosing the disease, the treatment for pneumonia through the early part of the twentieth century was largely symptomatic and consequently ineffectual with a consequent high associated mortality rate. Therapy included emetics, use of counterirritants, cathartics, gastric irritants, digitalis, sedatives and hypnotics, respiratory stimulants, and finally oxygen.[5] Probably oxygen represented the only therapeutic agent that may have temporarily prolonged life.

A major step forward in the treatment of pneumonia occurred with typing of the pneumococcus. The initial work was performed by a research team at the Rockefeller Institute in 1912 and was followed by more precise classification of pneumococcal types by F. Griffith, an English bacteriologist. Griffith utilized the information provided by the Rockefeller Institute team and succeeded in developing a pneumococcal classification by types from sputum samples collected between 1920 and 1928. However, therapeutic application of the typing of the pneumococcus by the development of antisera was delayed until 1944, which proved to be ill-timed because the clinical use of already discovered antibacterial agents was under way.[5]

The sulfonamides were first discovered in 1908 by a Viennese student, Paul Gelmo; but clinical application had to wait until 1935, when prontosil, an azodye, was shown to be effective in curing laboratory mice of deadly streptococcal infections. Soon the sulfonamides were used on a large scale beginning with the sulfonamide found in prontosil and progressing to other members of the sulfonamide family that had a higher level of bacteriostatic action.[5]

In September 1929 Sir Alexander Fleming, a Scottish bacteriologist working in St. Mary's Hospital in London, discovered penicillin by a combination of prodigious effort and serendipity. Fleming noted that a mold had appeared on one of his petri dishes and had engulfed and destroyed staphylococcal colonies on the same dish. The mold was erroneously identified as *Penicillium rubrum* initially but subsequently was correctly shown to be *Penicillium notatum*. This early error in identification was of little consequence, as the impact of the discovery would soon have a monumental effect on the treatment of pneumonia and a multitude of other infectious diseases. Because of the difficulties of extracting, purifying, and stabilizing penicillin, it was not used on a human subject until January 27, 1941 to treat the complication of a febrile reaction subsequently attributed to a pyrogen found in the material injected. Refinements in the penicillin preparations provided, including separation of pyrogenic contaminants by chromatography, soon led to mass production of the first bactericidal agent ever therapeutically employed in the treatment of disease.[5]

The appearance of penicillin introduced a revolutionary approach to the management of pneumonia. With the ongoing introduction of additional antibiotics, mortality rates dropped precipitously except in the elderly, the chronically ill, and those with debilitating diseases.

Modern Investigation

A tribute to the investigational abilities of modern "pioneers in medicine" can be seen in the elucidation of the causative agent of *Legionella pneumophila*. In July 21–24, 1976 a convention was held by the American Legion at the Bellevue-Stratford Hotel in Philadelphia. During the 2-week period after this meeting, 182 of the legionnaires contracted a mysterious respiratory ailment, with the death toll eventually reaching 29. Efforts were made to identify the causative organism without success.[6]

It is interesting to note how the adage "the more things change, the more they remain the same" was fortified and confirmed by the press speculations concerning this "mysterious killer." Note the "enlightened" reaction of the *Philadelphia Daily News* of August 9, 1976: The disease was attributed variously to (1) Polish Communists, who some theorized were hiding aboard the Polish tall ship on the Delaware River and making nocturnal forays to the Bellevue to spread a specially formulated killer disease; (2) magicians who held a conference at the Bellevue before the legionnaires and whose acts included birds and rabbits, which may have left contaminated droppings in the hotel; and (3) local drug companies accused by the Veterans of Foreign Wars of being part of a "possible conspiracy" in which lethal flu virus was seeded among legionnaires to create an epidemic and thus allow the drug companies to make a fortune selling vaccines.[7] On the basis of these commentaries, this twentieth century tabloid could justifiably have been labeled "The Inquisitional Gazette," as it represented the same type of impedimental thinking (and opposition) that the great innovative minds faced centuries ago.

When the outbreak occurred, initial speculation focused on the possibility of a highly lethal virus that had made an uncharacteristic early seasonal (prewinter) appearance as had the unidentified strain that caused the pandemic of 1918.[7] A bacteriologic Armageddon was soon predicted by a large number of prophets of doom. Sanity prevailed, among a small number of cooler heads within the world of medical investigation, however, and eventually the mystery was unraveled. The first chapter of this mystery dates back to 1943 during the epidemic of Fort Bragg fever. This infection was characterized by a pretibial rash that resembled erythema nodosum. During the outbreak Hugh Tatlock, one of the medical investigators studying the epidemiology of the problem, reported recovery of the first isolate of a *Legionella* species, a strain of *L. micdadei*. Tatlock eventually found that the primary causative agent was *Leptospira autumnalis*, and that the *Legionella* organism demonstrated when the blood of an afflicted soldier was cultured was a secondary invader. These observations were consistent with the subsequent clinical findings characteristic of *Legionella* infections, none of which described a pretibial rash. Outbreaks of acute respiratory disease caused by the *Legionella* organism have been traced back as early as 1959, with no success at attempts to track down the causative organism.[7]

The multifaceted nature of the organism was in retrospect poignantly demonstrated in July 1968, when a mysterious unexplained disease attacked the employees and visitors in a health department in Pontiac, Michigan. The illness, much milder than that seen in the Philadelphia epidemic, was characterized by upper respiratory and neurologic symptoms without pneumonia. There were no fatalities, and the entity was labeled "Pontiac fever." Extensive efforts were made to identify the organism without success, but an airborne mode of spread was demonstrated by exposing guinea pigs to the air-conditioning system and injecting them with water from the condenser; the test animals developed a nodular localized pneumonia.[7] It was not until the Philadelphia outbreak of 1976 that efforts to identify the organism met with success. Much of the credit for the eventual solution of the mystery belongs to a team from the Centers for Disease Control (CDC) in Atlanta and the Pennsylvania Department of Health. Ultimately, however, it was the unrelenting efforts of one man, Joseph McDade, that led to identification of the causative bacterium, subsequently named *Legionella pneumophila.*

McDade succeeded in identifying a gram-negative bacillus by injecting guinea pigs with infected lung tissue. Initially, there was some degree of disappointment in that McDade was unable to transmit the disease to other guinea pigs, and the organism could not be subcultured onto agar. Efforts to demonstrate the organism in embryonated eggs also met with failure because McDade was searching for a rickettsial source and the procedure included incorporation of penicillin and streptomycin to eliminate "contaminants." Finally, McDade decided to eliminate the antibiotics when infecting the eggs, and during the last week of December 1976 the culprit was identified and subsequently named *Legionella pneumophila.*[7] Hence a modern milestone in bacteriologic investigation had been achieved within a relatively short period.

Conclusion

The pathways and thought processes leading to the success in identifying *Legionella pneumophila* surely revert to the much earlier era when "peripneumonia" was first described by Hippocrates. The 1976 outbreak at the Bellevue-Stratford Hotel reawakened within the world of medicine a renewed respect for the potentially deadly consequences of infectious diseases. Indeed the current mortality rate of bacteremic pneumococcal pneumonia remains at the unacceptably high level of 30%. Accordingly, the threat of infectious disease in the form of yet undiscovered organisms or resistant mutations is as omnipresent today as it was centuries ago. To cope with this threat, medical investigators must be constantly vigilant and aware of the possibilities.

References

1. Perkins JF Jr: Historical development of respiratory physiology. In Handbook of Physiology. Vol. 1. Sect. 3. Respiration. Washington, DC: American Physiological Society, 1964, pp. 2, 5, 7–11, 13.

2. Major RH: Classic descriptions of disease, 3rd ed. Springfield, IL: Charles C Thomas, 1932, pp. 56e, 68, 69, 559–561, 565–567.
3. Garrison FH: An Introduction to the History of Medicine, 4th ed. Phila delphia: Saunders, 1913, pp. 110–112, 114, 129, 353, 432, 575–579, 641.
4. Massengill SE: A Sketch of Medicine and Pharmacy. Bristol: S.E. Massengill, 1943, p. 45.
5. McGrew RE: Encyclopedia of Medical History. New York: McGraw-Hill, 1985, pp. 29, 37, 38, 40, 151–153, 271, 319, 246–248.
6. Winn WC Jr: Legionnaires diseases: historical perspective. Clin Microbiol Rev 1988;1(1):60–81.
7. Miller LD: The ill-fated tripartite meeting of 1976. Surgery 1989;105:303–308.

2
Who Gets Pneumonia?

ROBERT D. BRANDSTETTER

Respiratory infections are the most common of all infections. The most serious respiratory infection, pneumonia, carries the highest mortality of all infectious diseases and is the fifth leading cause of death. Pneumonia is an inflammatory process of the alveolar space, with the diagnosis based on clinical findings and supporting laboratory data. Although pneumonia can be caused by numerous etiologic agents, infectious pneumonia depends on the presence of microorganisms and their biologic products. Indeed equally as true as "no acid—no ulcer," one can say, "no microbe —no infectious pneumonia."

It has been recognized that microorganisms of different species or different strains of the same species may vary in their capacity to produce disease. Furthermore, humans are not equally susceptible to the disease caused by a particular bacterium or virus. The protection of the lung parenchyma from such microorganisms results from a complex interaction between anatomic barriers and cleansing actions present in the upper airways and the cellular and humoral responses operant in the terminal air spaces[1] (Table 2.1). When one or more of these defenses fail, respiratory tract infection may occur.[2–4]

Inhaled particles may be deposited in the respiratory tract as a result of several mechanisms (impaction, sedimentation, brownian motion). The relative importance of each of these mechanisms in determining the retention of any given particle is related to whether the particle is inhaled through the nose or the mouth, as well as the size, shape, and density of the particle.

Impaction

The first line of defense is in the nasopharynx, where filtration begins. Particles larger than 10 μm and smaller than 0.5 μm are efficiently removed. After passing through a coarse filter of vibrissae just within the nares, which sifts out large particles, the inhaled stream of air containing

TABLE 2.1. Alteration of lung host defense mechanisms.

Altered host defense	Potential disorder or infection
Physical (airways) defenses	
Filtering dysfunction	
Ciliated and squamous epithelium in nasopharynx	Colonization with pathogenic gram-negative organisms
Altered reflexes	
Cough	Bronchitis, aspiration
Sneeze	Microateletasis, aspiration
Bronchoconstriction	Hyperactive airways
Mucociliary dysfunction	
Mucociliary clearance	Bronchiectasis
Cellular (alveolar) defenses	
Phagocytic disorders	
Macrophage	*Pneumocystis carinii*, *Legionella* sp., *Mycobacterium*
Neutrophil	Decreased inflammatory response, gram-negative infection, fungal infection
Humoral deficiency	
Defects of complement system	
C2, C3b inactivator	Encapsulated bacterial infections
C5, C6, C7, C8	Neisserial infections
Immunoglobulin Deficiency	
IgA deficiency	Sinopulmonary infection
IgG4, IgG2 deficiency	Pneumonia with encapsulated bacteria

gases and particulates smaller than 10–15 μm enters the nasal cavity, where it is intimately exposed to the large internal surface area of the nasal septum and turbinates. Most particles larger than 10 μm are removed in this stage. As the air stream changes direction in the nasopharynx, most of the remaining particles of about 10 μm impact on the posterior wall of the pharynx. Large collections of immunologically active tissue (tongue, tonsils, adenoids) are strategically located at the site of greatest impaction in the nasopharynx.[5]

Sedimentation

Sedimentation is the chief mechanism of deposition of particles in the size range 0.2–5.0 μm and occurs as a result of gravitational forces in lung regions of low flow. Droplets carrying infectious microorganisms are often smaller than 2.0 μm in diameter. The range of airflows required for sedimentation to occur may be found throughout the respiratory tract adjacent to the bronchial wall, but sedimentation occurs predominantly in the region of "slow laminar flow" between the 15th and 23rd bronchial generations.

Brownian Motion

Particles of 0.1 μm and smaller are deposited mainly as the result of brownian motion owing to their constant bombardment by gas molecules. Diffusion is characterized by a series of excursions of relatively high velocity and short duration, such that the smaller the particles the greater the effect and the higher the probability of particle deposition on both the upper and lower airway mucosa.

Should microorganisms enter the respiratory tract by any of these three mechanisms, they are mechanically removed by sneeze, cough, or bronchospasm or by their entrapment and cephalad transport via the mucociliary escalator.

Sneeze and Cough Reflexes

The sneeze and cough reflexes provide important mechanisms by which excess secretions and foreign bodies in the trachea or major bronchi can be removed from the airways and disposed of by expectoration or swallowing. Sneezing is a forcefully explosive exhalation triggered by recptors in the nose and nasopharynx. In people with normal lungs and intact neurologic pathways, the cough reflex represents the most effective means of expelling foreign bodies and secretions. In the presence of severe disease, such as chronic bronchitis, cystic fibrosis, and emphysema, cough can be remarkably inefficient. Patients with such neurologic disorders as Parkinson's disease, cerebral strokes, and amyotrophic lateral sclerosis may have an absent cough reflex, leaving them particularly vulnerable to aspiration and serious episodes of pneumonia.

Bronchoconstriction

Stimuli of various types can produce vagally mediated reflex contraction of the airway smooth muscle. Such stimuli may thus cause bronchoconstriction.[6] Reflex bronchoconstriction is characterized by an increase in airway resistance. The importance of bronchoconstriction as a protective mechanism may lie in the prevention of the deeper penetration of mechanical or chemical irritants into the lungs. Mediator interactions, such as mast cell degranulation, may also contribute to endogenous regulation of bronchomotor tone. Compromise of this reflex by altered vagal tone may thus be responsible for inhaled particulates reaching the more distal airways. At this level the importance of the defense mechanism rests in the escalator mucociliary system and the humoral defense system.

Mucociliary Dysfunction

The mucociliary system is one of the lung's primary defense mechanisms.[7] It protects the conducting airways by trapping and sweeping away bacteria, inhaled particles, and cellular debris. Particles deposited between the posterior two-thirds of the nasal cavity and the nasopharynx and from the larynx to the terminal bronchioles land on airways lined by mucus-covered, ciliated epithelium and are removed by means of mucociliary transport mechanisms.[8] The nasopharyngeal and tracheobronchial portions of the ciliated airways transport mucus toward the oropharynx, where it can be eliminated by expectoration or swallowing.[9,10]

Although mucous glands and goblet cells abound in the major airways, few goblet cells are seen at the level of the terminal bronchiole in normal humans. Each cilated cell accommodates approximately 200 cilia (5 μm long and 0.3 μm in diameter). Cilia have an ultrastructure consisting of two central and nine paired peripheral microtubules. Diseases of the mucous gland or ciliated cells leads to chronic respiratory conditions where recurrent infection is the rule.[11]

Under such pathologic conditions as chronic bronchitis, hypertrophy of the mucosal glands may result in a change in the ratio of gland to bronchial wall thickness from the normal 30% to 50% or more; and goblet cells may be found in terminal bronchioles, where they are normally rare or absent.[12] As mucous viscosity rises, impairment of mucociliary transport may be expected, particularly if the mucus is purulent. Volumes of mucus may then be in excess of the ciliated cells' ability to remove it. Mucous plugging and infection may result, which may in part be the cause of recurrent infection in patients with bronchiectasis, cystic fibrosis,[13] and other diseases of the bronchial mucosal membrane.[14]

Finally, the viscoelastic properties of mucus may also be altered in the presence of disease, with infection resulting.[15] This problem is noted specifically in cystic fibrosis patients who suffer from *Pseudomonas* and staphylococcal infections.

The cilia play an important role in removing microorganisms, but only in the presence of mucous—and normal mucus at that. Congenital cilial dysfunction was well described with recognition of the immotile cilia syndrome.[16,17] This disorder occurs when ultrastructurally either dynein arms or radial spokes are missing or there is transposition of two of the microtubules. Kartagener syndrome, where there is sinusitis, bronchiectasis, and frequently situs inversus, is the prototype of this disorder with recurrent bronchial and parenchymal lung infections.[18,19]

Finally, in addition to congenital defects, cilia may acquire abnormalities of structure, usually as a result of chronic respiratory infection. This problem can impair cilial beating and thus affect the propulsive action that clears the airways.[20]

Phagocytic Disorders

Should an infectious agent penetrate the local defenses, the phagocytic defense system is activated. Alveolar macrophages and neutrophils make up this host defense line.

Alveolar macrophages are normally present in the distal lumen of the lower respiratory tract, especially in the alveoli. Although alveolar macrophages are clearly bone-marrow-derived, their exact circulatory pathways are not so well defined. Elimination of foreign particles and microbes from the distal air spaces of the lung initially depends on the immediate phagocytic capability of the alveolar macrophage. Phagocytosis by macrophages is a complex procedure ranging from microbe recognition and adhesion of the plasma membrane to the particle to fusion of the pseudopodia. Opsonization of particles and microbes enhances their phagocytosis by macrophages. During phagocytosis macrophages generate highly reactive toxic products of oxygen (oxygen radicals) such as hydrogen peroxide (H_2O_2) or the hydroxyl radical (OH), which work in conjunction with hydrolytic and proteolytic enzymes from degranulating lysosomes to kill bacteria within the phagocytic vacuole.[21]

Macrophages are generally considered to be the first line of defense against facultative and obligate intracellular parasites, such as *Mycobacterium tuberculosis*. Alveolar macrophages are also responsible for clearing some gram-positive bacteria, such as *Staphylococcus aureus*, whereas other organisms such as *Pseudomonas aeruginosa* and *Klebsiella pneumoniae* usually require neutrophils for optimal clearance. A small group of microbes seem to be adapted to survive in macrophages, and containment or eradication can be difficult. These organisms include *Toxoplasma gondii*, *Legionella pneumophila*, *Pneumocystis carinii*, and cytomegalovirus.

The neutrophil is probably more important than the macrophage in terms of phagocytic function—if for no other reason than because we are more aware of its role in phagocytosis. Neutrophils are the key elements in the acute inflammatory response following their mobilization by chemotactic factors. The neutrophil exists in small numbers in the pulmonary interstitium, and when necessary it can be recruited in large numbers from the circulating and marginated pool of neutrophils.

It takes 10–14 days for a stem cell in the bone marrow to be released into the systemic circulation. Once in the vascular space, its life-span is only about 10 hours before it migrates between endothelial cells and enters tissue. Once bacteria are identified, the neutrophil may then successfully ingest and kill them. This process depends on many steps, such as adherence, chemotaxis, degranulation, oxidative burst, and digestion. Defects in any of these steps can result in serious, often fatal infection.

Movement toward a chemical stimulus is known as *chemotaxis*. Such chemical messages can come from bacterial factors, complement fragments, lymphokines, peptides, prostaglandins, leukotrienes, immunoglobulins, collagen fragments, and immue complexes. Should there be a failure of the neutrophil to migrate toward the stimulus as a result of these factors, phagocytosis cannot occur. This defect may be seen if pseudopods are deprived of their organized movement by cytosol protein activity.

Adherence depends on properties of the neutrophil cell surface and can be impaired by alcohol or glucocorticoids. There appears to be induction of an inhibitory plasma factor. Other reasons for decreased "sticking" include antiinflammatory agents, such as aspirin. Rarely, low levels of magnesium can interfere with the adherence of neutrophils to capillary endothelial surfaces. Accordingly, these events may functionally limit the number of neutrophils that can be mobilized to an inflamed site.

Ingestion depends on opsonization. Specific serum factors, such as immunoglobulin G (IgG) and complement function as opsonins. The opsonins coat the particle and bind to specific receptors on the phagocyte cell surface. As more opsonins bind to surface receptors, the bacterium is ultimately engulfed. Opsonization may be hampered by extracellular bacteria that produce antiphagocytic substances. These substances may be capsules (*Streptococcus pneumoniae*), M proteins (*Streptococcus pyogenes*), pili (*Neisseria gonorrhoeae*), protein A (*Staphylococcus aureus*), and cytotoxins (streptolysins S and O).

The killing of microorganisms occurs during ingestion. Bacterial killing involves several mechanisms, all of which are set in motion by two cellular events: degranulation and initiation of the respiratory burst. Degranulation is the process of fusion between the primary phagosome and the granules present in the cytoplasm of the phagocyte. The granules contain the material that participate in bacterial killing and degradation. During degranulation these materials are discharged into the vesicle containing the ingested microorganism. This antimicrobial system of the

TABLE 2.2. Inherited defects of oxygen-dependent bactericidal mechanisms.

Chronic granulomatous disease
Glucose-6-phosphate dehydrogenase deficiency
Myeloperoxidase deficiency
Glutathione peroxidase deficiency

neutrophil includes oxygen-dependent agents (myeloperoxidases) and oxygen-independent agents (acid, lysozyme, proteases).[22–24]

The respiratory burst describes a metabolic pathway, dormant in resting cells, whose function is to produce a group of highly reactive microbicidal agents by the partial reduction of oxygen. It is the elaboration of these oxidizing agents (oxygen, H_2O_2) provided by the respiratory burst coupled to the actions of the granule contents that results in killing.[25,26] Defects in these systems have been recognized and are believed to be responsible for recurrent infections.

Table 2.2 lists inherited defects of oxygen-dependent bactericidal mechanisms. With chronic granulomatous disease there is failure to show an increase in oxygen uptake and oxygen or H_2O_2 production.[27] Myeloperoxidase deficiency leads to the elimination of only a fraction of the oxygen-dependent bactericidal mechanisms.[28] Finally, glutathione peroxidase deficiency may also be associated with an increased susceptibility to bacterial infection by suppression of oxygen uptake and oxygen and H_2O_2 production.[29]

Humoral Deficiencies: B Cell Dysfunction and Complement Disorder

When the immediate phagocytic responses are inadequate, the humoral defense system is activated. Should this system fail, serious consequences may result. Humoral deficiencies are classified as disorders of B cells (immunoglobulin) or of the complement system. Humoral deficiencies generally lead to infection by extracellular encapsulated organisms and more episodes of bacteremia.

Immunoglobulin Deficiency

In the upper airways (nasal passages, oropharynx, conducting airways) local secretions contain the principal immunoglobulin, IgA. It is secreted by plasma cells in the bronchial mucosa but diminishes in relative concentration in distal portions of the lung. IgA thus forms part of the mucosal barrier that prevents adherence and absorption of foreign substances, including organisms. IgA can neutralize respiratory viruses and certain endotoxins, and it can agglutinate microbial organisms. Therefore absence of IgA or organisms that elaborate IgA proteases that destroy it can result in recurrent sinopulmonary infections, such as sinusitis and chronic bronchitis. Secretory IgA levels correlate better with respiratory immunity to specific infections than do serum levels.

Antibodies of the IgG isotype predominate in the lower respiratory tract. Whereas inactivation of IgA by bacterial proteases is an attractive hypothesis pertaining to bacterial colonization and chronic bronchitis, abnormalities in IgG are undoubtedly associated with infection. Respiratory tract infections (pneumonia and sinusitis) are usual manifestations of this immunoglobulin deficiency. Bacterial infections with encapsulated organisms that require opsonizing antibody (IgG) for efficient host phagocytosis are particularly common.

Immunoglobulin E is also secreted by plasma cells in the bronchial mucosa; like IgA, it is a mucosal antibody present in respiratory secretions. It is especially prominent in atopic individuals. IgE acts in association with local mast cells and enhances host defense by recruiting eosinophils, promoting smooth muscle contraction and mucous secretion, and increasing epithelial and endothelial permeability. IgE may thus function to protect the respiratory mucous membrane, perhaps against some parasites, but it is best known for its adverse effects as the reaginic antibody responsible for immediate (type I) hypersensitivity reactions.

Defects In Complement

Complement is a series of plasma proteins that act as sequential enzymes. They are triggered by antigen-antibody reactions (classic pathway) or by endotoxin or bacterial cell walls (alternate pathway). Complement activation is typical of IgG reactions but does not occur during IgA or IgE responses. Complement activation results in phagocytosis and lysis of infecting organisms and other foreign cells, regardless of whether antibody has been involved. These effects are produced by opsonization, a coating that enhances phagocytosis. Some complement components have powerful additional effects in many aspects of the inflammatory response (e.g., in chemotaxis and vascular permeability).

Immunoglobulin G (IgG1, IgG3, or IgM)-antigen-antibody complexes activate C1 of the classic pathway. Active C cleaves C2 and C4 into the proteolytic enzyme C4b2a. This C3 convertase cleaves C3 into a variety of proteins, including C3a, C3b, C3c, C3d, and C3e. The C3b formed functions in the alternative pathway or transforms the C3 convertase into a C5a and C5b. C5b, with the final complement proteins C6, C7, C8, and C9, inserts into the cell membrane, alters permeability, and causes osmotic lysis of the cell.

Isolated complement protein deficiencies do occur and may be responsible for life-threatening infections. Most complement functions (including opsonization cytolytic bactericidal activity) and recruitment of neutrophils to the site of inflammation are missing in the singular complement-deficient patient.

C3 deficiency is a rare disorder that leads to recurrent pneumonia, sinusitis, and otitis. Organisms most often associated with C3 deficiency are *Streptococcus pneumoniae*, *Staphylococcus aureus*, *Hemophilus influenzae*, and other gram-negative organisms.

C5 deficiency results in depressed chemotaxis, most likely due to decreased formation of C5a and impaired cytolysis. *S. aureus* and gram-negative infections may be a consequence of such a deficiency.[30]

Deficiencies of other components of the complement system, such as C2, C6, C7, and C8, may result in recurrent streptococcal and pneumococcal respiratory infections, as well as neisserial infections.[31,32] These infections, however are unusual.

Other Causes of Pneumonia

There are numerous other causes for lower respiratory tract infection with impairment of one or more of the host defense systems. There may be congenital deficiency or abnormality in cellular immunity. Acquired deficiencies include leukemia, myeloma, and other dysproteinemias, decreased cell-mediated immunity (lymphoma, diabetes), agranulocytosis and nonspecific interference by disease, splenectomy, or therapy (corticosteroid, cytoxic agents). Defects in cellular immunity (T cell function: DiGeorge syndrome) can result in *Listeria monocytogenes*, *Mycobacterium tuberculosis*, or *Toxoplasma gondii* infection. Other diseases, such as severe combined immunodeficiency, Wiskott-Aldrich syndrome, and ataxia-telangiectasia, may also result in serious infection due to opportunistic organisms as well as common bacteria (*S. pneumoniae*, *S. aureus*, and *H. influenzae*). The acquired immunodeficiency syndrome (AIDS) may find a patient with episodes of *Pneumocystis carinii*, cytomegalovirus, usual and atypical mycobacteria, and typical bacterial infections during the course of the illness.

References

1. Rhodin JAG: Ultrastructure and function of the human trachea mucosa. Am Rev Respir Dis 1966;93(Suppl)3:1–15.
2. Newhouse M, Sanchis J, Biennenstock J: Lung defense mechanisms. Part I. N Engl J Med 1976;295:990–998.
3. Newhouse M, Sanchis J, Biennenstock J: Lung defense mechanisms. Part II. N Engl J Med 1976;295:1045–1052.
4. Green GM, JaKab GJ, Low RB, Davis GS: Defense mechanisms of the respiratory membrane. Am Rev Respir Dis 1977:115:479–508.
5. Proctor DF: The upper airways. I. Nasal physiology and defense of the lung. II. The larynx and trachea. Am Rev Respir Dis 1977;115:97–129, 315–342.
6. Leff AR: Endogenous regulation of bronchomotor tone. Am Rev Respir Dis 1988;137:1190–1216.
7. Kinosita KH, Murakani A: Control of ciliary motion. Physiol Rev 1967;47: 53–82.
8. Sleigh MA, Blake JR, Liron N: The propulsion of mucus by cilia. Am Rev Respir Dis 1988;137:726–741.

9. Harada RN, Repine JE: Pulmonary host defense mechanisms. Chest 1985;87: 247–252.
10. Wanner A: Clinical aspects of mucociliary transport. Am Rev Respir Dis 1977;116:73–125.
11. Reid LM: Correlation of certain bronchographic abnormalities seen in bronchitis. Thorax 1955;10:199–204.
12. Reid LM: Measurement of the bronchial mucus gland layer; a diagnostic yardstick in chronic bronchitis. Thorax 1960;15:132–141.
13. Tomashefski JF, Christoforidis AJ, Abdullah AK: Cystic fibrosis in young adults. Chest 1970;57:28–32.
14. Sanchis J, Dolovich M, Rossman C, et al: Pulmonary mucociliary clearance in cystic fibrosis. N Engl J Med 1973;288:651–654.
15. Denton R, Forsman W, Hwang SH, et al: Viscoelasticity of mucus; its role in ciliary transport of pulmonary secretions. Am Rev Respir Dis 1968; 98:380–391.
16. Holley MC, Afzeluis BA: Alignment of cilia in immotile-cilia syndrome. Tissue Cell 1986;18:521–529.
17. Eliasson R, Mossberg B, Camner P, et al: The immotile-cilia syndrome. N Engl J Med 1977;297:1–5.
18. Malech HL: Abnormal neutrophil migration in Kartagener's syndrome. Ann Intern Med 1980;92:520–538.
19. James EF: Does Kartagener's syndrome exist? Lancet 1978:2:573–574.
20. Waite D, Steele R, Ross I, et al: Cilia and sperm tail abnormalities in polynesian bronchiectasis. Lancet 1978;2:132–135.
21. Klebanoff SJ: Oxygen metabolism and the toxic properties of phagocytes. Ann Intern Med 1980;93:480–489.
22. Zucker-Franklin D, Hirsch JG: Electron microscope studies on the degranulation of rabbit peritoneal leukocytes during phagocytosis. J Exp Med 1964; 120:569–576.
23. Sbarra AJ, Karnovsky ML: The biochemical basis of phagocytosis. I. Metabolic changes during the ingestion of particles by polymorphonuclear leukocytes. J Biol Chem 1959;234:1355–1362.
24. Klebanoff SJ: Myeloperoxidase; contribution to the microbicidal activity of intact leukocytes. Science 1970;169:1095–1097.
25. Babior BM: Oxygen-dependent microbial killing by phagocytes. Part I. N Engl J Med 1978;298:659–668.
26. Babior BM: Oxygen-dependent microbial killing by phagocytes. Part II. N Engl J Med 1978;298:721–725.
27. Berendes H, Bridges RA, Good RA: A fatal granulomatosis of childhood: the clinical study of a new syndrome. Minn Med 1957;40:309–312.
28. Mandell GL, Hook EN: Leukocyte bactericidal activity in chronic granulomatous disease; correlation of bacterial hydrogen peroxide production and susceptibility to intracellular killing. J Bacteriol 1969;100:531–532.
29. Holmes B, Park BH, Malawitsa SE, et al: Chronic granulomatous disease in females: a deficiency of leukocyte glutathione peroxidase. N Engl J Med 1968;278:976–980.
30. Miller ME, Nilsson UR: A familial deficiency of the phagocytosis-enhancing activity of serum related to a dysfunction of the fifth component of complement. N Engl J Med 1970;282:354.

31. Glovsky MM, Opelz G, Terasaki PI: Genetic opsonic, and bactericidal studies in a C2 deficient family. Clin Res 1976;24:327A.
32. Petersen BH, Lee TJ, Snyderman R, et al: Neisseria meningitidis and N. gonorrhoeae bacteremia associated with C6, C7 or C8 deficiency. Ann Intern Med 1970;90:917.

3 Pathophysiology of Pneumonia

MONROE KARETZKY

Pneumonia has been studied intensively as to its etiology, pathogenesis, clinical manifestations, laboratory findings, therapy, prognosis, and complications. It may be suprising therefore to discover the fragmentary knowledge available regarding its pathophysiology. Although great strides have been made, they have primarily focused on findings in the acute lung injury syndrome. The discussion in this chapter is limited to the classic parenchymal lesions of lobar and bronchopneumonia.

The cause of impaired lung function during pulmonary infection appears to be the result of a direct effect of microbial infection on lung tissue and an indirect effect due to alteration of the lung's surfactant system. Lung surfactant, a complex phospholipid, serves to decrease the surface tension of the alveoli and small airways without which lung inflation would require higher pressures and lung stability would be altered. Instability leads to the gradual reduction of surface area reflecting a changing equilibrium position between the forces necessary to maintain inflation and those promoting collapse and atelectasis.

Mechanical Abnormalities

Studies of pulmonary function in patients with pneumonia, similar to those more extensively reported for patients with tuberculosis, have demonstrated that values reflecting physiologic status relate poorly to the extent and nature of the disease process as assessed by the chest roentgenogram either before or after treatment. Vital capacity and total lung capacity are usually reduced, and residual volume is increased.[1] These values tend to return toward normal during treatment (Fig. 3.1). Associated acute endobronchial disease, depending on its severity, may significantly influence these measurements. Although there tends to be hyperventilation at rest, the maximum breathing capacity is initially decreased.

In patients with typical lobar pneumococcal pneumonia, the magnitude of the reduction in lung volumes exceeds what would be expected on the

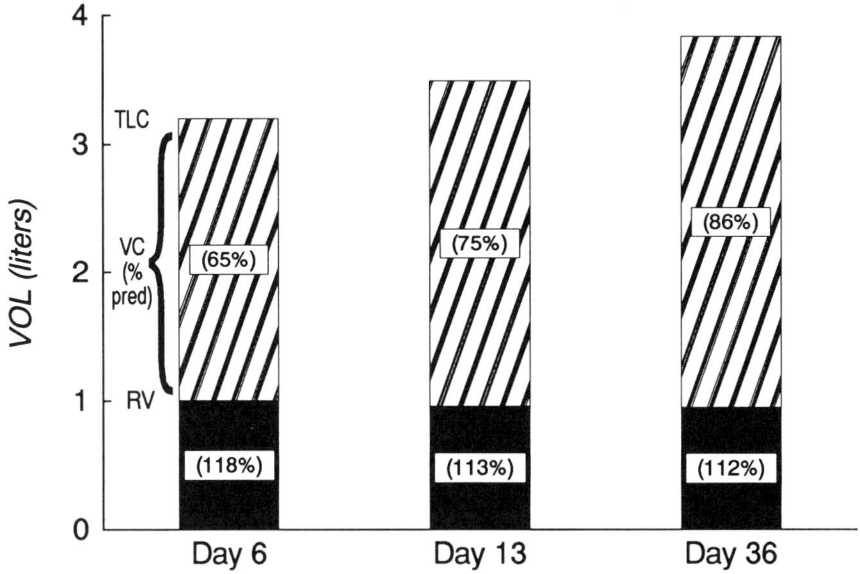

FIGURE 3.1. Pulmonary function tests in a patient with right middle lobe pneumonia as the chest roentgenogram showed partial and then complete clearing. (Data from Colp et al.[1])

basis of assessment of radiographic involvement. However, those with the most extensive radiographic changes have been observed to have the lowest vital capacity with subsequent increases tending to be preceded by radiographic clearing. The total lung capacity decreases to the extent of the fall in vital capacity, and the residual volume reflects the associated airway involvement. The observed decreases in flow rates are a result of both airway and parenchymal inflammation. The extent of endobronchial disease is variable and may manifest only during augmented ventilation when turbulence elevates resistance to such a degree that the distal lung participates less and less in the tidal volume. The limitations of the radiographic picture, which has been aptly termed the "shadowgram," are its inability to display "strategic" lesions and the true anatomic extent or severity of the observed lesions, which becomes readily apparent in autopsy studies of pneumonia patients.

It was suggested as early as the turn of the century that pneumonic lungs, because of their increased rigidity (retractile force), would require an increased negative pleural (distending) pressure to achieve expansion. It was subsequently shown in a dog model that these changes in the mechanical characteristics of the lungs preceded radiographic changes and were apparent only hours after infection.

The development of the technique of intraesophageal pressure measurement as a means of determining intrapleural pressure subsequently

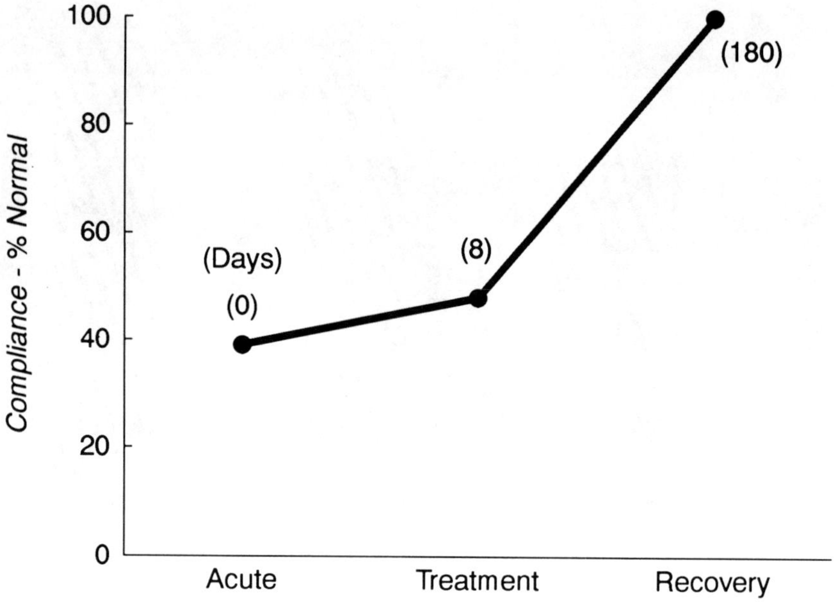

FIGURE 3.2. Change of complicance in a patient with pneumonia (right middle and lower lobe) in the absence of chest pain with treatment. (Data from Marshall and Christie.[2])

allowed confirmation of these findings in patients with lobar pneumonia.[2] With pneumonia there is an increase in lung rigidity due to generalized congestion of the lungs similar to that seen with other diseases such as heart failure. Marshall and Christie[2] found the expected decrease in compliance (the ratio of change in volume to change in pressure); but the magnitude of the increase in lung rigidity they demonstrated could not be explained by the apparent extent of consolidation shown by chest roentgenogram (Fig. 3.2). Furthermore, with recovery changes in the elastic properties of the lungs also bore no relation to the radiographic findings. These studies indicate the extent of involvement of radiographically silent areas of the lung by the pneumonic process. This study supported previous findings that the degree of impairment in vital capacity and lung volumes exceeded that which would be predicted by radiographic findings. The presence of concomitant pleurisy further decreases these values during tests of pulmonary function.

The total lung compliance consists of at least two components: (1) tissue compliance due to elasticity; and (2) surface compliance due to surface tension at the gas–liquid interface in the alveoli. The tension in the alveolae–air–water interface provides both a retractive force opposing lung inflation and an alveolar subphase pressure promoting the accumulation of fluid. Animal studies of pneumonia have demonstrated a

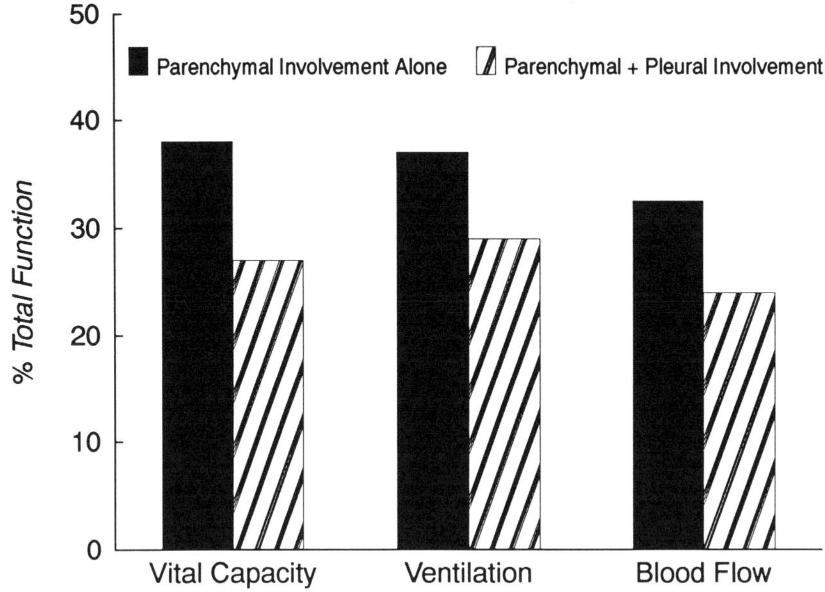

FIGURE 3.3. Differential function values for the affected lung in the presence of pneumonia with and without pleural involvement. (Data from Autio.[4])

decrease in compliance of a similar magnitude in grossly uninvolved areas of lung that even on microscopic examination shows no histologic evidence of an acute inflammatory process.[3] This finding suggests that the altered pulmonary function is due predominantly to an increase in surface forces, implying disruption of the surfactant system. In addition, the rigidty of the lung is increased as a result of the expected loss of tissue elasticity from the inflammatory process itself. Under normal conditions, lung recoil pressure is dominated by tissue forces as the surface tension approaches zero near functional residual capacity after an inflation to total lung capacity. In the presence of pneumonia, during prolonged tidal breathing at lower volumes, as the surface tension rises and volume falls, surface forces contribute increasingly to recoil pressure and promote pulmonary edema by lowering the hydrostatic pressure (more negative) of the alveolar subphase.

An additional consideration to the parenchymal disease is the extent to which pleural involvement influences ipsilateral lung function in comparison to the "unaffected" contralateral lung. The pleura can account for as much as 20% of the transpulmonary pressure at the functional residual capacity. Pleural complications have an unexpectedly large effect on the distribution of blood flow and ventilation. This excessive decrease in ipsilateral lung function has been demonstrated by bronchospirometric studies and has been attributed to the rigidity of the reactive pleura causing increases in both airway and vascular resistances.[4] The resulting differential decreases in both gas and blood flow to the underlying lung are reflected by the contributions of the affected side to the total oxygen uptake, vital capacity, and ventilation, which are decreased, in this order (Fig. 3.3). Thus the affected lung tends to be relatively hyperventilated relative to its blood flow, which is reflected by its diminished contribution to total oxygen uptake. This condition contributes further to the observed reduction of overall lung compliance during the acute phase, but the reduction is greater than can be accounted for by the apparent consolidation seen on chest roentgenogram. The influence of pleural pain exaggerates the shallow breathing characteristic of pneumonia and augments the adverse ventilation-perfusion relations that exist in low-compliance areas or in regions of airway narrowing.

Work and Pattern of Breathing

The viscoelastic properties of the lungs in pneumonia are readily altered. The work of breathing may be significantly augmented depending on the severity of the pneumonic process causing alteration of the thoracic wall and lung compliance and to a lesser extent airway resistance. The pattern of respiration established is such as to seek the necessary exchange of air at the least expenditure of muscular effort.[2] During the early phase of pneumonia the respiratory pattern is indeed found to be precisely what one would predict to maintain the least work of breathing for the altered compliance (Fig. 3.4).

The work of breathing is therefore minimized for any given alveolar ventilation by appropriate alterations in the respiratory pattern in the presence of disease as well as health. The optimal respiratory frequency and tidal volume are achieved that are most economical in terms of respiratory work. The rapid breathing characteristically observed therefore reflects not distress or fatigue but the body's ability to have adequate gas exchange for the least expenditure of muscular effort. The tachypnea of pneumonia is a well known clinical phenomenon; it occurs in the absence of pleuritic pain and is unaffected by the accompanying arterial hypoxemia.

The altered pattern and work of breathing are apt to be associated with unusual breathlessness (dyspnea), though patients with pneumonia in the absence of pleuritic pain seems to be extraordinarily unconcerned with their compromised ventilatory state. Unlike patients with heart failure, they can lie flat in bed; and except for those patients in extremis, their breathing seems effortless in contrast to that of patients compensating for metabolic acidosis or obstructive lung disease.

In addition to the altered elastic forces of the lung with pneumonia, there is also distortion of flow-resistive forces of the airways. With the

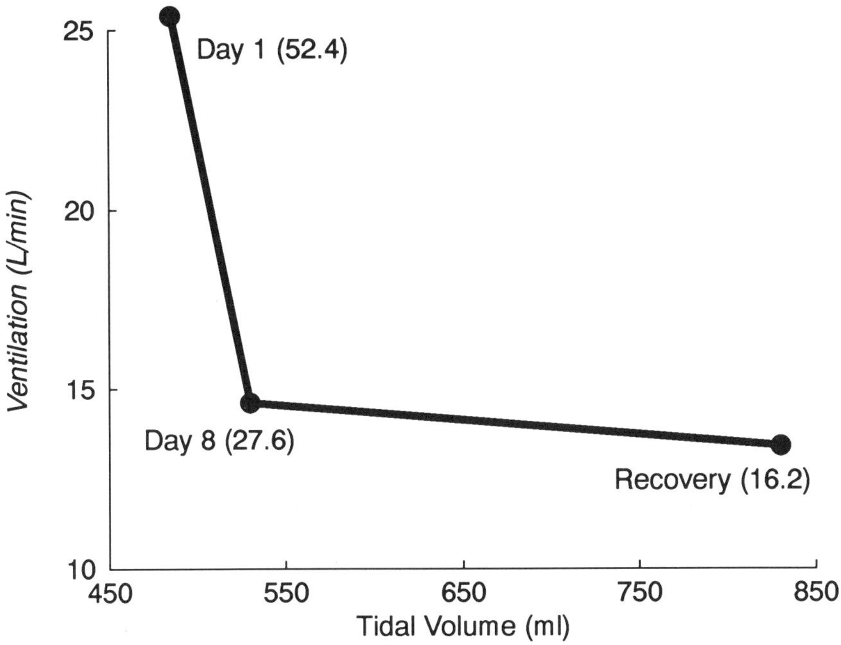

FIGURE 3.4. Changes in respiratory pattern with respiratory frequency (f) observed in patients with pneumonia. The optimal respiratory rates calculated for minimal work were 46, 25, and 17 for days 1, 8, and recovery, respectively. (Data from Marshall and Christie.[2])

inevitable associated bronchitis, airway diameter diminishes and resistance to flow increases according to Poiseuille's law: The force required for laminar air movement varies with the radius of the tube to the fourth power. The effect of elevated body temperature is yet another factor to be considered to alter the respiratory pattern but has not been studied in patients with pneumonia. In normal subjects with the alveolar PCO_2 held approximately constant, respiratory frequency and total ventilation rises slowly as the rectal temperature rises.[5] At constant but elevated body temperature, frequency increases at any given level of pulmonary ventilation; the effect is most marked at high levels of total ventilation. Caution has been suggested when assuming it is simply a manifestation of a residual panting mechanism in humans to effect evaporate heat loss. Instead, it has been suggested that, along with the associated rise in pulse rate, the tachypnea may exemplify a general increase in the frequency of rhythmic processes with unsteady-state characteristics more of carbon dioxide hyperpnea rather than of thermal panting.

These alterations in compliance and resistance increase the load for the respiratory muscles. The force the muscles can generate is related to a number of factors, including their length, velocity of contraction, fatigue, and contractility. Displacement of the resting position of the respiratory muscle fiber on its length–tension curve, as reflected by altered functional residual capacity, decreases the force-generating capability of the intercostal muscles and the diaphragm. Force of contraction, however, can be maximized at low velocities; and with maximum load, velocity falls to zero.

Excessive loads may lead to fatigue after a finite period and resultant ventilatory failure. In recent years various determinants of respiratory muscle strength and endurance have been studied and emphasized, including oxygen delivery as affected by both arterial oxygenation and cardiac function as well as its distribution as muscle blood flow. Hypercapnia and metabolic acidosis also impair respiratory muscle contracting ability and cause diaphragmatic dysfunction. In addition, sepsis in animal models has been shown to decrease muscle mass; but decreases in diaphragmatic contractability has also been observed without affecting the muscle mass. Moreover, the observed increases in diaphragmatic blood flow and oxygen consumption out of proportion to the load suggest the possibility of various defects, including a failure of excitation-contraction coupling and the uncoupling of oxidative phosphorylation.

Decreases in respiratory muscle strength have been demonstrated during apparent viral upper respiratory tract infections in otherwise normal healthy adults[6] (Fig. 3.5). Thus an acute myopathy causing respiratory muscle dysfunction may coexist with parenchymal disease, suggesting that patients with pneumonia are predisposed to develop respiratory failure. The proteolytic effects of interleukin-1 and other acute-phase circulating inflammatory mediators (including proteases, which increase peripheral muscle protein degradation) may be the responsible agents for the myopathy. This extensive muscle weakness, giving rise to fatigue or impaired endurance, may be of much greater significance than previously appreciated; symptomatically, it is reflected by the commonly recognized myalgias. Thus pneumonia increases the load on the respiratory pump, and the associated inflammatory process simultaneously impairs the respiratory muscles' pressure-generating capacity.

A given ventilation can be produced not only with a variety of combinations of tidal volume (V_T) and respiratory rate (f) but also with different mean inspiratory flow rates (V_T/T_I) and duty cycle, the ratio of inspiratory time to total cycle duration (T_I/T_{TOT}). To minimize inspiratory work (power output) for a given V_T and f, it is useful to inspire the tidal volume as slowly as possible to limit the nonelastic energy requirement. The oxygen cost of breathing, however, appears to be more closely related to mean pressure developed by the inspiratory muscles (respiratory force) than to mechanical power. Force is minimized by a high inspiratory flow (very high drive) and very low T_I/T_{TOT}. With pneumonia, loss of lung volume, and alteration of the pressure–volume curve,

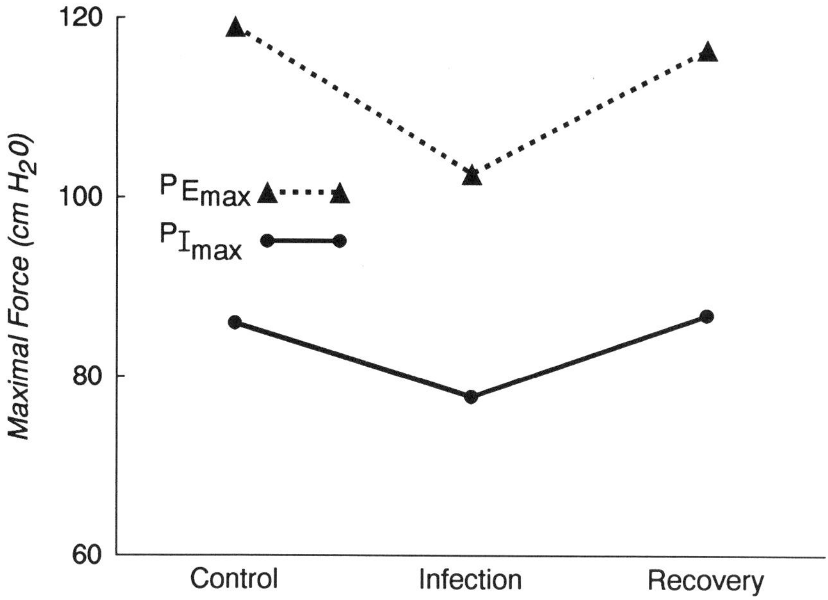

FIGURE 3.5. Effect of viral upper respiratory tract infections on respiratory muscle strength in 22 healthy adults. P_I = maximal inspiratory force; P_E = maximal expiratory force. (Data from Mier-Jedrzejowicz et al.[6])

the tidal volume is reduced so as not to encroach into the less-compliant upper range of lung volume but not too low so it goes into the high-resistance, lower-volume range. Thus it is possible from knowledge of the elastic and nonelastic components of pulmonary resistance to calculate optimum values for the rate and depth of breathing at any level of pulmonary ventilation that would involve the respiratory muscles in minimal work. Although agreement between calculated and observed values appear to reflect changes in mechanical properties of the lungs, the respiratory frequency usually approximates the value that requires the least average force rather than the least work of the respiratory muscles. The respiratory frequency is under vagal control; and, as a result, the work of breathing is increased when the vagus nerves are blocked.

In association with increased ventilation and the rapid respiratory frequency are a decrease in inspiratory time (T_I) and an increase in the inspiratory flow rate (V_T/T_I),[7,8] indicating increased respiratory center drive (Fig. 3.6). The duty cycle has been shown to be as important as the pressure generated during diaphragmatic contraction for determining fatigue. Increases in inspiratory time increase the duration of diaphragmatic contraction and decrease the expiratory (T_E) or recovery time available for relaxation between contractions. The shortened T_I is associ-

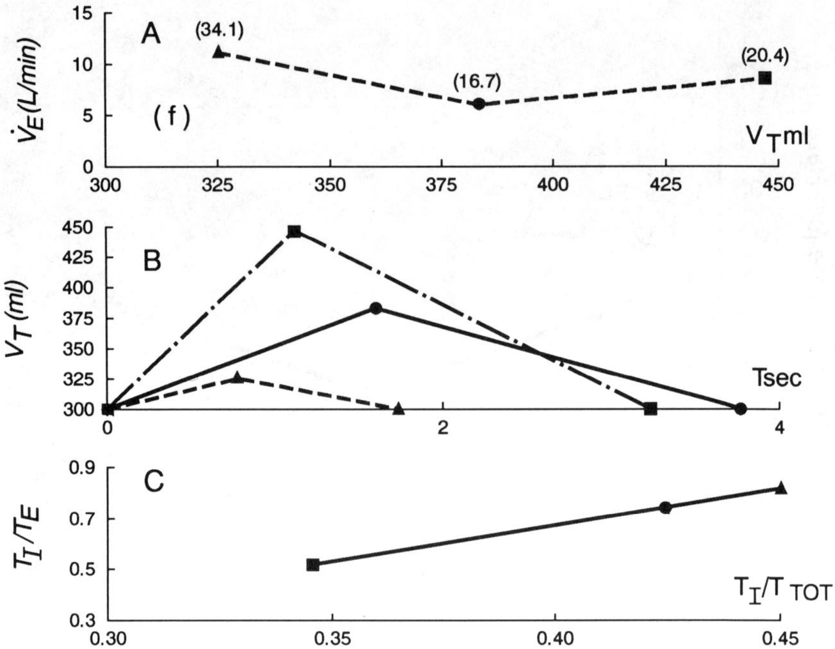

FIGURE 3.6. Breathing patterns measured without mouthpieces: normal subjects (circles), pneumonia patients (triangles), and COPD patients (squares).[7,8] (A) Hyperventilation with pneumonia is frequency-dependent in contrast to COPD where an increase in V_T occurs at rest. (B) The inspiratory flow rates (V_T/T_I) increase in both pneumonia patients (425 ml/second) and COPD patients (438 ml/second) in comparison to normal subjects (249 ml/second). (C) In pneumonia patients respiratory timing is essentially normal in contrast to the decreased T_I/T_{TOT} and T_I/T_E maximizing T_E in obstructive airway disease.

ated with an essentially normal T_I/T_{TOT} and a normal T_I/T_E, in contrast to that seen with true obstructive lung disease, where expiration is prolonged with respect to inspiration and T_I/T_{TOT} is decreased (Fig. 3.6C).

Respiratory muscle blood flow is influenced by both muscle tension and duty cycle. At moderate tensions, blood flow would become limited when the duty cycle exceeds 0.3.[9] With resolution of the pneumonia, these values return the respiratory mechanism to normal,[10] continually operating at maximal efficiency at a new level (Fig. 3.7). There is no consistent relation demonstrable between arterial oxgyenation and the rapid, shallow breathing present acutely or its normal resolution with recovery. Similarly, the respiratory pattern with sedation (i.e., morphine) resulting in depression of ventilation, which increases arterial desaturation, is unaltered by oxygen therapy.[8] Thus in contrast to the respiratory effects of ventilatory depressants, oxygen therapy is observed to have no effect

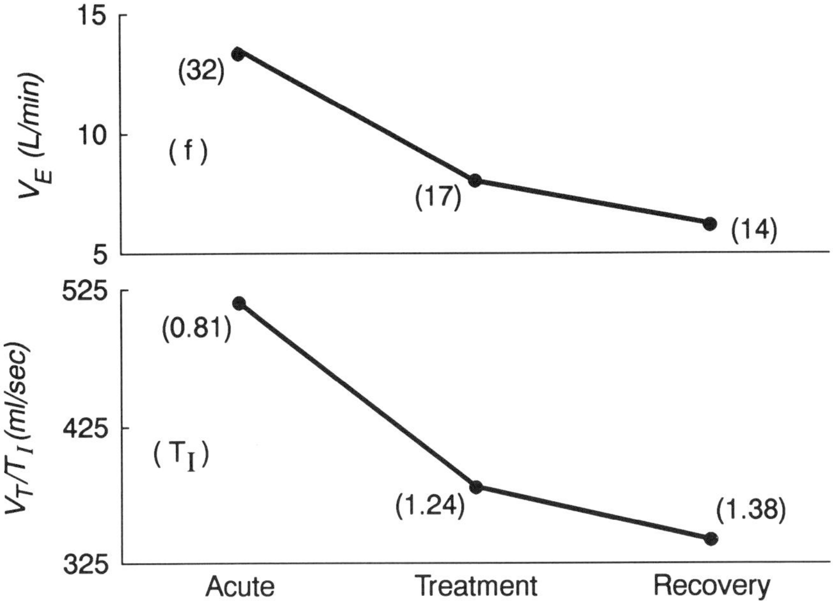

FIGURE 3.7. Resolution of the breathing pattern in one patient with lobar pneumonia from the acute stage to convalescence measured without a mouthpiece by plethysmography. (Data from Binger and Davis.[10])

on the respiratory pattern in patients with pneumonia, and hypoxia therefore is not responsible for the observed increased respiratory drive.

Gas Exchange

In 1919 Stadie demonstrated decreased arterial saturation in patients with pneumonia. There was wide variation observed, with a mean arterial oxygen unsaturation in the fatal cases of 32% compared to 13.9% in nonfatal cases. Similarly, venous desaturation was 57% in fatal cases and 36.3% in survivors. The hypoxemia was related to venous admixture of reduced hemoglobin, and arterial unsaturation of more than 20% was associated with a fatal outcome. Only 7 of these 33 patients had lobar pneumonia. Since these initial observations, a good deal of evidence has accumulated suggesting that the mechanisms of venous admixture in lobar and bronchopneumonia differ[11] and go beyond the simplest explanation of perfusion of consolidated, nonfunctioning, parenchymal tissue (Fig. 3.8).

With unilateral disease the unimpaired lung may be expected to become overdistended, which would be exaggerated with ventilator

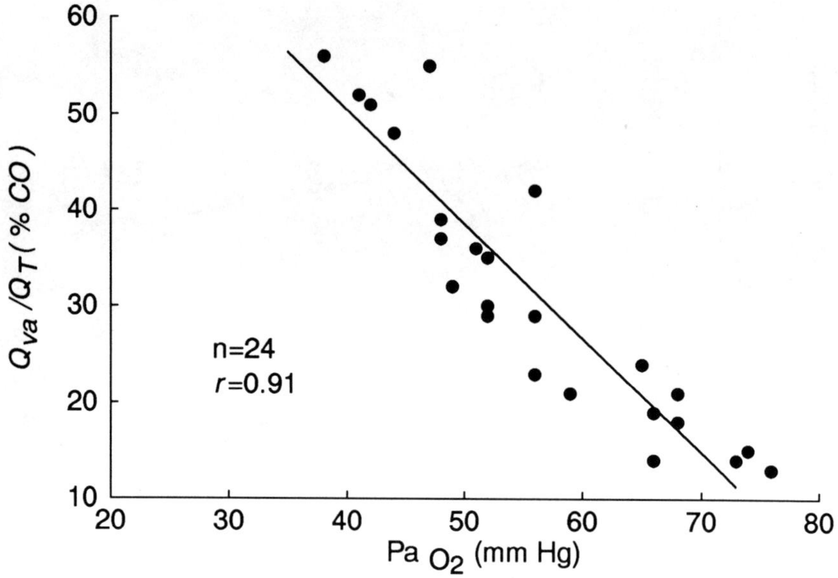

FIGURE 3.8. Arterial PO_2 in 15 patients with pneumonia during different phases of the disease and the calculated total venous admixture shown as the percent of total cardiac output. There is a close correlation between the combined physiologic and venoarterial shunt with arterial oxygenation. (Data from Mellemgaard.[11])

management. A disproportionate fall in diffusing capacity (D_{LCO}) may be seen if the diseased lung maintains patent pulmonary artery channels; and under these circumstances varying degrees of venous admixture (Qva) and arterial hypoxemia develop. Hypoxemia of pneumonia, although variable, is to a major degree determined by the magnitude of the mismatching of ventilation and perfusion in areas of the lung that are in fact not consolidated.

Depending on the volume of normal lung coexisting and ready to accommodate an increased fraction of the pulmonary blood flow through normally ventilated alveoli, the ventilation/perfusion (V/Q) ratio may be barely disturbed. Arterial oxygenation may remain normal in the resting state. Intrinsic autoregulatory mechanisms resulting in "in situ" thrombosis decreases the blood flow to the pneumonic lung. It results from anatomic narrowing of the pulmonary vessels in the diseased area caused by organic destruction of the vessels or vasomotor hypoxic vasoconstriction in response to local decreases in alveolar oxygenation (PAO_2), which serves to raise the vascular resistance and limit blood flow in order to maintain a normal V/Q relation.

With diffuse bronchopneumonia, the blood vessels are engorged with blood and are markedly distended. Thus the inflammatory process over-

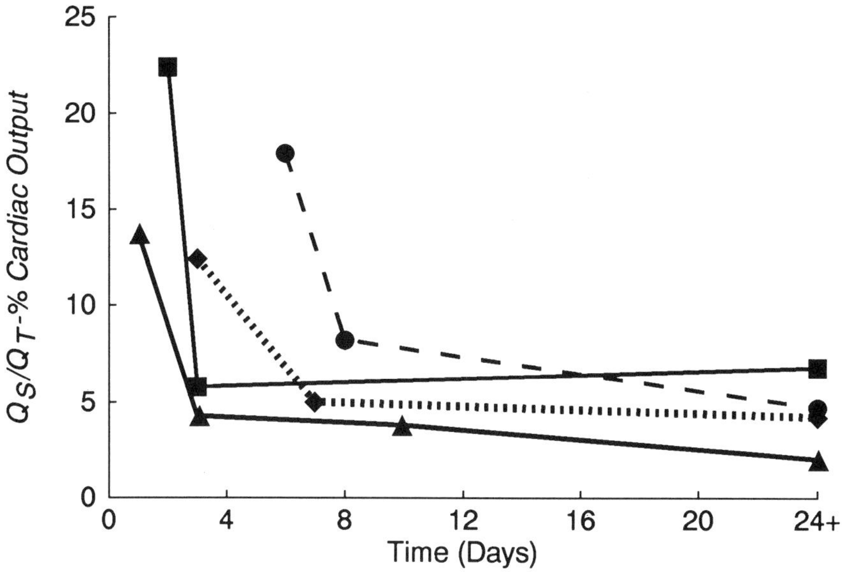

FIGURE 3.9. Time course of the right-to-left shunt in four patients with lobar pneumonia. (Data from Mellemgaard.[11])

whelms or destroys mechanisms of purposeful blood redistribution—in contrast to findings of postmortem injection studies of lobar pneumonia. The latter have shown that the small pulmonary vessels during early pneumonic hepatization are narrowed with decreased filling and are virtually obliterated with gray hepatization. Similarly, in vivo studies utilizing nuclear or angiographic techniques show a marked reduction in local perfusion in areas of pneumonic consolidation. Again, because no correlation exists between arterial desaturation and the extent of radiologic abnormality initially or with recovery, these observations suggest a redistribution of blood and inspired gas away from the parenchymal areas of pneumonic infiltration. Thus an anatomic basis exists for the physiologic demonstration that a pure (true) shunt tends to be the major mechanism of arterial hypoxemia during the first 48 hours of lobar pneumonia, and thereafter arterial desaturation is due primarily to the redistribution of blood to areas of low V/Q zones, as with bronchopneumonia (Fig. 3.9).

In patients with moderately severe pneumonia, virtually all of the shunt is pulmonary; but in patients with severe pneumonia, both the pulmonary and the postpulmonary component of the total shunt are markedly increased.[12] This increase in postpulmonary shunt has been attributed to an increase in the bronchial circulation and in the metabolism (oxygen extraction) of the lung tissue itself in the pneumonic area. Thus the cause

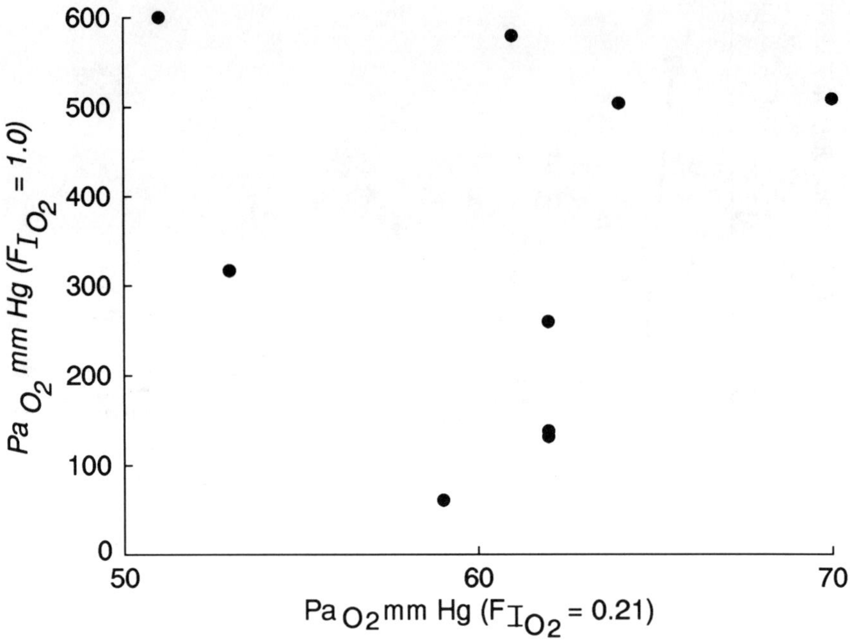

FIGURE 3.10. Arterial PO_2 in nine patients while breathing room air and 100% oxygen, showing the variable and unpredictable contribution of ventilation-perfusion mismatching and right-to-left shunt to the total venous admixture. (Data from Davidson et al.[13])

of hypoxia and its magnitude in pneumonia depend on both the severity and the duration of the disease.

At rest, during the initial phase of disease, ventilation is more disturbed than perfusion in the pneumonic area; and perfusion tends to be distributed to low V/Q units.[12] It results in a variable and unpredictable contribution of the shunt fraction to the venous admixture[13] (Fig. 3.10). If, however, blood flow is sufficiently augmented by exercise, the available normal lung tissue is markedly diminished by disease, or the "skip areas" of disease exceed the autoregulatory mechanisms capacity for control (as with bronchopneumonia in contrast to lobar pneumonia), the V/Q ratio may be seriously disturbed and arterial hypoxemia pronounced.

In support of regional airway obstruction and compliance alterations as mechanisms of relative overperfusion of hypoventilated areas is the demonstration that intrapulmonary gas mixing is grossly altered. The rapid, shallow breathing exhibited by patients in accordance with altered lung mechanics characterizing pneumonia promotes arterial desaturation even in normal subjects. This pattern of ventilation favors distribution of the tidal breath to the apical regions of the lung, whereas the distribution of perfusion remains basally oriented. Therefore the tendency for arterial hypoxemia to lessen after several days is presumably a result of return to a normal pattern of respiration and reduced blood flow in the consolidated areas.

Another measure of the efficacy of lung function is the deadspace ventilation, which represents that portion of the total ventilation that appears to take no part in gas exchange. It is termed the physiologic deadspace and is made up not only of the actual volume of gas contained in the anatomic deadspace but also of a virtual volume of gas arising from the contribution of all alveoli where ventilation is maintained but circulation is reduced or absent (alveolar deadspace). Thus just as venous admixture represents wasted perfusion, deadspace represents wasted ventilation. Deadspace expressed as a percentage of tidal volume (V_D/V_T), normally about 30%, increases acutely during pneumonia and normalizes with recovery. Hyperventilation at rest and with exercise in normals tends to reduce the V_D/V_T ratio and serves the same purpose of enhancing the efficiency of gas exchange in patients with pneumonia.

Carbon dioxide retention, except during infancy, is a rare occurrence with pneumonia in the absence of preexisting lung disease. Its rarity may be attributable to the state of hyperventilation and the shape of the carbon dioxide dissociation curve, allowing the areas of reasonably normal lung to eliminate more than its share of carbon dioxide.

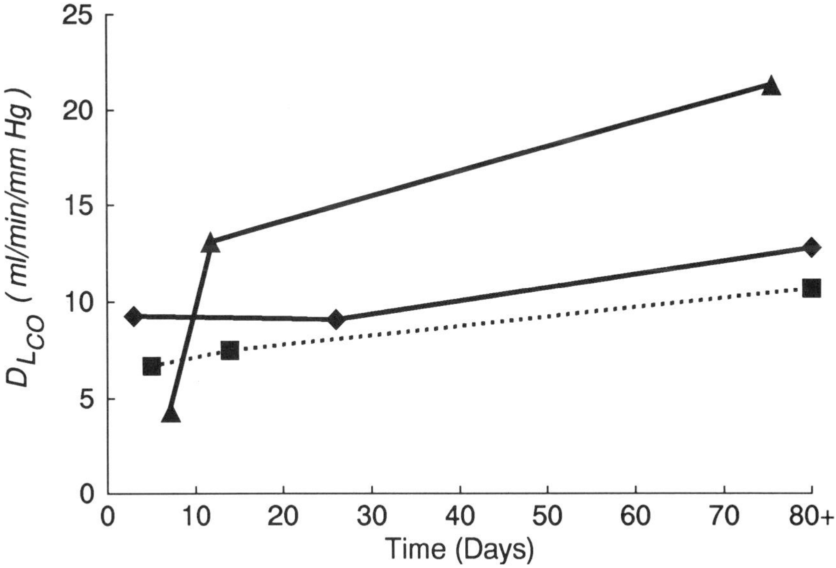

FIGURE 3.11. Resting D_{LCO} values in three patients with varicella pneumonia acutely and during convalescence. (Data from Bocles et al.[14])

The diffusing capacity is a complex measure of gas-exchanging capacity of the lungs, including such factors as the permeability of the alveolar-capillary membrane and the size of the total functional alveolar capillary interphase, or area available for exchange. Significant diffusion defects are present acutely with pneumonia and persist well after radiographic and blood gas findings return to normal[14] (Fig. 3.11). This pattern is particularly characteristic of viral pneumonias.[14] The subjective complaint of dyspnea, as with arterial blood gases, does not correlate with the degree of impairment of diffusing capacity. In addition, there is no significant relation with the degree of hyperventilation as reflected by the arterial PCO_2 with the observed diffusing capacity.

Acid-Base Balance

Hyperventilation with associated hypocapnia is the rule in patients with pneumonia. Respiratory acidosis is seen not uncommonly in infants[15] and patients with underlying preexisting lung disease. When acidosis is present, be it respiratory or metabolic, the increase in H^+ ion concentration serves as an additional stimulus to respiration. The relation between arterial PO_2 and PCO_2 is rather poor (Fig. 3.12), and hypoxia alone is therefore an inadequate explanation for the hyperventilation seen with pneumonia.

The infrequent occurrence of respiratory acidosis and the poor correlation between arterial PCO_2 and PO_2 in pneumonia patients has long been observed and related to the different shapes of the oxygen and carbon dioxide dissociation curves.[16] Overventilation of the noninvolved perfused lung may compensate for the diminished carbon dioxide clearance but not for the inadequate oxygen uptake of the pneumonic perfusate. Thus the mixed arterial PCO_2 is normal or low.

The primary mechanisms leading to hyperventilation in pneumonia patients appear to be complex. One is the stimulation of extra- and intrapulmonary mechanical stretch or propioceptors carried in myelinated vagal afferents. The other is "bronchial" and interstitial C-fiber irritant receptors, which via nonmyelinated vagal afferents stimulate the central controller directly. Data suggesting pulmonary C-fiber receptors as sensors of carbon dioxide in mixed venous blood further support implications of their role in patients with disease, pneumonia in particular, and in exercise hyperpnea. The introduction of organic acid into the right atrium causes a vagally mediated tachypnea, apparently through nonmyelinated fibers not affecting tidal volume. The tachypnea associated with pneumonia appears to be mediated by the parenchymal C-fiber receptors, also termed J receptors. These C-fiber receptor endings act as if they were located in the interstitial space between alveolar walls and pulmonary capillaries (juxtapulmonary capillary receptors). Thus not only

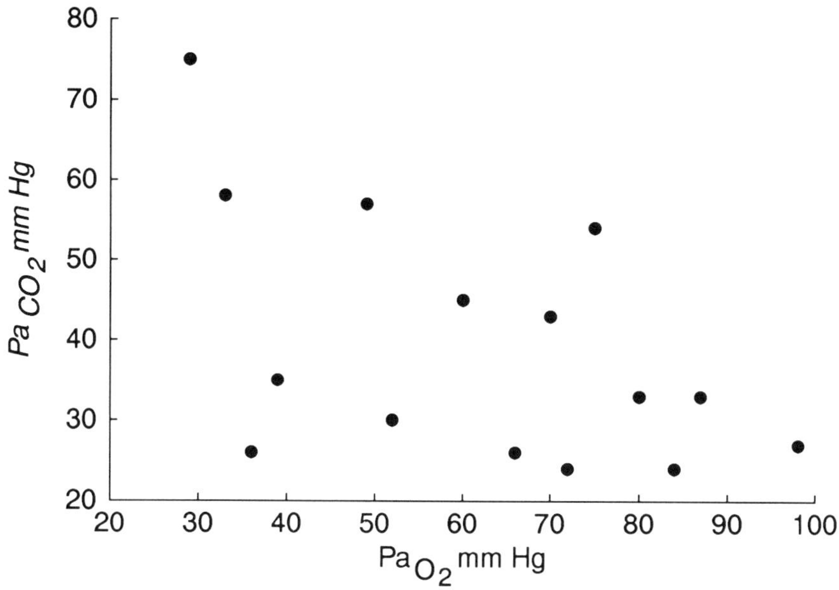

FIGURE 3.12. Relation between arterial PO_2 and PCO_2 values (r = 0.52) on admission in 15 patients with pneumonia while breathing room air. (Data from Simpson and Flenley.[15])

do they have great circulatory accessibility, they are readily exposed to the chemical mediators released during inflammatory processes. These chemical substances may readily depolarize the nonmyelinated nerve endings that appear to be exquisitely sensitive to and readily stimulated by inflammation.

The hypocapnia of pneumonia due to tachypnea has been observed only with intact vagi in the experimental animal and is not dependent on hypoxemia or elevated body temperature, as it is present after their alleviation or in their absence. Moreover, the volume and frequency patterns of ventilation are independently determined through vagal afferents.

As in normal subjects with purposeful variation of their pattern of ventilation under experimental conditions, it is not possible in patients with pneumonia to determine the level of their effective alveolar ventilation and accurately estimate P_ACO_2, utilizing clinical signs of respiratory distress. These objective assessments of respiratory rate and thoracic excursion as well as physical examination utilizing auscultation and percussion are found to be of no value as an indication of the blood gas levels or acid-base balance in patients with pneumonia.

Because hypoxemia does not serve as the respiratory stimulus, oxygen therapy does not cause ventilatory depression and carbon dioxide reten-

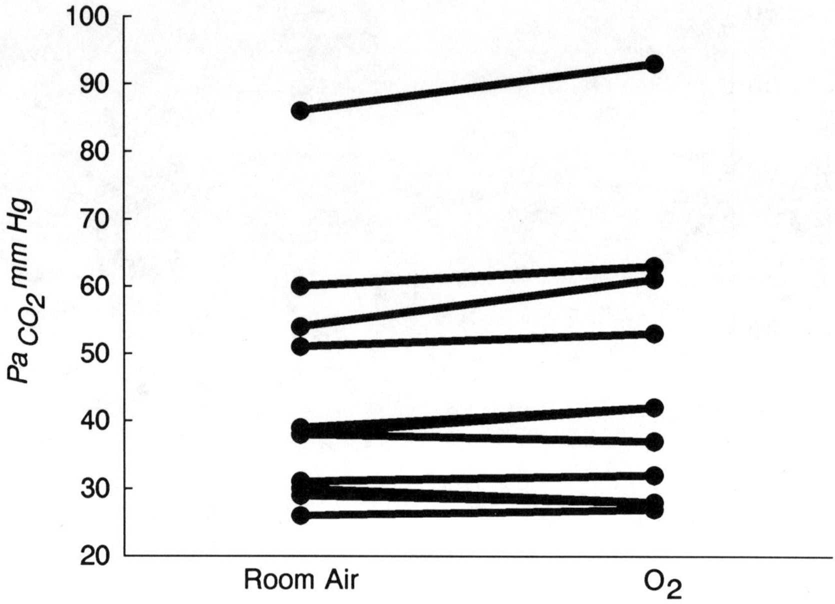

FIGURE 3.13. Arterial PCO_2 values initially present in 11 patients with pneumonia while breathing room air and after treatment with an enriched inspired oxygen concentration. (Data from Herzog et al.[17])

tion, nor does it worsen respiratory acidosis and carbon dioxide narcosis when hypercapnia exists initially.[17] The patients demonstrating an increase in arterial PCO_2 following the initiation of oxygen therapy, especially in those in whom it is initially raised (Fig. 3.13), do so as a result of the Haldane effect (oxyhemoglobin is a poorer buffer than reduced hemoglobin) and alleviation of hypoxic vasoconstriction. As in patients with chronic obstructive lung disease, this effect occurs with no significant change in minute ventilation.

Patients presenting with metabolic acidosis do not restore their base deficit with oxygen therapy. The acidemia does not correlate with the arterial PO_2 and therefore is not strictly of anaerobic origin. The acidemia does represent an adverse prognostic factor, be it metabolic or respiratory in origin. Although respiratory acidosis is more immediately amenable to treatment with intubation, assisted ventilation with a mechanical device has not been shown to affect prognosis.

Hemodynamics

The efficiency of the lungs as a gas-exchange mechanism depends on proper functioning of the vascular plumbing and the parenchymal bellows. As first suggested by in vivo and in vitro opacification studies of

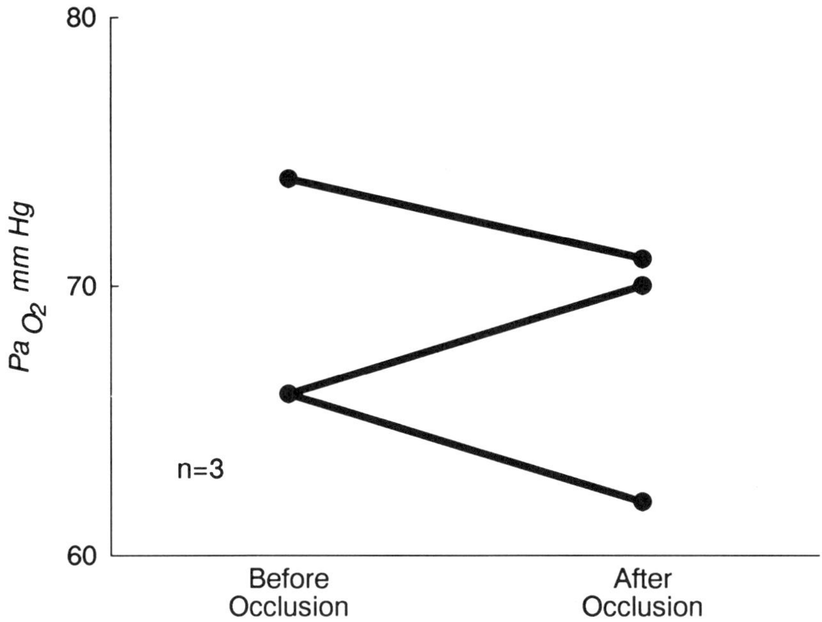

FIGURE 3.14. Arterial oxygenation in three patients with pneumococcal lobar pneumonia before and after pulmonary artery occlusion on the affected side. (Data from Alexander et al.[20])

tuberculous alterations of the vascular bed, major physicopathologic alterations are present in the lesser circulation with inflammatory disease of the lungs.[18]

In the usual "atypical" interstitial pneumonia, as in miliary tuberculosis, there is little evidence of circulatory impairment at rest or with exercise, nor is there pronounced orthostatic lability.[19] With lobar pneumonia the cardiac output and metabolic rate are increased. The increased blood flow is primarily rate-dependent and the increased oxygen delivery (DO_2) exceeds the increase in oxygen uptake (VO_2) with a decreased arteriovenous oxygen difference [$(a-v)O_2$]. Both systemic and pulmonary vascular beds accommodate to the increased flow with no significant elevations in mean pressure. Bronchospirometric studies show an ipsilateral decrease in ventilation, vital capacity, and oxygen uptake. The perfusion of the pneumonic lung is decreased to a greater extent than what would be predicted from the decrease in vital capacity.[20] Temporary complete occlusion of the pulmonary artery supplying the consolidated lung by inflation of a balloon results in no significant change in arterial oxygenation (Fig. 3.14). This finding supports the concept of diminished blood flow to the involved lung in patients with lobar pneumonia, with the venous admixture being primarily due to ventilation-perfusion mismatch of the contralateral lung or increased bronchial flow to the involved lung.

If reduction of the pulmonary vascular bed is extensive, with a hyperdynamic circulation due to toxicity, pulmonary hypertension and cor pulmonale may appear acutely. Furthermore, the adage concerning digitalizing the elderly patient with pneumonia reflects the decreased reserve of the elderly in time of increased demand and the implied impairment of ventricular function that has been postulated to occur with infection and has been documented with sepsis.

Much of the persistent mortality due to pneumonia has been attributed to cardiovascular collapse. The usual hyperdynamic response is often not seen in patients dying of pneumonia, reflecting their inability to respond to the excessive metabolic demands of infection. Moreover, hypodynamic responses, aside from representing preexisting diminished reserve, appear to represent a direct toxic effect of infection on the myocardium—just as generalized sepsis has been described to result in ventricular dysfunction.[21] Unlike septic patients, however, those with classic bacterial lobar involvement and low cardiac output have an elevated total peripheral vascular resistance rather than an associated decrease in afterload.

In the absence of an anatomic or physiologic systemic shunt, as found with the acute lung injury syndrome, a normal or narrowed arteriovenous oxygen difference is considered an indication of adequate tissue perfusion and a physiologically intact circulation. In one series of pneumonia patients, as many as 35% behaved aberrantly and had a widened arteriovenous oxygen difference unrelated to arterial oxygenation, suggesting inadequate tissue perfusion for the increased metabolic demand requiring increased extraction to meet tissue needs.[22] In contrast to the usual course of events, the cardiac output increased in these patients, as did their blood volume in the face of a decreasing oxygen consumption during convalescence (Fig. 3.15), with normalization of the arteriovenous oxygen difference. These changes were associated with a decrease in total peripheral vascular resistance, which was significantly elevated during the acute phase.

Lobar inflammation is associated with a reduction or elimination of local pulmonary blood flow, whereas bronchial circulation in the same region expands. This change is due in part to differential effects of inflammatory mediators on the two circulations, allowing teleologically for maximum preservation of gas exchange and ventilation-perfusion relations while providing the necessary substrate for nutrition and inflammation. Thus, as with chronic fibrosing pulmonary disease, the collateral blood supply of the lungs gains in relative importance in the presence of acute inflammatory disease of the lung as well.

The C-fiber receptors in the tracheobronchial airways seem to have a prevalent chemoreceptor function, whereas the pulmonary C-fiber receptors (J receptors) have been presumed to be mechanosensitive. In

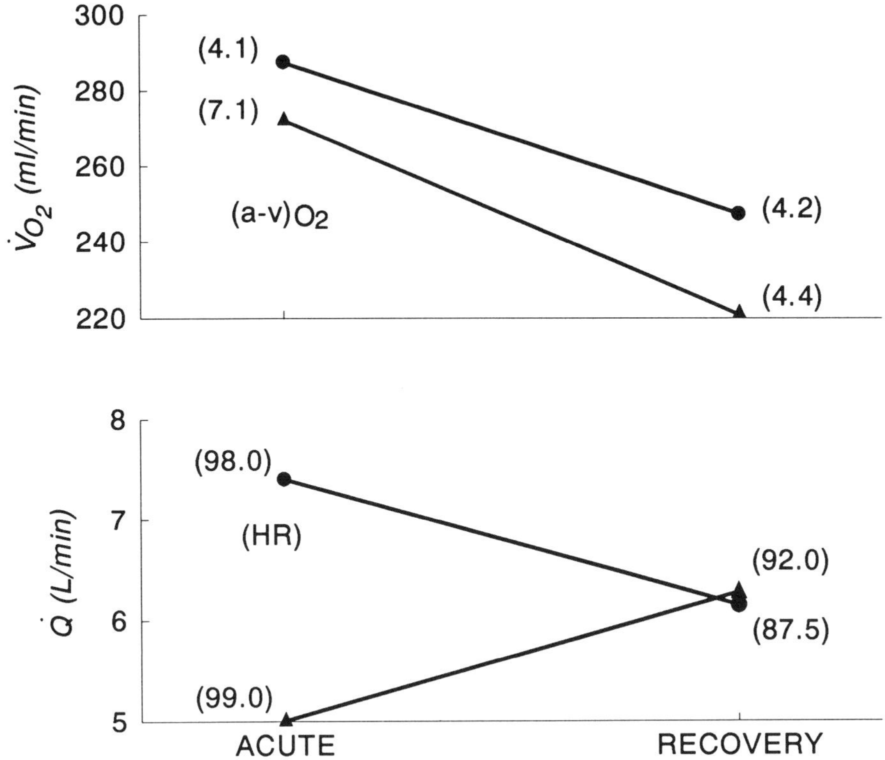

FIGURE 3.15. Hemodynamic status of 17 patients with pneumonia during acute and convalescent stages. The normal circulatory response ($n = 11$) is represented by circles, and the atypical response ($n = 6$) by triangles. (Data from Benson et al.[22])

general, pulmonary C-fiber receptors show a greater response to mechanical events than do bronchial C-fiber receptors. Many stimuli affecting the pulmonary circulation (e.g., congestion, edema, embolism) serve to excite the endings of the pulmonary C fibers, and they have been implicated in mechanisms that limit the intensity of exercise (J reflex). The J receptors are also excited by various pharmacologic agents, including inflammatory chemical mediators as previously mentioned (p. 41) such as cytokines, prostaglandins, and bradykinin. They are thought to serve as an integral link in the integration of cardiovascular and ventilatory function through a complex of cardiovascular and reflex interactions resulting in inhibition of vagal cardiomotor output. Although such a relation between cardiopulmonary function is of obvious functional utility, similar responses have not been demonstrated in disease states such as pneumonia.

Finally, one can also speculate that the tachypnea resulting from J-receptor stimulation in pneumonia patients also serves to increase diaphragmatic blood flow. This redistribution of cardiac output occurs with increases in frequency of diaphragmatic contraction with a constant duty cycle up to respiratory rates of 80 breaths/minute.[23] In addition, as would be predicted because muscle blood flow is impaired during contraction, diaphragmatic blood flow increases with decreasing duty cycle (increased duration of relaxation period) at all respiratory rates.[23] It may therefore be concluded teleologically that pulmonary C fibers serve to influence respiratory frequency and duty cycle to effect a ventilatory strategy of maximizing diaphragmatic blood flow and respiratory force.

References

1. Colp CR, Park SS, Williams MH Jr: Pulmonary function studies in pneumonia. Am Rev Respir Dis 1962;85:808–815.
2. Marshall R, Christie RV: The visco-elastic properties of the lungs in acute pneumonia. Clin Sci 1954;13:403–408.
3. Somerson NL, Kontras SB, Pollack JD, Weiss HS: Pulmonary compliance: alterations during infection. Science 1971;171:66–68.
4. Autio V: The reduction of respiratory function by parenchymal and pleural lesions: a bronchospirometric study of patients with unilateral involvement. Acta TubercBelg 1959;37:112–125.
5. Hey EN, Lloyd BB, Cunningham DJC, et al: Effects of various respiratory stimuli on the depth and frequency of breathing in man. Respir Physiol 1966;1:193–205.
6. Mier-Jedrzejowicz A, Brophy C, Green M: Respiratory muscle weakness during upper respiratory tract infections. Am Rev Respir Dis 1988;138:5–7.
7. Sackner MA, Krieger B: Noninvasive respiratory monitoring. In Scharf SM, Cassidy SS (eds): Lung Biology in Health and Disease. Vol. 42. Heart-Lung Interactions in Health and Disease. New York: Marcel Dekker, 1989, pp. 663–805.
8. Tobin MJ, Chadha TS, Jenouri G, et al: Breathing patterns: diseased subjects Chest 1983;84:286–294.
9. Hussain SNA, Magder S: Respiratory muscle function in shock and infection. Semin Respir Med 1991;12:287–297.
10. Binger CAL, Davis JS Jr: The relation of anoxemia to the type of breathing in pneumonia. J Clin Invest 1928;6:171–185.
11. Mellemgaard K: The mechanism of hypoxemia in lobar pneumonia. Scand J Respir Dis 1967;48:109–116.
12. Lampron N, Lemaire B, Teisseire B, et al: Mechanical ventilation with 100% oxygen does not increase intrapulmonary shunt in patients with severe bacterial pneumonia. Am Rev Respir Dis 1985;131:409–413.
13. Davidson FF, Glazier JB, Murray JF: The components of the alveolar-arterial oxygen tension difference in normal subjects and in patients with pneumonia and obstructive lung disease. Am J Med 1972;52:754–762.
14. Bocles JS, Ehrenkranz NJ, Marks A: Abnormalities of respiratory function in varicella pneumonia. Ann Intern Med 1964:60:183–195.

15. Simpson H, Flenley DC: Arterial blood-gas tensions and pH in acute lower-respiratory-tract infections in infancy and childhood. Lancet 1967;1:7–12.
16. Hastings AB, Neill JM, Morgan HJ, Binger CAL: Blood reaction and blood gases in pneumonia. J Clin Invest 1924–1925;1:25–45.
17. Herzog H, Staub H, Richterich R: Gas-analytical studies in severe pneumonia: observations during the 1957 influenza epidemic. Lancet 1959; 1:593–597.
18. Cicero R, Celis A: Ante-mortem and post mortem angiography of the pulmonary arterial tree in advanced tuberculosis. Am Rev Tuberc 1955; 71:810–821.
19. Berven H: Studies on the cardio-pulmonary function in the course following the acute stage of "atypical" pneumonia. Acta Med Scand Suppl 1962; 382:7–47.
20. Alexander JK, Takezawa H, Abu-Nassar, Yow EM: Studies on pulmonary blood flow in pneumococcal pneumonia. Cardiovas Res Center Bull 1963; 1:86–92.
21. Abel FL: Myocardial function in sepsis and endotoxin shock. Am J Physiol 1989;257:1265–1281.
22. Benson H, Akbaiuan M, Adler LN, Abelmann WH: Hemodynamic effects of pneumonia. I. Normal and hypodynamic responses. J Clin Invest 1970; 49:791–798.
23. Buchler B, Magder S, Roussos C: Effects of contraction frequency and duty cycle on diaphragmatic blood flow. J Appl Physiol 1985;58:265–273.

4 Pathogenesis of Pneumonia

MONROE KARETZKY

Community-Acquired Pneumonia

Community-acquired pneumonia causes large numbers of hospital admissions each year. Although the incidence varies greatly in different geographic and socioeconomic settings, in the United States it has been found to cause 10–15 cases per 100,000 population annually, predominating in the very young and the elderly. Hospitalization may be required in as many as 25% of cases. It is this group from which all the mortality data have been recorded, in contrast to the ambulatory group with "walking pneumonia." Thus adult community-acquired pneumonia occurs in more than 3 million persons per year in the United States; and even though most are treated as outpatients, the disease still accounts for more than 50,000 hospital admissions annually. Major determinants of hospitalization and a complicated course in patients not initially admitted to the hospital include the existence of comorbid conditions, age greater than 65 years, and high grade fever (>101°F). Social factors and patient reliability are also prominent triage considerations that classically account for the high admission rates for patients with pneumonia to municipal institutions.

Various pathogens show seasonal and clustering patterns. Although a definite causative agent is identified in fewer than 50–70% of cases, most of those identified continue to be bacterial, with *Streptococcus pneumoniae* predominating[1] (Fig. 4.1). The distribution of etiologic diagnoses varies greatly among community, municipal, and military institutions. *S. pneumoniae* is responsible for as many as 60% of cases in adults hospitalized with pneumonia in city hospitals but more typically 15–30% in community hospitals, followed in frequency by atypical organisms. The term atypical pneumonia is used to describe community-acquired pneumonias that do not respond to penicillin but to antibiotics such as tetracyclines and erythromycin. Most commonly these pneumonias are caused by *Mycoplasma*, *Chlamydia*, and *Legionella* species. Viral infections are uncommon, with influenza virus the classic pathogen predisposing to secondary bacterial pneumonias. The spectrum of infectious agents has

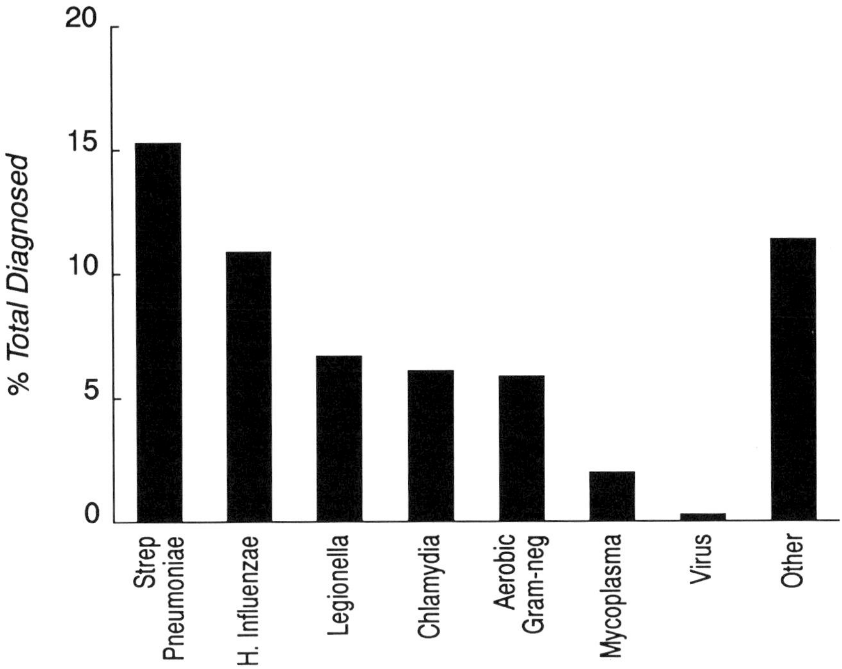

FIGURE 4.1. Etiology of 359 cases of community-acquired pneumonia. The specific organism was unidentifiable in 32.9% of cases. (Data from Fang et al.[1])

continuously broadened during the antibotic era, influencing initial empiric antibiotic therapy. Primary gram-negative bacillary infections have become a growing concern as a cause of community-acquired pneumonia.

The means by which organisms enter the body and invade the lung varies with the pathogen. Most patients developing bacterial pneumonia are predisposed by age and underlying disease, including alcoholism (Fig. 4.2). Bacteria from endogenous flora are classically aspirated as "bronchial emboli," and atypical and viral organisms enter by inhalation of infected droplets from other patients, animals, and a variety of environmental sources. The nasooropharyngeal airway has a complex microbial flora consisting of more than 215 species of aerobic and anaerobic organisms that serve no known purpose and usually cause no ill effects. The oropharyngeal flora, as a rule, does not include aerobic gram-negative rods. Elderly patients, however, who are debilitated are frequently colonized with aerobic gram-negative rods and have an incidence of a "primary pneumonia" due to enteric organisms variously reported to range from 10% to 60%. Colonization has been found to correlated with the general health status in the elderly. The oropharyngeal ecology presumably

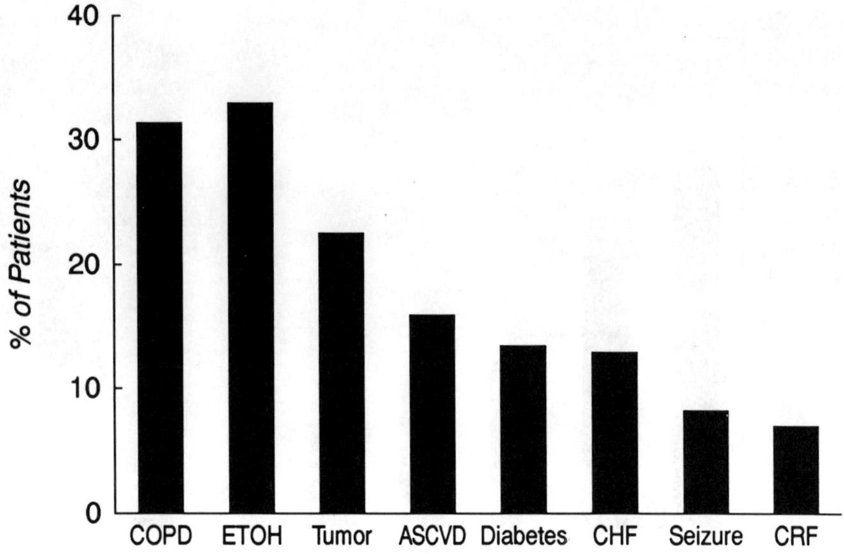

FIGURE 4.2. Most common predisposing conditions in 359 cases of community-acquired pneumonia. There was no underlying disease in 30.6% of episodes, and 36.2% of the patients were immunocompromised. COPD = chronic obstruction pulmony disease; ETOH = alcohol abuse; ASCVD = arteriosclerotic cardiovascular disease; CHF = congestive heart failure; CRF = chronic renal failure. (Data from Fang et al.[1])

reflects the distribution and density of bacterial adhesins and epithelial cell receptors.

Numerous combinations of animal models and organisms have been studied since the turn of the century, reflecting efforts to delineate the nature and progression of the inflammatory response in bacterial pneumonia. However, our knowledge of the biology of oropharyngeal colonization remains in the early stages of development. It has been shown that bacterial attachment to mucosal surfaces normally involves interaction of bacterial lipoteichoic acid with fatty acid-binding sites of fibronectin deposited on mucosal epithelial cells.

It has been clearly demonstrated that most bacterial pneumonias are the result of microaspiration of nonsterile upper respiratory secretions into the lungs, and they are in fact a form of aspiration pneumonia. Aspiration is a routine occurrence in normal individuals during sleep; and depending on the volume of aspirate, the number and virulence of organisms contained, and host defenses, infection may result. Sixty years ago Loeschke related the apparent influence of gravity on the location of pneumococcal pneumonia to secretions aspirated during sleep. These normal nocturnal "bronchial emboli," when facilitated by underlying disease, damaged mucosal integrity, impairment of the mucociliary escalator, or other environmental or host factors, allow tissue invasion. Cold exposure, drugs (sedatives, anesthetics, alcohol), and chronic bronchitis impair ciliary function and are common precipitating events. The elderly and cigarette smokers, possibly responsible for the observed male predominance, are also predisposed to an increased incidence of pneumonia.

Thus a decade after the centennial celebration of the first isolation of *S. pneumoniae*, the organism remains undiminished in frequency, with a static mortality during the postantimicrobial era of up to almost 30% in elderly or concurrently debilitated patients. Studies indicate no significant decline in the incidence of pneumococcal pneumonia from the preantibiotic era, although the mortality of bacteremic pneumococcal pneumonia has fallen from approximately 80% to 20%. This decrease is entirely a result of antibiotic therapy, with no significant effect demonstrated that can be attributable to advances in ventilatory management. Various well known mortality risk factors exist, such as age and heart failure, giving rise to the clinical adage of starting the elderly patient with heart failure on both digitalis and penicillin.

Because of the frequent occurrence of symptoms of upper respiratory tract infection preceding pneumococcal pneumonia, the belief that viral infection often preceded bacterial pneumonia was propagated. The virus was thus credited with weakening the host defense mechanisms. This concept has been repeatedly disproved except for classic influenzal pneumonia. Another exception to this suggestion appears to be the mechanism for the spread of *S. pneumoniae* among normal family contacts. Findings suggest that the enhanced production of respiratory secretions with presumed viral colds may play a role in the transmission of *S. pneumoniae* from carriers to other susceptible family members and presumably even other patients, accounting for institutional outbreaks of pneumococcal pneumonia. Rhinoviruses and clustering of specific types of *S. pneumoniae* were frequently found simultaneously in individual families, suggesting that the viral infection led to dissemination of the bacterial invader.[2] The receptive properties for bacteria in these virus infected host cells appear to altered by different mechanisms. In addition, the extensive desquamation of mucosal epithelium resulting from viral infection exposes the basement membrane to bacterial invasion. Thus as classically illustrated by postinfluenza bacterial pneumonia, not only is the mucosal barrier compromised, but with the loss of ciliated cells "pulmonary toilet" is impaired and the bacterial population of the lower respiratory tract increases, further promoting infection.

Others have shown a circadian periodicity of susceptibility to pneumococcal infection, and animal studies have further suggested that survival patterns could be altered by environmental lighting conditions. Interestingly, survival is adversely affected by nocturnal challenge, presumably the most likely time for aspiration to occur in humans.[3] This point correlates with studies showing that environmental light is important for synchronizing the periodicity of the host response to infection, presumably related to endogenous steroid responses to infectious challenge.

The substantial persistently high mortality found with community-acquired pneumonia is not limited to those with *S. pneumoniae* but extends to other etiologies with single species of pathogens as well.[4] The high mortality has been attributed to several factors, including irreversible physiologic damage prior to the administration of the appropriate antibiotic(s) and the onset of action. Others have also shown that these pneumonias may be caused by combinations of aerobic respiratory pathogens, including atypical and gram-negative organisms.[5] This concept of polymicrobial infection has been well established since the 1970s, especially for anaerobic pleuropulmonary infections and nosocomial pneumonias. There are no distinctive features of etiology in terms of the symptomatology, physical signs, radiographic features, or laboratory data. Findings classically defining "atypical" pneumonia are now found to be obsolete, and greater efforts are needed to utilize laboratory advances to identity the specific causative agents.[6] Early identification of a gram-negative etiology is important because of the increased morbidity and mortality of these pneumonias and the favorable effect on outcome of appropriate initial antibiotic therapy.

Nosocomial Pneumonia

Nosocomial infections are those that occur in an institutional setting, such as a hospital, convalescent center, or skilled-nursing facility. Pneumonia represents about 10–25% of all nosocomial infections and carries the highest mortality rate. Mortality rates of 30–50% have been reported; confounders include age greater than 60, severity of underlying disease, and bilateral pneumonia. Nosocomial bloodstream infections are recognized as an important cause of excess mortality, and bacteremic nosocomial pneumonia has been observed to carry a mortality rate of up to 60%. The microbial causes of nosocomial pneumonia, similar to community-acquired pneumonias, have significantly changed since the 1970s. Aerobic gram-negative bacilli still predominate, with reported incidences usually in the range of 60% or more of such infections. However, there has been a greater variety of gram-negative organisms and an increasing number of atypical etiologic agents, including viruses (e.g., herpes simplex but particularly *Legionella* species) and fungal species (primarily *Aspergillus* and *Candida*). Antibiotic-resistant gram-negative species and coagulase-negative and penicillin (methicillin)-resistant staphylococci are other growing problems.

Technologic advances have also brought new routes of transmission, including contaminated intravenous fluids, invasive catheters for medications or hemodynamic monitoring, and other delivery systems, particularly ventilators (their nebulizers in the past but primarily their circuit tubing today). The role of those involved in "infection control" in hospitals has grown; but despite vigorous surveillance and control efforts, predisposing host factors and technologic "advances" have ensured new and old microbial pathogens the "security" to maintain their share of hospital morbidity.

Many control practices have added to health care costs, whereas surveillance studies have succeeded in abating others particularly in regard to pneumonia. One such classic study demonstrated that mainstream nebulizers served as vectors for nosocomial pneumonia via their aerosols, which were heavily contaminated with gram-negative bacilli. Once recognized, decontamination was readily achieved with the routine use of acetic acid; and presently mainstream nebulizers are no longer used. This study, however, led to a good deal of attention being given to the entire ventilator circuit, and protocols were introduced to change the tubing every 24 hours and to use disposable equipment to minimize the incidence of aerosol inoculums causing pneumonia from contaminated circuits. Subsequently, changes of ventilator circuits every 48 hours was found to be as or more effective than the 24-hour ritual. Most recently, not changing ventilator circuits at all during mechanical ventilation has been shown to have no adverse effect on the rate of nosocomial pneumonia or on patient and circuit colonization.[7] Presumably, less manipulation of tubing decreases the incidence of spillage of contaminated condensate into the tracheobronchial tree (Fig. 4.3). The problem is of special significance in these patients because of the high incidence of pneumonia in ventilator-dependent patients and associated high mortality rate.

The risk and mortality of nosocomial pneumonia in the elderly are increased; and aspiration of oropharyngeal or gastric secretions is an especially obvious risk factor in both the acute and long-term care settings. Difficulty with oropharyngeal secretions, the presence of nasogastric tubes, and the onset of an unusual event such as increased confusion or agitation have been directly associated with the prodrome of pneumonia in the elderly. Poor nutritional status has also been identified as a risk factor in the elderly, possibly by enhancing gram-negative oropharyngeal colonization and depression of cellular immunity.[8]

The continued high frequency of aerobic gram-negative pneumonias has been attributed to the high prevalence of their colonization in the oropharynx of hospitalized debilitated patients. The incidence of colonization increases with the duration of hospitalization and the severity of underlying illness.

The impairment of normal cleaning processes, such as inhibition of cilial beating or of salivary flow, predisposes to colonization. Tissue invasion by bacteria is preceded by colonization of the airways, facilitated by attachment of the mircoorganism to the airway mucosal lining surface. Such adherence allows the bacteria to obtain nutrients from the epithelial

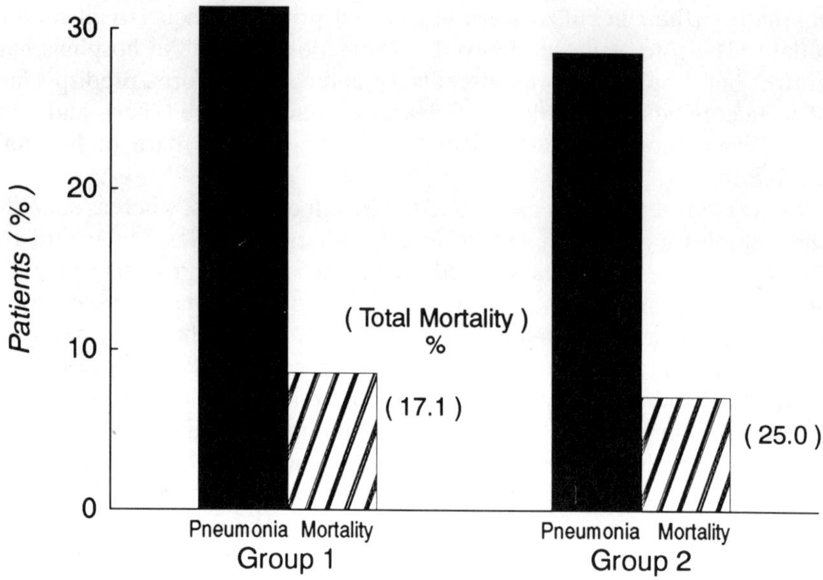

FIGURE 4.3. Incidence (solid bars) of nosocomial pneumonia and deaths (diagonal bars) in patients mechanically ventilated with circuit changes every 48 hours (group 1; $n = 35$) and in patients having no circuit changes (group 2; $n = 28$). Both groups had similar durations of mechanical ventilation: Gp1 = 10.1 days; Gp2 = 9.1 days. (Data from Dreyfuss et al.[7])

lining cells and induce synthesis of proteins essential for continued adherence and tissue invasion while establishing protected glycocalyx-coated microcolonies. Bacteria have proteinaceous ligands or adhesive antigens on their surface that allow stereochemical attachment in a selective manner to receptors of epithelial cells and their cilia. In an acutely or chronically ill host this process requires undefined metabolic changes that affect mucosal cells and facilitate bacterial attachment or colonization.

Normal oropharyngeal flora, like other microbes, need to be attached to a surface to grow, which appears to be regulated by selective adherence to cells via a variety of binding mechanisms. Normal cells prevent such attachment to binding sites by forming antibodies to the adhesins and secretory glycoproteins (e.g., fibronectin) that inhibit bacterial adherence to cell surface receptors and colonization by gram-negative bacilli and select for adherence of gram-positive organisms. Fibronectin and human salivary mucins act as soluble receptors exhibiting "molecular mimicry" of epithelial tissue receptors; they constitute an important host defense mechanism that interferes with bacterial attachment to tissue surfaces. The buccal or pharyngeal epithelial cells of acutely ill patients in the intensive care uint contain less fibronectin and sialic acid on their surface. Elastase, a salivary protease derived from polymorphonuclear cells, digests the fibronectin, allowing colonization not found in normal individuals. Oral secretions from such patients exhibit an elevated protease activity that is responsible for the enhanced receptivity and colonization of the oropharyngeal epithelial cells by *Pseudomonas* and other facultative gram-negative bacilli.

There are a number of binding mechanisms, among which are bacterial saccharide or nonglycosylated binding sites located on filamentous appendages called fimbriae in gram-positive organisms and pili in gram-negative bacilli. The affinity and number of adhesin molecules on the bacteria and the distribution and number of epithelial receptors determine the propensity of a species to colonize. Protein, lipoteichoic acid, and polysaccharide adhesins have been described, each organism appearing to have its principal adhesin, though a single bacterium may contain more than one type of adhesin and fimbriae. Bacterial adhesins serving specialized roles have been described, such as those designed to bind to extracellular matrix proteins, basement membrane constituents, and lectins that bind to carbohydrate residues at sites on "target" cells. Thus even normal microaspirated volumes of highly contaminated innoculums of piliated gram-negative bacteria in the face of impaired defense mechanisms may result in pneumonia in the hospitalized "immunocompromised" host. Other, even less clearly defined processes predispose to colonization and tissue invasion by other encapsulated species and by airborne pathogens introduced by aerosol.

The incidence of nosocomial pneumonia is increased by well documented predisposing pharmacologic factors, such as the inappropriate use of prophylactic antibiotics, corticosteroids, and other immunosuppressive therapy, especially in patients immunodepressed by their primary disease. Other factors predisposing to pneumonia in the hospitalized patient are immobility and a nasogastric tube, making the esophagogastric sphincter incompetent. Enteric feeding can be performed without added risk using a small-bore feeding tube.

The microaspiration of gastric flora has been suggested as a primary mechanism of pneumonia, especially in intubated patients on ventilatory support. The stomach may serve as a reservoir of bacteria when its hydrochloric acid is neutralized or its secretion is impaired or absent. Not only do the bacterial numbers increase when the pH lethal to microorganisms is not achieved, the number of species multiply.[9] If bacteria reach the lung as a liquid bolus, fewer organisms are needed to cause infection than if they arrive by aerosol. Such bacterial overgrowth appears to be controlled with a lower incidence of nosocomial pneumonia in patients treated with sucralfate, which preserves the gastric acid protective mechanisms ($pH < 4$) compared to ventilator patients treated with antacids or histamine type 2 blockers[10] (Fig. 4.4). Mortality is increased by superimposed nosocomial pneumonia to the same degree regardless of the prophylaxis regimen.

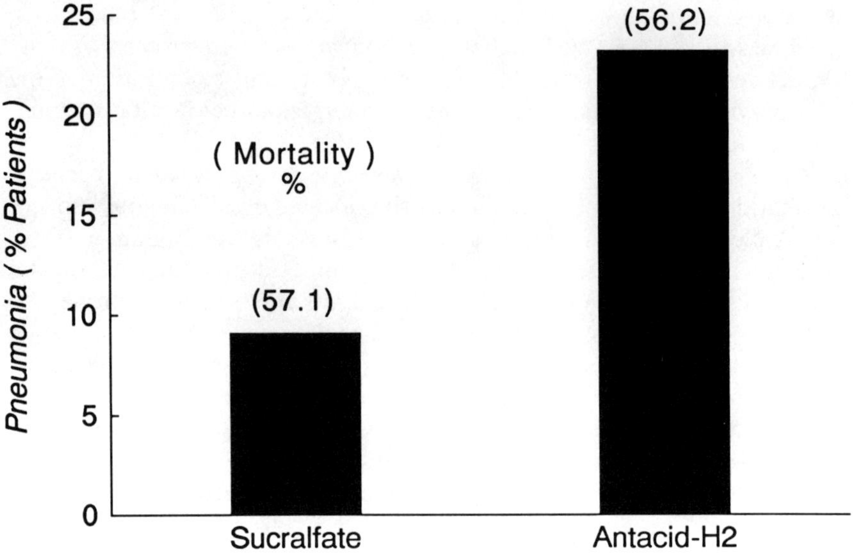

FIGURE 4.4. Incidence of nosocomial pneumonia in patients with mechanical ventilation receiving prophylaxis against stress-induced upper gastrointestinal tract bleeding. Antacids or H2 blockers (cimetidine or ranitidine) alone or together, $n = 69$; sucralfate alone, $n = 55$. (Data from Driks et al.[10])

Criteria for diagnosing nosocomial pneumonias vary but usually include the following after 72 hours of hospitalization.

1. Appearance of a new or progressive infiltrate on chest roentgenogram
2. Fever
3. Leukocytosis
4. Purulent sputum

It has become increasingly apparent that the diagnosis of nosocomial pneumonia in mechanically ventilated patients, particularly those with preceding diffuse radiographic abnormalities such as are seen with acute lung injury, is difficult on the basis of such clinical criteria. Studies based on autopsy findings in patients with the acute lung injury syndrome (adult respiratory distress syndrome; ARDS) have shown the increased risk of pneumonia and that it is the most common complicating infection. Moreover, clinical findings were found to have almost no predictive value, not only for identifying specific etiologic pathogens but most importantly as to which patients had nosocomial pneumonia at the time of death.

With ARDS the problem of overdiagnosis and underdiagnosis of superimposed infectious pneumonia exists. Studies have revealed as much as 36% false-negative and 20% false-positive diagnoses of pneumonia based on clinical criteria.[11] There is no correlation of clinical findings, duration of ventilation, or the apparent response to antibiotic therapy to the histologic diagnosis of pneumonia.[11] This finding casts considerable doubt on the accuracy of estimates of the frequency of pneumonia based on clinical criteria alone. Even with a correct diagnosis, gram-negative bacilli are routinely isolated from airway specimens, rendering their clinical significance difficult to evaluate: are they invasive, causative agents or simply colonizing commensal inhabitants? Various approaches have been suggested, including quantitative cultures of specimens obtained by bronchoscopy using the protected specimen brush, or bronchoalveolar lavage (BAL) supplemented by microscopic grading of BAL samples.

Another area of controversy is the prophylactic use of poorly absorbed, topical antibiotics given by inhalation or direct oropharyngeal application and enteric administration with or without a parenteral drug for selective digestive decontamination. The advantage is that topical administration of antimicrobial agents results in high concentrations but has the disadvantage of the emergence of drug-resistant bacterial strains. This strategy, utilized especially for preventing nosocomial pneumonia in ventilated patients, has been widely studied in Europe. Published reports on the efficacy of such regimens for preventing pneumonia and reducing mortality continue to be contradictory.[12,13] The thesis promoting this approach is in part that the concentration of a systemically administered antibiotic is much lower in mucosal secretions than in serum. However, because bacterial adhesins are proteins, even low concentrations of antibiotics impairing protein synthesis may effectively diminish adherence and allow the body's defense mechanisms to suppress bacterial colonization. Thus it is not an antibiotic's ability to inhibit bacterial growth alone that determines its efficacy but its ability to prevent the bacteria from "hanging on" as well.

Postoperative Pneumonia

Advances in preoperative management, intraoperative technique, and postoperative surveillance have failed to diminish the incidence of postoperative pneumonia. Such lower respiratory tract infections are by definition nosocomial in nature and account for 50% of hospital-acquired pneumonias. Over the past half-century various risk factors were suggested that have recently been clarified (Table 4.1). Age and sex were found to be factors only dependent on site and duration of surgery rather than an innate predisposing respiratory pattern, such as predominant abdominal rather than thoracic breathing.[14] Obesity was a factor only when it was exogenous (>200% predicted weight) (Fig. 4.5).

Preoperative evaluation of pulmonary function has been stressed,[15] but assessment of its predictive value continues to be discouraging for both nonpulmonary thoracic surgery and upper abdominal surgery. The appro-

TABLE 4.1. Risk factors for postoperative pneumonia.

Age: Elderly
Sex: Male > female
Weight: Obesity
Smoking history: Increased secretions
Operative site: Upper > lower abdominal
Time of surgery: Duration of anesthesia
Lung function: Chronic lung disease
Nutrition: Serum albumin
Duration of hospitalization (pre- or postop): Gram-negative colonization and inactivity

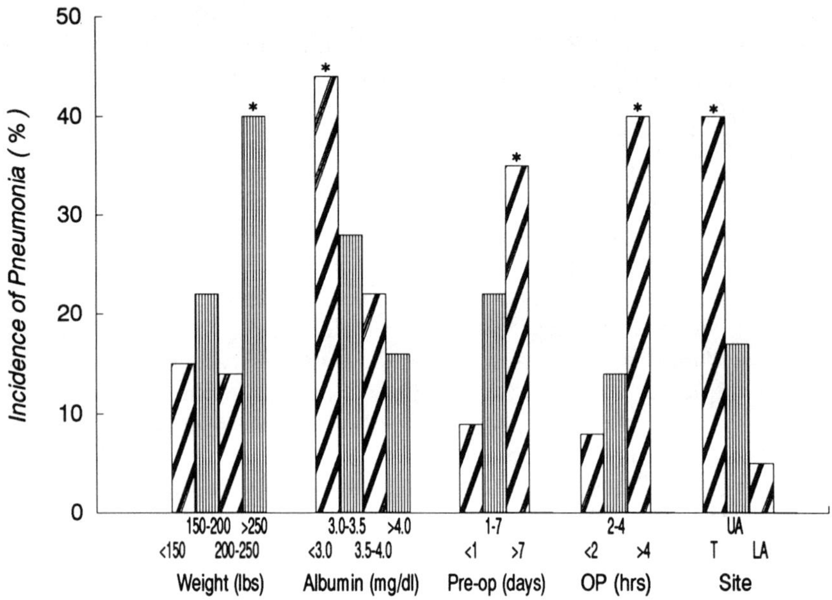

FIGURE 4.5. Relation between predisposing factors and incidence of postoperative pneumonia including body weight, serum albumin concentration on admission, duration of preoperative hospitalization, duration of the surgical procedure (OP), and the site of surgery: T = thoracic; UA = upper abdominal; LA = lower abdominal; * = $p < 0.05$. (Data from Daritaldi et al.[14])

priate tests of lung function that constitute an adequate screening profile for predicting postoperative pulmonary complications remain in question.[16]

Spirometry alone does not appear to be sufficient, and concepts of nuclear and stress testing to supplement clinical assessment for determining which patients undergoing nonresectional thoracic and abdominal surgery are at increased risk are now being explored.[15] The importance of the severity of preexisting pulmonary disease and the value of prophylactic measures remain to be clearly documented.

Postoperative atelectasis and pneumonia, if not used synonymously, share, as inferred by the term "hypostatic pneumonia," a closely related pathogenesis. The former is marked by hypoxia with or without radiologic findings and the latter always by an infiltrate on roentgenogram. In contrast to pulmonary collapse, atelectasis does not necessarily exist as a well localized or radiographically visible entity giving rise to qualifying terms such as miliary, micro, and macro to infer the size and extent of the lung units collapsed. The pathogenesis of the atelectasis that characteristically follows upper abdominal surgery is multifactorial, promoted by the decrease in vital capacity, functional residual capacity (FRC), and tidal volumes that are observed postoperatively. This restrictive pattern of lung mechanics is attributable to pain and the resulting splinting of an abdominal wall whose anatomic integrity and functional capacity have been impaired due to increased intraabdominal pressure from distended aperistaltic bowel, which both displaces the diaphragm upward into the chest and impairs its descent.

Aside from altering the resting position of the fibers (increased length) of the prime inspiratory muscle of ventilation to a presumably more favorable position on their length-tension curve, the diaphragm at this expiratory level behaves as if it has been traumatized and is variably dysfunctional. Thus compartmental displacement is modified, and the diaphragm's contribution to the tidal breath after upper abdominal surgery is reduced. Total pain relief only partially corrects the restrictive defect. This ventilatory defect is similar to that seen in patients with muscle weakness or paralysis of the diaphragm; and over the past century diaphragmatic failure was suggested as a potential mechanism for postoperative pulmonary atelectasis. It has been suggested that the apparent postoperative diaphragmatic dysfunction is secondary to direct local irritation or trauma, the result of the abdominal wall incision and the surgical procedure. Moreover, postoperative visceral gaseous distension and pneumoperitoneum may contribute. Investigators have also proposed that reflex inhibition of phrenic nerve output is responsible for the observed impairment of diaphragmatic contraction.[17] It is therefore of interest to speculate on the effects on lung mechanics and gas exchange that occur during sleep in postoperative patients. In those with severe diaphragmatic paresis normal REM (rapid eye movement sleep stage) induced paralysis of the intercostals and accessory respiratory muscles would effectively remove all inspiratory activity.

The contracted abdominal expiratory muscles are best treated with muscle relaxants. These agents, as reflected by the relief of associated wheezing expiration, may potentially act as "functional" bronchodilators. This mechanism of atelectasis and postoperative hypoxia is reproducible in normal subjects made to tidal breath with normal volumes in an expiratory position (decreased FRC).[18] The resulting hypoxemia is not immediately alleviated by normal or deep breathing (Fig. 4.6), which is in

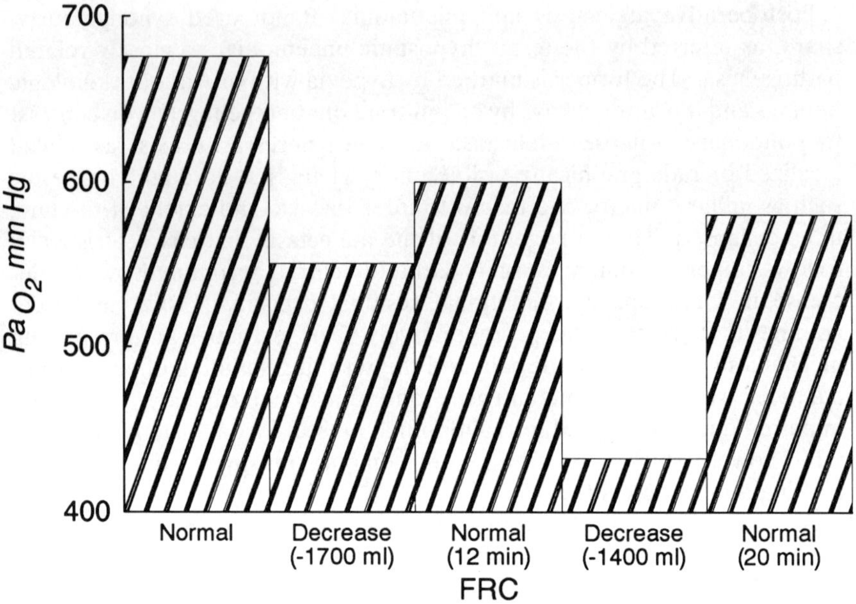

FIGURE 4.6. Effect of repeated episodes of breathing at decreased FRC on arterial oxygenation in a normal subject while breathing 100% oxygen in the upright position. The tidal volume and $PaCO_2$ were unchanged. The change in volume is indicated, as is the time of normal FRC breathing after which the PaO_2 was determined. (Data from Nunn et al.[18])

contrast to the salutory effects of such sigh maneuvers after the promotion of alveolar collapse with purposeful alveolar hypoventilation.[19] The concept of atelectasis resulting from increased surface tension and alveolar instability due to the inactivation of surfactant has become firmly established in the literature. The surfactant is inactivated as a result of its not being renewed by periodic reexpansion, as accomplished by normal sighing and changes in posture. Analgesics (e.g., morphine) have been shown to inhibit such spontaneous deep breathing as well as the cough reflex. In addition, high inspired oxygen concentration with loss of the splinting effect of the inert gases (nitrogen) in room air promotes absorption (diffusion) atelectasis. Whatever the pathophysiologic mechanism(s) for postoperative atelectasis, it is presumably additive, and increased muscle force is necessary for reexpansion and the effort required to avoid progression.

Factors identified to limit atelectasis are lateral transverse (rather than vertical midline) incisions, separate abdominal and thoracic incisions (diaphragm not divided) rather than a single thoracoabdominal incision, and sitting postoperatively rather than lying in the supine position. Additionally, energy and resources have been devoted to the development of respiratory and chest physiotherapy techniques to prevent and minimize postoperative airway occlusion and atelectasis. Such therapies have their origins from the respiratory physiologist Yandell Henderson, who concluded more than six decades ago that a functional element predisposing to postoperative pneumonia such as atelectasis "can be combated from the side of the physiology of respiration."[20] He suggested developing breathing techniques that promote drainage, restore the FRC, and prevent "obstructive" pneumonia.

It has been suggested that clapping and thumping is ineffectual in patients with previously normal lungs, and that at a minimum a physiotherapist's valuable time should not be wasted on nonbronchitic patients. Much of the controversy over the efficacy of breathing devices, such as positive-pressure breathing (IPPB) instruments, has subsided with the relatively simplistic acceptance of incentive spirometry (IS) in its place or simple old-fashioned unsupervised voluntary or coached deep breathing exercises.

Studies have shown that IPPB is of little or no value and that IS has equivalent results. Despite the glaring absence of demonstrable success for either prophylaxis or treatment of atelectasis, IS continues to be widely used and essentially all hospitals' limited resources continue to be expended in this fruitless endeavor.[21] Continuous positive airway pressure (CPAP) has also been advocated on theoretic grounds to increase FRC. Its benefit remains in doubt and is not indicated in patients with chronic obstructive pulmonary disease (COPD). With such equivalent "nonresults" we are left with no scientifically demonstrated benefit from current modes of prophylaxis or therapy, particularly in patient at high risk. Most recently, as an outgrowth of experience in the treatment of obstructive sleep apnea (OSA), lobar collapse has been successfully treated with nasal CPAP. It acts as an aerodynamic strut of the upper airway in patients with OSA and presumably has a similar therapeutic mechanism of action on the lower proximal airways in postoperative patients.

In conclusion, factors predisposing to the development of postoperative atelectasis are thought to be numerous, and little benefit has been demonstrated from current prophylactic techniques. The significance of such failure is believed to be the continued high incidence of the natural consequence of impaired airway drainage, infection, or postoperative pneumonia, which has not decreased over the decades.

Immunocompromised Host

In reality, a discussion of the pathogenesis of pneumonia is synonymous with a presentation of impaired host defense mechanisms—physical, physiologic, and systemic. Consideration of the immunocompromised host classically focuses on impaired cellular and humoral responses to environ-

TABLE 4.2. Pneumonia in the immunocompromised host.

Immunologic impairment	Opportunists	Predisposition
Granulocytopenia (functional or absolute)	Gram-negative bacilli	Myeloproliferative disorders
	Fungi: *Aspergillus*	Corticosteroids
	Gram-positive cocci	Cytotoxic agents
Humoral dsyfunction	Gram-positive cocci: *S. pneumoniae*	Lymphoproliferative disorders
	Gram-negative bacilli *P. aeruginosa* *H. influenza*	Corticosteroids, cytotoxic agents
Cellular dysfunction	Protozoa: *Pneumocystis, Toxoplasma, Cryptosporidium*	AIDS
	Mycobacterium	Lymphoma
	Nocardia	Renal failure
	Legionella	Corticosteroids
	Listeria	Cytotoxic agents
	Fungi (cryptococci) and viruses (CMV, herpes)	Immunosuppressives

mental organisms, including those classically presented as pathogens but emphasizing an otherwise ubiquitous population of commensal bystanders now able to cause "opportunistic" infections (Table 4.2). Defects are rarely pure, but one disorder is usually predominant.

The creation of iatrogenic diseases has more than kept pace with the pharmaceutical industries' technology in developing new generations and classes of antibiotics designed to eradicate infection. Drug-induced pulmonary disease resulting from drugs used to treat the primary diseases of the immunocompromised host are considered in a subsequent section. This section refers to the patient with malignancy, especially lymphoma and leukemia, and the consequences of chemotherapeutic agents; tranplant patients and the consequences of immunosuppressive agents; other diseases and consequences of treatment with corticosteroids; and primary neutropenia. The lungs almost invariably become infected in these patients, and pneumonia carries a mortality exceeding 50%. In patients with hematologic abnormalities who develop pneumonia and respiratory failure, requiring admission to the intensive care unit, mortality approaches 100%.

Although opportunistic infections are common, "usual" bacterial pneumonias are most frequent. Much emphasis has been placed on the increasing incidence of fungal pneumonias, especially aspergillosis and candidiasis, the difficulty of making a diagnosis short of autopsy, and the importance of empiric therapy. With transplant patients specific infectious agents have a frequency distribution according to the stage of immunosuppression; but with bone marrow transplantation, cytomegalovirus is always the infection to be listed first when determining a "most likely"

TABLE 4.3. Pulmonary infiltrates in acute myelogenous leukemia.

Pneumonia
Infections
Radiation
Drug toxocity
Nonspecific
Leukemic infiltrations
Parenchymal
Nonparenchymal
Pleural
Vascular
Hemorrhage
Infarction
Pulmonary edema

list of specific causative agents. Pneumonia therefore is the most common life-threatening infection for the immunocompromised host. Compounding the diagnostic problem is the fact that about 25% of the infiltrates seen on chest radiograph are noninfectious in nature and may be accompanied by fever.

Noninfectious pulmonary complications in particular pose a real problem of differential diagnosis in leukemic patients. There are many causes of pulmonary infiltrates in leukemic patients, but the autopsy incidence of pleural or pulmonary involvement in acute myelogenous leukemia (AML) ranges from 20% to 35%, with 64% cited in one series.[22] Most parenchymal abnormalities are attributed to infection, hemorrhage, or pulmonary toxicity secondary to chemotherapeutic agents (Table 4.3).

Tryka et al.[23] described yet another AML pulmonary entity they termed leukemic cell lysis pneumopathy, where leukemic blast cells presumably damaged by chemotherapy release cytokines and other inflammatory mediators. The patients have characteristic reversible radiologic abnormalities and fever resulting in dyspnea (Fig. 4.7). The recognition of this noninfectious entity causing inflammatory parenchymal disease, pneumopathy, requires clinical differentiation from infectious pneumonia, which is responsible for most pulmonary infiltrates in leukemic patients and is the primary cause of death.[24] Tryka et al. suggested that their findings were similar to the nonspecific pneumonias frequently seen in patients with hematologic malignancies after chemotherapy.[23] They attributed this response of "diffuse alveolar damage" to release of intracellular chemical mediators or metabolic products of lysed blast cells rather than simple leukostasis. Their patients had patchy alveolar or nodular bilateral infiltrates seen on chest radiographs. This distribution of the lesions suggest a uniquely limited release of soluble mediators with successful localization

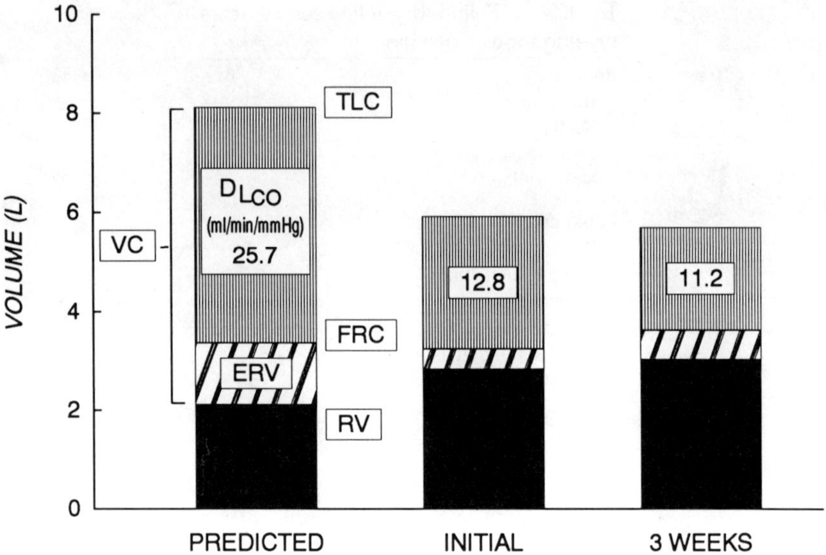

FIGURE 4.7. Pulmonary function tests of a patient with leukemic cell lysis pneumopathy. The tests were performed when the pulmonary changes were first observed and subsequently when they were no longer radiologically apparent. The decreased diffusing capacity reflected the patient's anemia and elevated carboxyhemoglobin level due to cigarette smoking, which was also thought to be responsible for the apparent gas trapping. VC = vital capacity; ERV = expiratory reserve volume; TLC = total lung capacity; FRC = functional residual capacity; RV = residual volume; D_{LCO} = diffusing capacity.

of the injury to lung parenchymal cells. Biopsies were performed in these patients an average of 23 days after the start of chemotherapy. The chest roentgenograms began to resolve 3–17 days after biopsy in four patients; the remaining patient had only partial clearing with remnant scarring. Few patients with hematologic malignancy survive hospitalization following open lung biopsy for evaluation of pulmonary infiltrates. Therefore it is important to be aware of this additional entity of leukemic cell pneumopathy in order to adequately consider the probability of a noninfectious process as the cause of a new pulmonary infiltrate.

Most studies of pulmonary infiltrates in leukemia have included heterogeneous groups of patients with different underlying diseases, various immunosuppressive drug regimens, and most recently allogenic bone marrow transplantation. Leukemic infiltration occurs primarily in a focal distribution at three sites in the lung; the most common is invasion of the alveolar septum followed by nonparenchymal locations, including peribronchial or perivascular collections, and lastly subpleural infiltration. This involvement is usually apparent only microscopically, being clinically and radiographically silent. It has been shown that for determining specific infectious etiologies for pulmonary infiltrates not only transbronchial biopsy but even open lung biopsy can be diagnostically misleading in patients with acute leukemia. Moreover, the use of BAL in patients with acute leukemia treated with antineoplastic agents is not useful for detecting causative pathogens of pneumonia,[25] which is in contrast to the favorable reports of BAL in more severely immunocompromised patients such as those having had bone marrow transplants where *Pneumocystis carinii* or CMV pneumonia is common. The findings at autopsy in patients with acute leukemia where these and other viral pneumonias are uncommon show infiltrates attributable to *Candida*, *Aspergillus*, or nonspecific pneumonia, further supporting the arguments for empiric therapy. Autopsy examination is the only definitive diagnostic procedure, and even then a significant number of cases have a nonspecific diagnosis of interstitial pneumonitis. It has been shown repeatedly that, despite residual leukemia at autopsy, pulmonary parenchymal involvement by leukemia cells is rare.

Vascular occlusion by leukemia cells occurs but is also rare and, in contrast to diffuse cellular infiltrative pulmonary involvement, tends to correlate with the peripheral white blood cell (WBC) count and can result in infarction. Tumor cell emboli and leukostasis with vascular obstruction in the absence of radiographic findings have been reported in autopsy studies of acute leukemia. Rapid, even fatal pulmonary edema was initially reported in acute leukemia patients without regard to the occurrence of WBC sequestration or leukostasis, now considered to initiate nonspecific mechanisms of pulmonary damage. The latter is thought to be a result of WBC activation, as is seen in leukoagglutinin transfusion reactions and the numerous other conditions predisposing to acute lung injury (ARDS). In contrast, others have reported respiratory distress due to intravascular leukostasis in a hyperleukocytic phase of AML requiring emergency chemotherapy, with dramatic regression of symptoms in parallel to the fall in the peripheral WBC count. At autopsy vascular leukostasis in the lung was the predominant finding without parenchymal infiltration.

With transplantation, allowing for problems of function and rejection, infection is the most important problem particularly during the first 3 months. The lung is the most common site of infection in heart–lung transplantation. CMV is a particularly troublesome problem, as it is in bone marrow transplants, and presents the additional problem of graft-versus-host reaction, suggesting an interaction of infection with rejection. Immunosuppression is the most obvious predisposing factor to infection, and unique to transplantation is the use of cyclosporine. Its main focus appears to be inhibition of the antigen-directed elaboration of interleukin-2 by T-helper cells. The use of antilymphocyte serum or antithymocyte globulin further enhances the occurrence of pneumonia, particularly that due to CMV. Important sources of infection include endogenous flora, reactivation of latent infections in the host and the donor organ, and the usual environmental airborne and contact contaminants. Fever is an undependable signal of infection in transplant patients, because even if it occurs it may be a manifestation of organ rejection rather than infection. The transplant patient is prone to another common noninfectious cause of fever: drug reactions, such as with antithymocyte globulin.

Patients with bone marrow transplants have the unique noninfectious entities of diffuse pulmonary alveolar hemorrhage (DAH) and graft-versus-host disease to differentiate from infectious pulmonary infiltrates.[26] This attempt by immunocompetent donor lymphocytes to reject the recipient may be complicated by bronchiolitis obliterans and a lymphocytic bronchitis that must be differentiated from nonspecific interstitial pneumonia, which is probably a manifestation of CMV or other viral infection. Noninfectious interstitial pneumonia, a major complication of transplantation, is a significant cause of death after bone marrow transplantation, where it has been attributed to the cumulative toxic effects of irradiation and chemotherapy on the lung. This idiopathic pneumonitis also appears to be a predisposing factor in the pathogenesis of DAH.[27]

Lung transplantation is the setting for other noninfectious complications of the immunocompromised host. With combined heart–lung transplantation, early experience suggesting that pulmonary rejection occurs only in concert with cardiac rejection proved false. The acute rejection process has been shown by many investigators to have a distinct histologic picture that can be differentiated from infection, and chronic rejection is probably represented by bronchiolitis obliterans.

Chronic idiopathic neutropenia has many causes; but whatever its pathogenesis, unlike the course of recurrent infection seen in neutropenic patients with leukemia or drug-induced granulocytopenia, its natural history is often benign, unmarked by lower respiratory tract infections. Thus qualitative and quantitative aspects of neutrophil function exist. In association with disease or secondary to therapeutic interventions, the incidence and severity of infection are inversely proportional to the absolute polymorphonuclear neutrophil (PMN) count. A threshold level of approximately 5000 cells/ml is suggested, but bacteremias are almost invariable associated with PMN counts of fewer than 1000 cells/ml. More importantly, the more rapid the decline (rather than the absolute nadir) and the greater the duration of neutropenia, the more inevitable is the occurrence of microbial invasion. Time is also important with respect to the likelihood of a particular nosocomial agent having an enhanced opportunity for achieving predominance and then colonization. This course of events classically occurs in the debilitated chemotherapy-treated patient in a hospital environment with alteration of resident flora or reactivation of latent foci of infection. Compromise of physical and natural defense barriers, such as endotracheal intubation, further ensures the occurrence as well as the site of infection to be in the pulmonary parenchyma.

Bacterial infections account for more than 50% of opportunistic infections in the immunocompromised host. The usual nosocomial agents predominate, and the pneumonia is frequently polymicrobial. *Legionella* is an opportunistic agent in the immunocompromised host especially in the renal transplant patient. As in acquired immunodificiency syndrome (AIDS) patients, those with T-cell deficiencies have an increased incidence of tuberculosis. CMV pulmonary infection is one of the most common complications in the transplant patient, usually occurring within the first 4 months after transplantation. CMV infection results from transmission of the virus from seropositive donor to a seronegative recipient via the allograft or by reactivation of latent CMV in the recipient, who was seropositive before transplantation. The association between seroconversion and the development of CMV pneumonia presumably exists because seroconversion serves as an indication of infection, and not primarily because it predisposes to pneumonia. However, this association illustrates the relative unimportance of antibody in defense against CMV infection. CMV infection further suppresses T-cell-mediated immunity and may cause severe neutropenia, predisposing to superinfections with *Pneumocystis* and *Aspergillus*.

Herpes simplex and varicella viral infections, like CMV infections, occur as a complication of T-cell deficiency states and rarely present as primary pneumonia. Pneumonia occurs more frequently in both children and adults who are immunologically compromised or otherwise at special risk. This group includes those with AIDS or malignancies (especially leukemia or lymphoma) and patients receiving immunosuppressive drugs, including corticosteroids. Varicella pneumonia has been reported to occur in 16–50% of adult cases of chickenpox. Pregnant women also appear to be predisposed. Varicella pneumonia has been reported to be more severe and to produce higher mortality in otherwise healthy pregnant women, but the pathogenesis of this phenomenon remains unexplained. An association between cigarette smoking has not been clearly shown with varicella as it has been with influenza. The differential diagnosis includes other viral diseases, especially herpes simplex, secondary bacterial infections, and the gamut of opportunistic organisms. Although it usually exhibits a benign course, this complication can cause considerable morbidity and mortality in predisposed groups, including pregnant women and immunosuppressed patients. In these patients the use of antiviral drugs, most notably acyclovir, has been shown to lessen the morbidity of both herpes simplex virus and varicella-zoster infections (Fig. 4.8).

The concept of "cellular dysfunction" broadly implies impaired activation of the foot soldiers of cellular immune function, the macrophage or monocyte— the killers of intracellular pathogens. Often the defect lies in the proximal limb of this defense, the T4-helper lymphocyte, and its failure to respond to antigen stimulation and release of cell-derived lymphokines, including tumor necrosis factor, interleukin-2, and granulocyte-

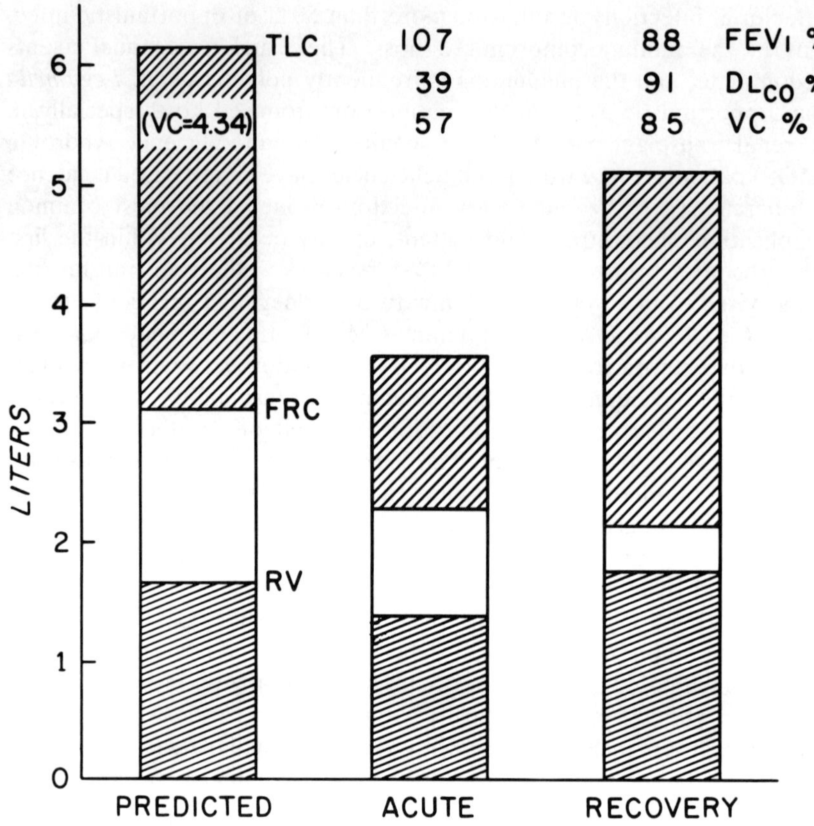

FIGURE 4.8. Pulmonary function testing in a patient with varicella pneumonia treated with acyclovir. TLC = total lung capacity; FRC = functional residual capacity; RV = residual volume; $FEV_1\%$ = FEV_1/VC; $D_{L_{CO}}\%$ = diffusing capacity % predicted; VC = vital capacity; VC% = % predicted. The acute restrictive ventilatory defect resolved when measurements were repeated 3 months later. Arterial oxygenation increased to 74 mm Hg. The patient continued to smoke, with a HbCO level of 6.7%.

macrophage colony-stimulating factor (GM-CSF). Each predisposition in some way favors a particular opportunist, and knowledge of this characteristic influences empiric therapy. Patients with humoral immune dysfunction are predisposed to infection with encapsulated pyogenic bacteria. The deficiency of opsonizing antibodies impairs the activity of all phagocytic cells. A well recognized determinant of humoral immunocompetence is hyposplenism resulting from either splenectomy or infarction, in most cases secondary to sickle cell anemia. Regardless of underlying predisposition, constant surveillance and ongoing analysis of alterations in clinical responsiveness and expeditious initiation of the most appropriate empiric antimicrobial regimen while awaiting yields of diagnostic efforts are critical factors in the achievement of a successful therapeutic outcome.

Acquired Immunodeficiency Syndrome

The pulmonary complications associated with AIDS have continued to characterize these patients' clinical course. Their paralyzed immune system, predisposing them to invasion by opportunistic organisms, was subsequently found to result from infection with a retrovirus, the human immunodeficiency virus (HIV). Various agents, including mycoplasmas, have been suggested as possible cofactors in cell death caused by HIV infection. In New York City AIDS is the leading cause of death among young male adults and black female subjects aged 15–44 years. Opportunistic pulmonary diseases are the most common cause of acute illness and death in patients with HIV infection.

The specific subset (CD4+) of helper T lymphocytes is the main target of the virus, reducing their number and function while causing a cascade of other immunologic deficits, including associated CD8+ T-lymphocyte, macrophage, natural killer (NK), and B-cell abnormalities. The T-helper lymphocyte plays a central role in regulating the immune system through the production of a variety of cytokines. These cytokines regulate T and B lymphocytes, NK cells, macrophage-monocytes, and probably polymorphonuclear cells.

AIDS is diagnosed in HIV-seropositive patients who develop an opportunistic infection or characteristic malignancy. AIDS occurs in more than 3% of seroconverters per year. The lungs are involved in as many as two-thirds of patients, *Pneumocystis* being the most common infectious agent, found in more than 50% of pneumonias. As many as 15% of the pulmonary complications of AIDS are noninfectious in etiology; they include Kaposi's sarcoma and lymphoma. Multiple simultaneously occurring pulmonary infections are commonplace; and when the pneumonia is not satisfactorily responding to specific treatment for an identified pathogen, others should be considered as well. *Pneumocystis carinii* pneumonia (PCP) is frequently associated with CMV infection; however, CMV coinfection does not appear to alter survival or the severity of the PCP of AIDS. Presently, the routine use of prophylactic therapy has decreased the incidence of PCP with a corresponding increase in the other opportunistic infections. Tuberculosis caused by typical and atypical organisms and the usual pyogenic community-acquired pneumonias are other common infectious agents.

AIDS patients with tuberculosis have typical clinical features but do not have characteristic roentgenograms. The cavitary disease is unusual but should not delay diagnosis.[28] Nontuberculosis mycobacteria, especially *Mycobacterium avium* complex, though frequently isolated from pulmonary secretions, were initially thought to produce little evidence that an additional burden of disease was being imposed by the coinfection. Subsequent studies have shown that *M. avium* is not merely a colonizer but that the disseminated infection contributes substantially to both morbidity and mortality in patients with AIDS.[29]

The major risk factor for tuberculosis and pneumocystosis is the level of immune dysfunction, as reflected by the CD4+ cell count. Infection is rare in patients with more than 100 CD4+ cells per cubic millimeter. Data indicate that tuberculosis is acquired by ubiquitous environmental exposure. There are predominant serotypes (i.e., serogroups 4 and 8 in the United States) that are more likely to cause infection and that are more virulent in AIDS patients. Because CD4 cells have a central role in antimycobacterial defenses, dysfunction of these cells places patients with HIV infection at high risk for primary tuberculosis or reactivation of the disease. Tuberculosis in patients with AIDS results from reactivation of a previous focus of infection, whereas disseminated *M. avium* appears to result from primary acquisition of the pathogen through either ingestion or inhalation. The gastrointestinal tract appears to be a more common portal of entry than the respiratory tract. Focal pneumonia caused by *M. avium* may present with or without dissemination, but local containment is rare and dissemination usually ensues. In patients with HIV infections plus tuberculosis, there is also a high incidence of extrapulmonary infection but usually with concomitant pulmonary tuberculosis.

Characteristically, after successful treatment for *Pneumocystis* the infection recurs (i.e., reinfection or relapses from indolent colonization) when the drug is stopped. Thus recovery from *P. carinii* infection does not confer effective immunity. Because of the observed persistence of *P. carinii* in posttreatment bronchoscopic specimens, caution is advised about assumming it to be the etiologic agent of a recurrent pneumonitis in such patients.

Survival significantly diminishes with each episode, and patients usually die within 2 years of their first major pulmonary infection. Pneumonia with respiratory failure requiring mechanical ventilation has been reported to have a mortality of at least 85%, and difficult ethical and economic questions have been raised regarding the appropriateness of their care in an intensive care unit. On further analysis, however, prognosis for patients requiring intubation with the first episode of PCP is better and, if treated early, they may have the same prognosis as those with PCP who did not require intubation.[30] Serum lactic dehydrogenese (LDH), PaO_2, and "hospital familiarity" with treating AIDS patients as well as the vigor of diagnosis and monitoring (i.e., use of the critical care unit) are now thought to influence survival significantly.[31,32]

Pneumocystis carinii maintains an extracellular existence in the lung and does not have an intracellular stage in its life cycle. *Pneumocystis* is characterized by the intraalveolar accumulation of trophozoites, cysts,

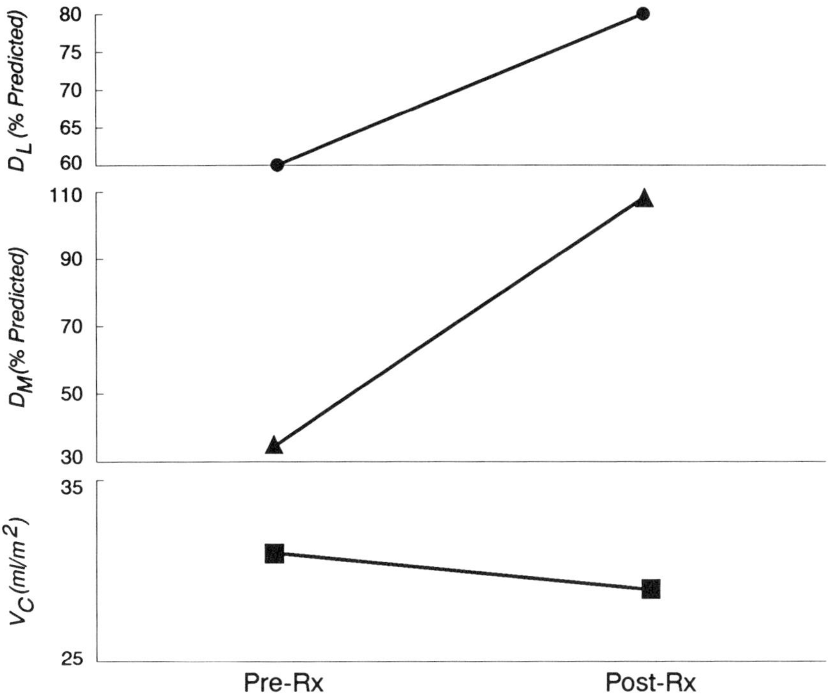

FIGURE 4.9. Mean values for diffusing capacity (D_L) and its membrane (D_M) and pulmonary blood volume (V_C) components in 20 AIDS patients with *P. carinii* pneumonia before and after antiparasitic treatment. (Data from Sankary et al.[33])

inflammatory cells, and cellular debris, including foamy, eosinophilic, proteinaceous material. Most dramatic, however, is the reported attachment of the trophozoites preferentially to type 1 alveolar epithelial cells. This tight adherence is accomplished through the use of parasitic "hooks," "anchors," and "pincers." They cluster between the air space and epithelial cells, presumably accounting for the reported efficacy of pentamidine administered by nebulization and for the characteristically early decrease in diffusing capacity.[33] Until late in the course of experimental infection the intraalveolar abnormalities occur with preservation of pulmonary capillaries. The reduction of diffusing capacity in patients with AIDS and PCP has been shown to be due to a selective decrease in membrane diffusion (D_M). This selective increase in the thickness of the diffusion pathway without a parallel change in the volume of blood in pulmonary capillaries (V_C) gives rise to a true alveolar-capillary block, causing the observed decrease in lung diffusing capacity (D_L) that is reversible with treatment (Fig. 4.9). Surfactant abnormalities accompanied by the expected alterations in compliance and lung mechanics have been described; others

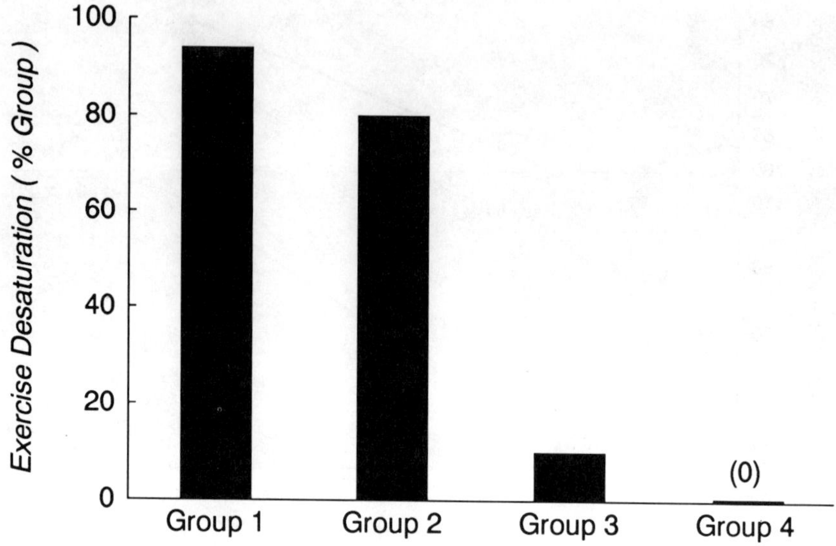

FIGURE 4.10. Exercise testing in patients with AIDS and pneumonia. Group 1: *Pneumocystis* with resting hypoxemia ($n = 16$). Group 2: *Pneumocystis* with normal resting arterial oxygenation ($n = 20$). Group 3: other causes of pneumonia with normal resting arterial oxygenation ($n = 19$). Group 4: healthy normal subjects ($n = 12$). The percent of each group with a positive desaturation test—defined as a decrease in saturation to less than 90% using a pulse oximeter—is shown. (Data from Smith et al.[34])

have emphasized the interstitial cellular reaction to be responsible for the restrictive ventilatory pattern. Exercise exaggerates the underlying defects, causing impairment of gas exchange and readily inducing arterial desaturation[34] (Fig. 4.10).

Serum LDH levels, presumably from lung parenchyma, are elevated; and as with the decrease in arterial oxygenation after exercise, the LDH level has been found to correlate with severity of disease, unlike the radiographic findings.[35] Radiologic presentation is varied and nonspecific, with more extensive disease associated with spontaneous pneumothorax. Pneumothorax is also seen as a complication of BAL and fiberoptic bronchoscopy[36] and is observed as well with tuberculosis infection in both AIDS and non-AIDS patients presumably related to infectious interstitial emphysema resulting from parenchymal destruction.[37] The role of nutrition in the pathogenesis of HIV infection and its complications has not been resolved. Anorexia, hypermetabolism, and malabsorption are important aspects of the malnutrition and cachexia observed. Weight loss and thinness have come to characterize "slim disease," but there is no evidence that aggressive enteric or parenteral feeding regimens alter the course of the disease.

Pulmonary infiltration seen on roentgenogram, with negative cultures, may be caused by a congestive cardiomyopathy. Such dilated cardiomyopathies may result from opportunistic or HIV infections of the myocardium itself. As many as 30% of AIDS patients also develop parenchymal inflammatory processes that lack an identifiable etiologic agent. These processes may have a more destructive pattern termed lymphocytic interstitial pneumonia whose pathogenesis has been related to a more active immune response to CMV infection and a milder nonspecific pneumonitis. The pathogenesis of the lung damage in severely immunosuppressed patients has been related to the HIV agent itself or directly to the cytopathogenic effects of CMV, related to the extent of virus replication.

There is no convincing evidence for the causative agent of these entities or why lymphocytic interstitial pneumonia, whose cells of origin appear to be T cells, is predominantly found in children. The clinical presentation is diverse and indistinguishable from that of identifiable opportunistic pulmonary pathogens. Nonspecific pneumonitis, which is associated with a normal roentgenogram in 50% of patients, is usually self-limited and requires no specific therapy; its role in predisposing to other infections is unknown.

Both CD8 lymphocytic alveolitis and chronic interstitial pneumonitis may occur in patients with HIV infection without associated radiographic signs or symptoms of pneumonia. These indolent infections present potential explanation for the observed deterioration of pulmonary function and even emphysematous changes reported in HIV-seropositive patients in the absence of recognized preceding pulmonary infections. Lymphocytic interstitial pneumonia appears to improve with corticosteroid therapy, but most recently antioxidant therapy including vitamin E, *N*-acetylcysteine, and ascorbic acid has been suggested because of reports implicating reactive oxygen species in the pathogenesis of HIV infection. Moreover, reports of decreased glutathione levels have been suggested to further predispose prednisone-treated HIV-infected patients to oxidant-mediated pulmonary damage. Because of potential deleterious effects such therapies must await further clinical investigation.

Toxic Lung Injury

Drugs

The panoply of drugs recognized to be capable of producing diffuse pulmonary injury is continuously increasing, and the most frequent problems of this type are a result of treatment with chemotherapeutic agents (Table 4.4). The pathologic changes in the lungs show varying degrees of organizing alveolar exudate and inflammatory cell infiltration with desquamation of necrotic type I and proliferation of type II alveolar lining cells. A

TABLE 4.4. Drugs producing diffuse pulmonary injury.

Cytotoxic drugs
Carmustine (BCNU)
Bleomycin
Cyclophosphamide
Busulfan
Mitomycin C
Methotrexate
Chlorambucil
Melphalan
Azathioprine
Procarbazine
Cardiac drugs
Amiodarone
Tocainide
Antimicrobials
Nitrofurantoin
Acyclovir
Sulfasalazine
Antirheumatics
Gold
Anticonvisulsants
Diphenylhydantoin
Carbamazepine

dose-response relation is often suggestive. Many of these agents' effects appear to be enhanced by synergism with other cytotoxic drugs (with which they are often given in combination) and irradiation or oxygen therapy; their effects are also affected by increased age, preexisting lung disease, and duration of administration.[38] Progression may occur, as with BCNU, even years after the drug is discontinued. Because the patients are immunocompromised, infection is an invariable entry in the differential diagnosis.

The mechanism of drug-induced lung injury is in all likelihood related to the ingredient that gives them therapeutic efficacy as a chemotherapeutic agent. Thus the therapeutic cytotoxic effect of bleomycin works against both cancer cells and healthy lung cells, causing cleavage and impaired synthesis of DNA; it is mediated by oxygen radicals generated by the formation of an unstable metal–drug complex. Bleomycin appears to chelate iron, which is than capable of donating and accepting electrons as it undergoes cyclic oxidation and reduction, facilitating single-electron transfer particularly to electrophilic molecules such as oxygen. Furthermore, the drug concentrates in the lung, which is relatively deficient in the hydrolase enzyme that inactivates the drug.

Pulmonary toxicity due to amiodarone is reported to occur with variable frequency; and as with other drug toxicities, it may be related to dose as well as preexisting lung disease. It too concentrates in the lung; and like the delayed reaction to nitrofurantoin, it is thought to cause direct toxic damage to the alveolar-capillary membrane by generating oxygen-derived reactive species within lung cells, particularly the endothelial cells, that overwhelm the cells' antioxidant defense mechanisms. It too has a pathogenetic mechanism of cyclic reduction-oxidation similar to that of bleomycin and the herbicide paraquat.

The toxicity of amiodarone has been further related to its lipophilic properties, promoting both intracellular concentration and delayed elimination, which allows the toxic effects to continue well after discontinuation of the drug. Such sequestration, even when extensive, remains reversible; but it results in an acquired lipid storage disease with a phospholipidosis in the alveolar macrophage and type II pneumocyte. Impaired phospholipid degradation through inhibition of lysosomal phospholipase A, rather than induction of reactive oxygen species, has been favored to be primarily responsible for the observed pathophysiology; it is characterized by the presence of lamellar inclusions on ultrastructural examination. This situation has been shown to lead to a decline in D_{LCO} even in the absence of histologic findings of "amiodarone pulmonary toxicity." These observations have led many to the general conclusion that a drug may have both direct (toxic metabolic) and indirect (inflammatory immunologic) mechanisms operating alone or in concert, one triggering the other.[39]

Allergic types of fulminant and reversible "hypersensitivity" reactions have been postulated for many of these drugs, particularly methotrexate and nitrofurantoin, inferring a greater role for inflammatory cells and mediators other than oxygen species in causing lung damage. In most cases of interstitial pneumonitis, the lymphocytes are of T-cell lineage. In studies of amiodarone drug toxicity, CD8+ suppressor/cytotoxic T lymphocytes are increased in BAL fluid, whereas with methotrexate-induced lung injury a T-helper lymphocyte response has been reported.[40] These different mechanisms may well coexist, differentiating acute and chronic toxicities as with nitrofurantoin; or they may be related and interdependent, contributing to the pathogenic spectrum of the nonspecific pneumonitis lung injury. The difference between the primary site of formation of reactive oxygen metabolites may differ (i.e., epithelial or inflammatory cells), but the end results of the action of the oxidant are similar whether the alteration in the protective detoxification pathways are overcome by primary biochemical reactions or preceded by an imbalance between effector and suppressor cells in the lung.

Finally, it has been proposed that the common final link of the various toxic mechanisms is a rise in the intracellular calcium concentration, causing irreversible cell injury. It has been suggested that the lung is uniquely susceptible to injury and becomes the target organ for these drugs because it has the highest oxygen concentration in the body, facilitating the formation of oxygen radicals and because some drugs or their metabolites (e.g., amiodarone and bleomycin) are concentrated in the lung.

Radiation Injury

Therapeutic irradiation results in a pneumonitis that, like chronic toxic pulmonary drug reactions, is delayed for 2–4 months and is related to dose, cytotoxic drug therapy, and oxygen therapy. The dose is a complex function of the amount of radiation, the volume of lung irradiated, and the rate at which the radiation is delivered. It is associated with the typical histologic findings of the alveolar-capillary unit in ARDS, limited to the area of exposure, though changes outside the field have been reported that are unexplained. Corticosteroids are thought to be effective treatment, but their withdrawal during irradiation is considered a predisposing factor for the development of "recall radiation pneumonitis."[41]

Radiation energy generates free radicals that interact with protein molecules, causing dysfunction of cell processes. The delay in manifestation of injury is attributed to impaired chromosomal DNA-regulated synthesis that is subsequently revealed when cell renewal and mitosis are required; the latter is reflected by the cytologic atypia of the alveolar epithelial stem cells, type II pneumocytes. "Nongenetic" macromolecules are also affected, which may account for the more acute forms of pneumonitis; these molecules are the result of damage to the cell membrane of endothelial and type I epithelial cells with a resultant increase in capillary permeability and the accumulation of intraalveolar fluid.[42] The effects are most readily discernible by the appearance of perfusion defects and impairment of the D_{LCO}, which may persist years after completion of therapy.

Another mode of tissue injury due to radiation exposure is the evolution of inflammation with lymphocytosis observed in nonirradiated as well as irradiated lung.[43] This appearance of immune effector cells, which cause "nodular infiltrates" (seen on radiographs) as the result of local confinement of inflammatory mediators, accounts for radiation changes outside the field of irradiation. Inhalation of β-emitting radionuclides may also cause injury; and it has been suggested that inhalation pneumonitis will be seen more frequently as radionuclide aerosols are increasingly used.

Radiation pneumonitis is usually associated with high-dose therapeutic irradiation of solid chest tumors. However, the lower total body irradiation doses now used for marrow transplantation to reduce the leukemia recurrence rate and failure of remission reduction has been associated with pulmonary toxicity and an increased risk of idiopathic interstitial pneumonitis. Various dosing and fractionation studies have not led to a consensus on either the role of irradiation or the optimum approach to it. The clinical, epidemiologic, and histopathologic pictures of radiation pneumonia and idiopathic interstitial pneumonia are similar, suggesting that interstitial pneumonitis is most likely a morbid manifestation of the cumu-

TABLE 4.5. Inhaled agents causing acute pneumonia.

*Aldehydes: acetaldehyde, acrylic aldehyde (acrolein), formaldehyde
*Ammonia
*Sulfur dioxide
*Chlorine, phosgene, hydrogen chloride, methylene chloride
*Nitrogen oxides (Nitrogen dioxide): "silo-fillers disease"
Metals especially oxides and salts
Methylisocyanate: "Bhopal pneumonia"
Mineral oil
Petroleum distillates
Fungal toxins: "organic-dust syndrome"
Hydrogen sulfide: "dung lung"
Welding (metals and polymers): "fume fever"
Trimellitic anhydride: "epoxy lung"

* Gases associated with fires.

lative effect of radiation and radiosensitizing chemotherapy, their respective toxicities acting synergistically on the lung.[44]

Inhalation Injury

The efficiency of the upper airway in dissipating heat usually limits thermal injury of the lower respiratory tract, where except for steam accidents the contents of the inhaled smoke are the pathogenic determinants of the lung injury. The history and occupational exposure are therefore critical for diagnosis of pulmonary injury from inhalation (Table 4.5).

Smoke inhalation from fires is the major cause of burn mortality, and death frequently occurs without surface burns. The morbidity and mortality that result from the effects of the toxic gases produced (e.g., "poison" war gases) is determined by their dose, the duration of exposure and the concentration of the gas. The gaseous composition of smoke is a mixture of irritants, cell poisons, and asphyxiants, the composition of which is a function of the material burning, the availability of oxygen, and the temperature of the fire. The increasing use of plastics has been thought to be a major factor in the rising incidence of pulmonary complications as a result of the thermal degradation of such compounds to hydrogen cyanide. The more incomplete the combination, the greater is the toxicity of resulting chemical products.

Airway involvement extends from the most proximal locations of airway exposure with laryngeal edema to the most peripheral with refractory bronchospasm as a manifestation of both thermal and chemical injury. The lung parenchymal involvement is most vividly apparent by the development of the acute lung injury syndrome. The immediate anoxic effect of a low oxygen environment is greatly enhanced by the associated formation of carbon monoxide, which exhibits high affinity for hemoglobin

(HbCO), decreasing the oxygen capacity of hemoglobin. Similarly, exposure to nitrogen oxides may result in methemoglobinemia. The metabolic acidosis frequently seen in victims of severe smoke inhalation is usually attributed to tissue anoxia caused by both environmental oxygen depletion and impaired oxygen transport to the tissue due to the formation of HbCO. In addition, there is frequently coexisting cyanide poisoning from cyanide inhalation, which acting together with CO inhibits cellular respiration, causing a conversion to tissue anaerobic metabolism and contributing to the observed lactic acidosis. Thus smoke inhalation has become an increasingly important cause of mortality after burn injuries as the management of fluid balance and infection have been advanced.[45] The HbCO level has until recently been erroneously thought to be a sensitive indicator of associated gaseous toxic products of combustion and to correlate adequately with the blood cyanide concentrations.[46,47] In the absence of severe secondary infection, survival from the acute toxic effect of smoke (and the similar war gases, chlorine and phosgene) on the lungs is usually followed by full recovery.

Symptoms of respiratory distress from chemically mediated acute lung injury are preceded by a symptom-free interval of 8–12 hours but may be delayed for more than 48 hours. The degree of injury is directly correlated to the degree of smoke exposure and the level of HbCO reached in the blood. The water solubility of a gas determines its primary site of deposition. The less water-soluble the gas (e.g., nitrous oxide), the higher is the concentration in more distal airways. Even with highly soluble gases, such as ammonia and sulfur dioxide, distal deposition and damage increases with decreased contact time proximally (i.e., high inspiratory flow rates). Inhaled water-soluble gases and particles between 0.5 and 3.0 μm in diameter reach the distal airways and alveoli. The sensitivity of pneumocytes to the cytotoxic effects of the noxious gas is a primary factor in determining the extent of lung injury. Epithelial injury initiates the cascade of inflammatory events, causing further damage to and impairment of the integrity of the alveolar-capillary membrane. The increase in microvascular premeability that results from mediator damage to epithelial and endothelial cells serves as the final common denominator. Cellular injury further impairs the mucociliary elevator mechanism, predisposing to secondary infection.

Aspiration Injury

Another frequent cause of chemical pneumonitis is aspiration of toxic materials that are either accidentally or intentionally ingested. Petroleum distillates (e.g., kerosene) are the most frequent toxic agents in this category. Gasoline, particularly high octane aviation fuel, frequently leads to acute intoxication; and death from respiratory failure and suffocation almost always occurs when workers enter tanks containing high concentrations of vapor. The gases of the volatile liquids have negligible pulmonary toxicity and produce their adverse effects acutely as asphyxiants and central nervous system (CNS) depressants. There are occasional reports of such catastrophes when an individual has primed a hose when siphoning a gas tank. Because gasoline vapor is heavier than air, concentrations rapidly fatal to humans can form in enclosed spaces when the air is displaced by the heavier vapors. Lower concentrations not high enough to cause acute distillate intoxication have been reported to produce toxic acute fatty changes in the liver and respiratory failure due to massive pulmonary fat emboli.

More commonly, in cases of acute intoxication, the acute pulmonary edema and "pneumonitis" seem to be associated with aspiration of distillate (especially kerosene) after ingestion by children, rather than inhalation of vapor. Pulmonary toxicity may also be a result of blood-borne dissemination of absorbed hydrocarbon in the absence of aspiration. Similarly, mineral oil may produce an intense pneumonitis when aspirated or inhaled aside from the more commonly known lipoid pneumonia with chronic aspiration. Other, more dramatic examples of pneumonitis exist, such as "fire-eaters lung" where performers have accidentally aspirated the petroleum used as ignition fluid for a flame-blowing act. Polyacrylamide, a synthetic polymer with various industrial uses, has been reported to produce asphyxia following aspiration. The substance's high viscosity causes both a chemical pneumonitis and airway obstruction, which can be worsened by lavage of the airway because the polyacrylamide solidifies when mixed with saline.

Drug Abuse

The pulmonary manifestations of illicit drug use require differentiation of infectious and noninfectious processes that are dependent on the specific drug used and its route of administration. Septic pulmonary embolism is common with intravenous drug abuse; and although there is a classic radiologic picture, this pattern may also be representative of a more classic bronchopneumonia. Acute lobar pneumonia must be differentiated from entities not of primary parenchymal origin, including a ruptured mycotic aneurysm and acute cardiogenic pulmonary edema due to destruction of the mitral, aortic valvular apparatus by bacteral endocarditis.

Any substance that can be dissolved or crumbled and insoluble "fillers" such as talc may be injected and trapped in the pulmonary sieve. Granulomatous foreign body reactions occurring in both the vascular and parenchymal lung tissue are a response to these agents and their soluble "fillers." Extravascular migration occurs, and the inflammatory response is characterized by a macrophage and granulomatous response.

The primary noninfectious manifestation to be considered is noncardiogenic "permeability" pulmonary edema epitomized by intravenous

TABLE 4.6. Drugs causing noncardiogenic pulmonary edema.

Heroin
Opium
Cocaine
Naloxone
Methadone
Propoxyphene
Chlordiazepoxide
Ethchlorvynol
Paraldehyde
Codeine
Meperidine
Barbiturates
Chlorpromazine

heroin abuse but associated with most drug overdoses. Abuse of analgesics, such as aspirin and other nonsteroidal agents, as well as tranquilizers and sedatives, most notably ethchlorvynol (Placidyl) have also been reported to precipitate noncardiogenic pulmonary edema (Table 4.6). The severity of this complication in addicts is clearly indicated by its place as the leading cause of sudden death. This point is emphasized by the graphic description of an autopsy finding of mortality due to acute narcotism: "Death overtakes the addict during the intravenous injection procedure and the needle of the syringe is found in the vein when the body is discovered, the striking finding is the tremendous pulmonary congestion and edema."[48] The edematous lung may be hemorrhagic and, along with microscopic findings and clinical manifestations (fever, leukocytosis) of acute inflammation, in survivors, suggests a fulminating bronchopneumonia that proves to be noninfectious. Its repeated description for more than 100 years suggests that it is not specific for heroin or impurities acquired during the "cutting" process.[49] Its appearance may be delayed as well as recurrent.

The mechanism of capillary leakage has been related to both the severe hypoxic damage to the alveolar-capillary membrane resulting from the dose-related hypoventilation due to CNS depression and the associated severe tissue acidemia of combined metabolic and respiratory origin. This phenomenon has been considered by some to be the urban clinical counterpart of "high altitude pulmonary edema." Other mechanisms include possible occurrence of "silent" aspiration and, finally, an acute immune reaction perhaps to associated "impurities" such as the "filler." The frequently associated inflammatory alveolitis may be related, but its role in pathogenesis is not considered primary. A neurogenic mechanism has also been postulated and has been related to (1) the increased intracranial pressure that is invariably associated with an acute respiratory acidosis and (2) nonspecific CNS injury, perhaps reflecting dysfunction of central opiate receptors.

Heroin readily passes through the blood-brain barrier and probably enters the brain tissue 10–20 seconds after the usual intravenous injection by addicts. The resulting pulmonary hypertension, increased pulmonary blood volume, and systemic vasconstriction manifest as pulmonary edema, having the characteristics associated with increased permeability. Preexisting granulomatous angiitis or angiothrombotic pulmonary hypertension (blue velvet disease)[50] is not a predisposing factor.

Cocaine, whether inhaled (sniffed, smoked) or injected,[51] has been associated with classic noncardiogenic pulmonary edema. A syndrome of diffuse pulmonary hemorrhage has also been reported with "free-basing"[52] and has been attributed to diffuse vascular injury and resulting ischemia, possibly secondary to vasoconstriction. The parenchymal hemorrhage may present with fulminant hemoptysis or occultly as diffuse infiltrates seen on the chest radiograph. Transient pulmonary infiltrates attributable to a hypersensitivity reaction to the drug or its adulterants have also been reported.[51] Various other syndromes occasionally resulting in pulmonary infiltrates have been related to "huffing and sniffing" various hydrocarbons. A dramatic lower airway thermal injury has been reported as due to either inhalation or intratracheal ignition of the ether vehicle used when free-basing cocaine, which also results in associated pulmonary edema.[53]

Aspiration/Chemical Pneumonitis

The term aspiration pneumonia has created a problem of semantics over the years, as at least three distinct clinical entities having a similar pathogenesis but differing in pathophysiology have been described. The adverse and occasionally fatal consequences associated with the aspiration of food or liquid vomitus have been recognized and described since antiquity. The sequela emphasized prior to Mendelson's astute clinical observations and those found in original animal experimentation were sudden death from suffocation due to airway occlusion and the development of pneumonia and abscess formation due to secondary bacterial invasion.

Although asphyxiation is uncommon and has been termed the "café coronary," the other consequences of aspiration may not depend on host and environmental factors. The altered states of consciousness that cause aspiration outside the hospital lead to community-acquired pneumonia from commensal organisms or, in predisposed hosts with poor oral hygiene, more indolent polymicrobial anaerobic or mixed aerobic-anaerobic necrotizing pneumonias. The altered state of consciousness may be brought on by drugs or the state that occurs during normal sleep. Numerous studies involving colored and radiopaque dyes and radioactive tracers have shown

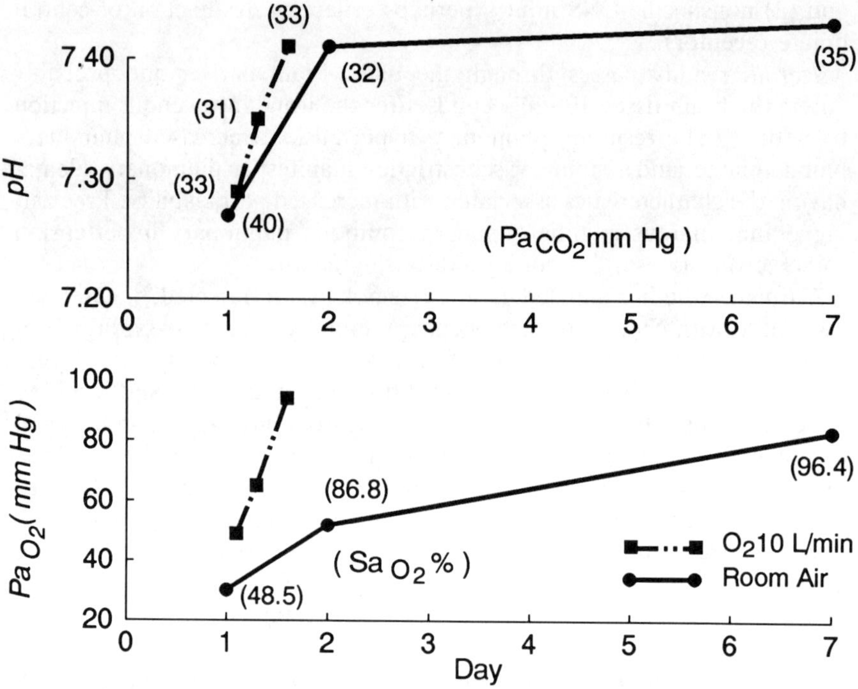

FIGURE 4.11. Acid-base and blood gas changes while breathing room air. The patient is a 38-year-old woman who developed the acid-aspiration syndrome during emergency cesarean section. The initial values, obtained in the operating room, illustrate the metabolic acidosis associated with severe hypoxemia, which was alleviated with oxygen therapy by face mask. There was no carbon dioxide retention, and mechanical ventilation was not instituted. The pulmonary edema seen on the initial chest roentgenogram cleared after 24 hours.

that aspiration is a routine nocturnal event even in normal individuals. Aspiration infection in the hospital typically results in the nosocomial gram-negative pneumonias caused by facultative enteric bacilli. The acute clinical manifestations that result from the aspiration of acidic gastric contents has been termed Mendelson syndrome.[54] This syndrome is one of the group of entities with distinct etiologies but displaying similar pulmonary pathophysiology that fall under the all-inclusive term adult respiratory distress syndrome (ARDS). It is the purpose of this section to illustrate the clinical presentation, review the pathophysiology, and discuss the pathogenesis of acid aspiration (Fig. 4.11).

The clinical settings for aspiration pneumonia (including old age, debilitation, and impaired swallowing function due to anatomic or functional defects present during altered states of consciousness) have been recognized for many years and emphasized repeatedly. It is also clear that vomiting is frequently occult, and it is often neither observed prior to nor is it a prerequisite for the development of aspiration pneumonia.[55] With the introduction of iodized oil into the mouths or nasopharynges of sleeping patients, Amberson was able, by means of roentgenography, to demonstrate its presence in bronchi and alveoli the following morning. The same procedure yielded similar results in patients in alcoholic stupor.[55] Subsequently, Gardner showed that after adding barium sulfate to all the beverages of 94 ambulatory, hospitalized, postoperative adult patients for a period of 2–4 days barium reached the lung in 10 patients, in none of whom was it suspected clinically. In nine cases the barium was demonstrated on radiographic examination, but in one case it was seen only on bronchoscopy.[56] Mardner repeated the study in a similar series of 51 patients, but this time he placed the barium directly into the stomach by tube. Under these conditions, daily radiographs demonstrated barium in only one patient.[56]

Thus it is apparent that regurgitation or vomiting is unnecessary for aspiration and that an impaired swallowing mechanism is a common phenomenon leading to aspiration in hospitalized patients. These observations are further supported by a report showing that 50% of postoperative patients who developed aspiration pneumonia were awake and alert when aspiration occurred. Regarding the diagnosis of aspiration, caution must also be exercised when interpreting autopsy findings. The postmortem findings in the airways are inconclusive evidence of antemortem aspiration because gastric contents may reach the bronchi after death.

If an impaired swallowing mechanism is relatively commonplace, why is it that the aspiration syndrome is not more prevalent? The answer to this question was initially suggested by Mendelson, who supplemented a retrospective clinical survey of obstetric patients with the first experimental approach to this problem. He differentiated between the clinical consequences of the aspiration of solid and liquid materials, the former giving rise to signs of suffocation and the latter to an asthma-like syndrome. As a result of his experiments with rabbits, he was able to attribute the bronchoconstriction and accompanying hemorrhagic pneumonitis and pulmonary edema to the acid content, rather than to the enzyme content, of gastric secretions. He thought that the chemical pneumonitis resulting from acid aspiration was analogous to that shown to result from chlorine and phosgene gas poisoning. The damage from the chemical burn is so rapid and extensive that a methylene blue indicator can be seen on the pleural surface of a dog model within 12–18 seconds of aspiration. Thus, as discussed previously, although aspiration of oral contents is a relatively frequent occurrence, stomach contents are only rarely found in the lungs of ambulatory patients, accounting for the low incidence of the acid-aspiration syndrome in such patients. This low incidence has been attributed not only to the integrity of host defense mechanisms but to a dose-response relation as well, the dose being a function of the bacterial load, the hydrogen ion concentration, the volume of aspirate, and the content of particulate matter in the aspirate.

Following Mendelson's report, it was shown that aspiration pneumonitis followed aspiration of gastric contents only if the pH was less than 2.5, that the enzyme content was not contributory, and that the role of bacterial infection was secondary.[57] More recent studies in dogs demonstrated that with a large enough volume of fluid aspirate hemorrhagic pneumonitis results even with solutions at pH 5.67.

In animals, experimental aspiration of any material, liquid or solid, regardless of pH, results initially in bronchospasm as a result of an "air closure reflex." The resulting arterial hypoxemia and fall in lung compliance can be relieved in sheep (but not in dogs) by administration of atropine at 25 times the routine dosage. Cervical vagotomy, however, is uniformly observed to diminish this reflex bronchoconstrictive response to aspiration.[58] Presumably, on the basis of this fragmentary evidence for parasympathomimetic vagal stimulation, atropine and antihistamines have been recommended, as have sympathomimetics, for the initial routine management of aspiration pneumonia in humans. The initial decrease in arterial oxygen tension following aspiration is progressive owing to the development of interstitial and alveolar edema and a necrotizing bronchitis. As with the anatomic gross pathology and micropathology, the degree of arterial desaturation has been observed to be proportional to the acidity of the aspirate. The severe hypoxemia is accompanied by only a transient elevation in the arterial PCO_2 and by normal right atrial and pulmonary artery pressures. The extent of the edema formation resulting from the passage of water from the intravascular compartment is reflected by decreased blood volume and an elevated hematocrit level.

Mendelson reported a 0.15% (n = 66) incidence of aspiration among 44,016 pregnant women. Most of the patients (70%) had an afebrile course, which led the author to emphasize that infection is only an occasional secondary complication and that routine antibiotic prophylaxis is unnecessary.[54] Subsequently, other studies also stressed that infection is not the primary problem, and that routine antibiotic therapy has not been shown to be efficacious; hence it is not a recommended intervention.

Although the desirability of *immediately evacuating* grossly visible material from the airways is apparent, vigorous suctioning and lavage with neutral or alkaline solutions have also been suggested. Such therapy has been shown to increase airway resistance and decrease lung compliance significantly, which further impairs gas exchange. Moreover, not only is such treatment ineffective in reducing the extent of the hemorrhagic pneumonitis and resulting arterial hypoxemia, it has been shown to make them worse. Therefore minimal volumes (10 ml) should be utilized to evacuate material from the major airways, and it should be done only two or three times. The initial outpouring of fluid from the bronchial epithelium in response to the acidic insult is so vigorous the acid is rapidly neutralized; hence lavage, especially with bicarbonate solutions, is superfluous.

Because of their actions as antiinflammatory agents, *systemic steroids* were used empirically to treat aspiration pneumonia; and they subsequently became a routine mode of therapy. Local steroid therapy has also been recommended because of observations made in dogs that immediate instillation of hydrocortisone had an ameliorating action on the pulmonary lesions that developed from aspiration of hydrochloric acid. A subsequent study showed that such endobronchial administration of corticosteroids is of no benefit and is perhaps detrimental.

The evaluation of systemic steroid therapy has been limited and controversial. Some investigators have shown favorable effects after experimental aspiration, with smaller decreases in arterial oxygen tensions and more circumscribed areas of pneumonitis, whereas others have been unable to demonstrate either physiologic or pathologic benefits, or they showed that systemic steroid therapy only delayed and did not prevent death of the animal models. Thus although systemic steroid therapy has not been shown to influence gas exchange adversely, its use for routine management of aspiration pneumonia is without clinical foundation; moreover, based on experience in other areas, it should be suspected of acutely increasing the potential morbidity due to infection.

A major therapeutic dilemma and area of controversy is *fluid therapy*. With other forms of ARDS, it is apparent that excessive fluid administration is detrimental.[59] Vigorous fluid therapy promotes loss of water in the lungs and causes fluid accumulation if similar mechanisms are operative after aspiration. Thus a balance must be struck in the efforts of fluid resuscitation to restore hemodynamic stability in order to treat the initial hypotension. This associated hemodynamic instability has been attributed to hypovolemia resulting from blood pooling in the pulmonary circulation and fluid (plasma) moving from the vascular compartment to the interstitial and alveolar spaces as a result of necrosis of types I and II pneumocytes, endothelial cells, and the intervening basement membrane, completely (and perhaps irreversibly at times) destroying the alveolar capillary barrier[60] (Fig. 4.12).

In Mendelson's study, all the patients with liquid aspiration survived; they were stabilized within 24–36 hours and had radiographic clearing of pulmonary infiltrates within 7–10 days.[54] Thus in otherwise healthy women of childbearing age, the prognosis is excellent and long-term effects on pulmonary function are either undetectable or minimal. The immediate prognosis in debilitated patients, however, is poor. In one study, mortality of 62% was reported.[60] If only one lobe was involved, 41% of the patients died; with more extensive pneumonitis, the mortality was a dramatic 90%.[61] The damaged epithelial barriers predispose to bacterial invasion, and an infectious, frequently polymicrobial, anaerobic pneumonia[62] develops in approximately 30% of patients (Fig. 4.13). In patients who survive the initial hypoxia and go on to develop secondary bacterial infection, the mortality rate has been reported to be in the range of 25–35%, with deaths occurring primarily among debilitated patients with

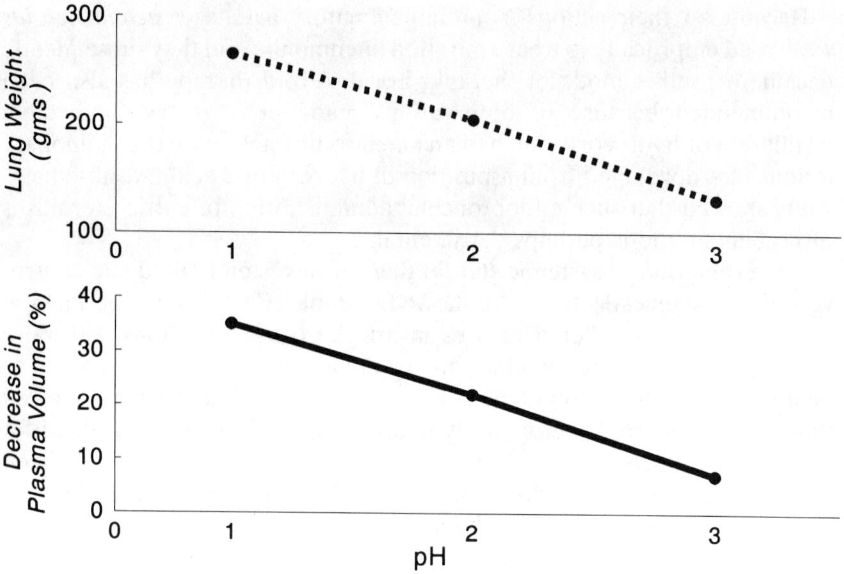

FIGURE 4.12. Effect on plasma volume and lung weight of increasing pH of aspirate in dogs. (Data from Awe et al.[60])

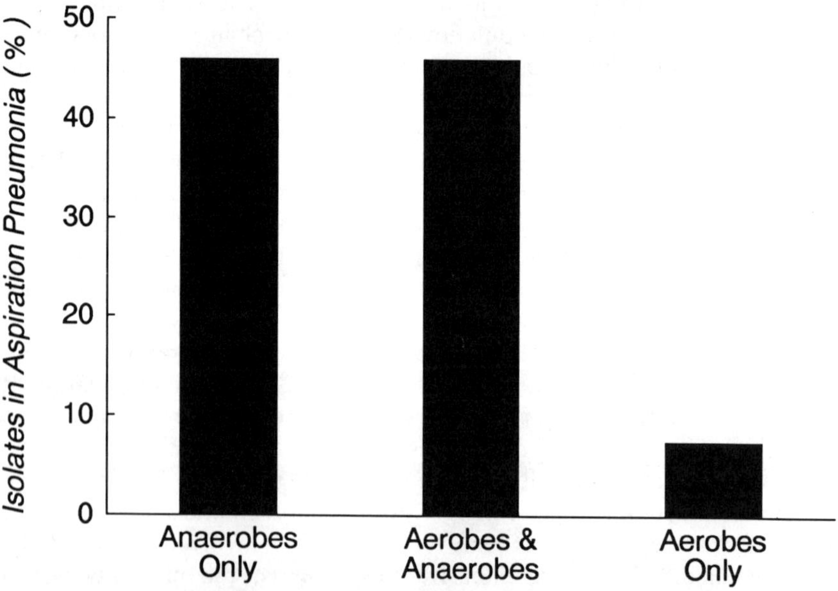

FIGURE 4.13. Infection of 54 cases of aspiration pneumonia were found to be polymicrobial in 40, with an average of 1.0 aerobic or facultative and 2.6 anaerobic isolates per episode. Gram-negative enteric organisms were predominant in hospitalized patients, but anaerobes were found concurrently in all but four cases. (Data from Bartlett et al.[62])

underlying significant disease processes. For this high risk group of patients, prophylactic antibiotic therapy also appears to be unwarranted because, as with steroid and ventilatory therapy, it has not been shown to affect the outcome even in this predisposed population.[60]

Thus aspiration results in a continuum of pulmonary consequences that depend on pH and the size of the particulate matter. Small nonobstructing particles of food may cause a prolonged inflammatory reaction. Classic aspiration pneumonia is a form of ARDS resulting from an acid-induced injury of the lung; it is primarily a problem of arterial hypoxemia that requires adequate oxygen therapy. Other modes of therapy have been shown not to alter survival in humans. In the otherwise healthy individual, the immediate and long-term prognoses are excellent. In debilitated patients with significant underlying disease processes, however, the rates of both immediate and delayed death are high. The late deaths reflect the significance of secondary infection due primarily to anaerobic organisms.

Pregnancy

Pneumonia complicating pregnancy and the puerperium was a major problem during the preantibiotic era, when almost 10% of pneumococcal pneumonia patients were pregnant and 0.6% of all obstetric patients had pneumococcal pneumonia. At Boston City Hospital, 1.2% of all cases of pneumonia were complications of pregnancy. The pneumonia caused high death rates among the mothers and an almost 60% peripartum fetal death rate.[63]

The absence of current literature on bacterial pneumonia during pregnancy is attributable to the efficacy of antimicrobial therapy. Viral infections, including influenza, CMV, and especially varicella, have replaced bacterial pathogens as a source of concern. The incidence of varicella pneumonia shows that approximately 10% of reported cases occur during pregnancy, with approximately 45% mortality. Most recently, several types of fungal infection have been reported during pregnancy, with coccidioidomycosis generating the most interest because of its tendency to disseminate during pregnancy, with 100% maternal mortality in the untreated patient. The risk has been attributed to the effects of estradiol-stimulated growth of fungal phases (arthroconidia, endospores, and spherules), rather than to impaired host immune factors. A variety of alterations of the immune system preventing rejection of the fetal allograft have been reported; and though they appear to be mild, they may well account for the virulence reported for specific infectious agents.

Alternatively, others have related increased maternal morbidity and mortality to alterations in pulmonary function, which are also relatively mild.[64] The decrease in FRC observed during pregnancy is attributable to

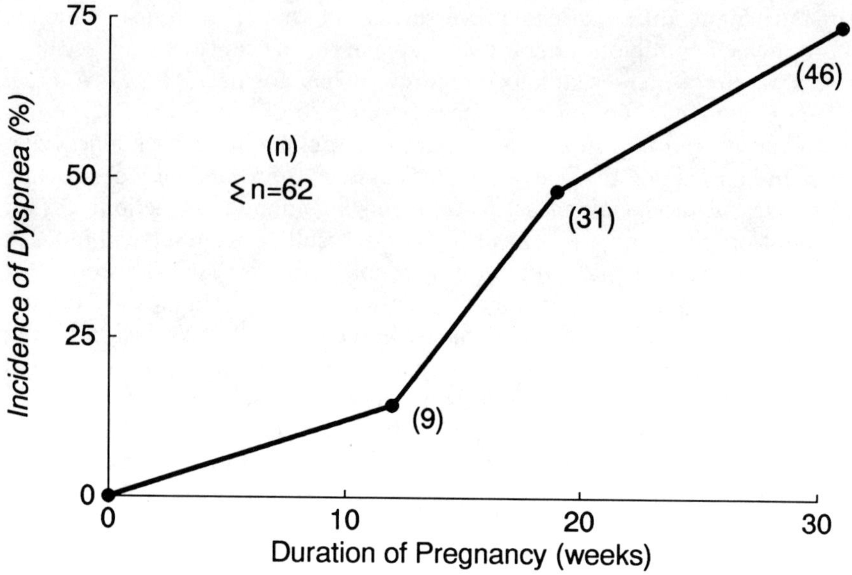

FIGURE 4.14. Incidence and time course of dyspnea during pregnancy in 62 women. (Data from Milne et al.[65])

the reduction in expiratory reserve volume as a result of the additional gravitational effects of abdominal contents altering the balance of the elastic recoil forces of the lung and chest wall. Thus both the intraabdominal and intrathoracic pressures become less negative, and the resting position of the diaphragm is elevated. Alterations of thoracic configuration with augmentation of the rib cage transverse diameters and lower thoracic perimeter upward tends to diminish diaphragmatic displacement. This increased abdominal girth places the expiratory muscle fibers on a more favorable portion of their length–tension curve, giving rise to the preservation or sometimes observed increase in vital capacity and reduced residual volume because of this increase in inspiratory capacity. Others have observed no change in lung compliance, with an increase in airway conductance due to possible hormone-related relaxation of bronchial smooth muscle. This finding has supported the concept of a physiologic rather than a mechanical cause for the dyspnea experienced durng pregnancy[65] (Fig. 4.14). The hyperventilation producing hypocapnia is a result of an increase in tidal volume rather than respiratory frequency.[65] The increase in ventilation observed at rest and with exercise is in excess of that which can be attributed to the associated rise in metabolic rate (increased $\dot{V}O_2$ and $\dot{V}CO_2$), thereby lowering the arterial PCO_2 at rest and increasing the ventilatory equivalent for oxygen. The alveolar ventilation increases to a lesser degree because of an increase in physiologic

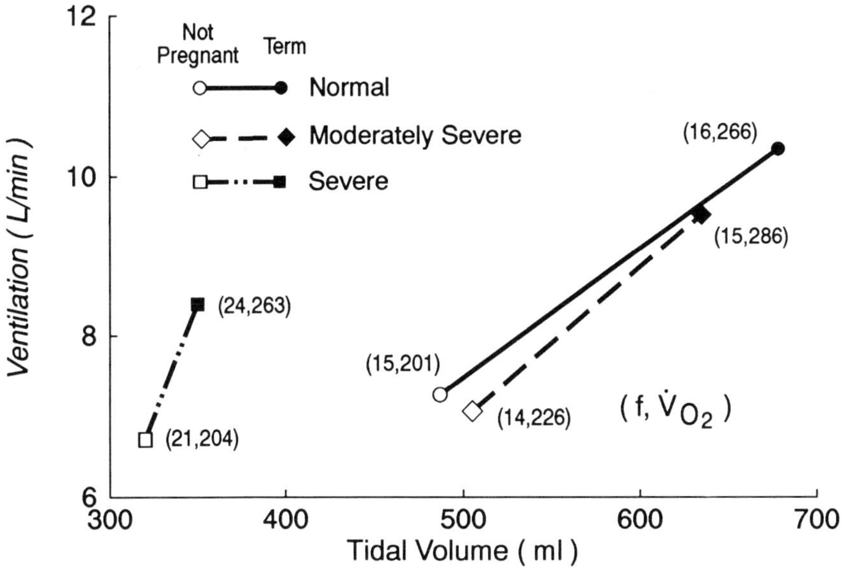

FIGURE 4.15. Mean values of the resting respiratory pattern of 19 normal women not pregnant and at term. Also shown are mean values of women with moderately severe ($n = 4$) and severe ($n = 5$) restrictive lung disease. The respiratory frequency (f) and metabolic rate ($\dot{V}_{O_2}$ ml/min) are shown. (Data from Cugell et al.[64] and Gaensler et al.[66])

deadspace that occurs with pregnancy. It suggests a progressive increase in the sensitivity of the respiratory center to carbon dioxide with advancing pregnancy that appears to return to normal immediately post-partum. The reported increment in inspiratory flow rate (V_I/T_I) further supports the concept of enhanced respiratory drive. The altered position of the diaphragm, with increased resting length and decrease in the radius of curvature allows more effective force development for a given efferent neural input.

The stimulus of the altered *milieu interieur* has classically been attributed to the increased serum progesterone concentration and its central effect (similar to that of aspirin) on the respiratory center and a metabolic effect of uncoupling oxidative-phosphorylation, which is also reflected in part by the increase in metabolic rate. The hyperventilation, dyspnea, and widened (A-a)DO_2 gradient must be differentiated from underlying disease before a simple physiologic explanation is given to dismiss the onset of dyspnea. Interestingly, the presence of a pleural effusion is not helpful, as it occurs frequently during the first 24 hours after delivery unrelated to the dyspnea and is a consequence of the intrathoracic pressure changes associated with delivery that may also cause barotrauma. Pneumonia represents

10% of all pulmonary complications but is the second commonest cause of maternal mortality and morbidity, exceeded only by cardiac disease. It is an especially threatening complication in patients with preexisting lung disease who are already compromised by the "physiologic" effects of pregnancy on gas exchange[66] (Fig. 4.15).

More recently, the acid-aspiration syndrome as described by Mendelson[54] has again focused attention on the predisposing factors of pregnancy in causing pneumonia. Mendelson suggested that, in comparison to preoperative preparations in other patients, obstetric patients are peculiarly susceptible to aspiration because of feeding practices during labor. Mendelson's commentary also serves today as the most important consideration of therapy, that is, prevention. In addition, gastric emptying may be delayed during labor, as reflected by the findings of more than 40 ml in the stomachs of 55% of obstetric patients compared to similar amounts in only 10% of other preoperative patients.[67] Others have attributed this apparent predisposition during pregnancy to displacement of the stomach by the uterus, thereby pressing the pyloric portion of the stomach upward and backward and impairing emptying. The more suspect etiology, however, is the high incidence of emergency procedures for obstetric patients. A previous study showed it to be true for 93% of obstetric patients whose deaths resulted from regurgitation or vomiting during anesthesia.[68]

The mortality rate in Mendelson's series (0% in acid-aspiration patients) and the prominent finding of bronchospasm is in contrast to the much higher mortality and incidence of infection without initial signs of hyperreactive airway in current published series of aspiration pneumonia. These differences have been attributed to the young, otherwise healthy population whom Mendelson reported. Others, however, have suggested that Mendelson's patients did not have Mendelson syndrome. This thesis is becoming more and more attractive as emphasis is given to the incidence of premature labor as the cause for emergency procedures and the acknowledged high incidence of unobserved and probably nonoccurring episodes of aspiration. Most important is the increasing appreciation of the high concentrations of chemical mediators, many of which are associated with the parenchymal inflammatory response and airway bronchospasm, such as platelet activating factor (PAF) present in high concentrations in the placenta and amniotic fluid. The placenta has been previously indirectly associated with the pathogenesis of Mendelson syndrome in that it is responsible for adrenal insufficiency: It serves as a sponge that absorbs the natural maternal corticosteroids, thus predisposing the mother to hypoadrenalism and rendering her unable to respond to the stress of acid aspiration—thus the basis for the proposal to treat the resulting pulmonary edema with corticosteroids. Similarly, amniotic fluid embolism is a well recognized entity that involves the embolism of fluid or particulate matter into the maternal circulation, causing acute cardiopulmonary collapse

TABLE 4.7. Spirometric, lung volume, diffusing capacity, and arterial blood gas values of a woman with acute pulmonary edema after delivery[a].

Measurement	Predicted	Actual value			
		Day 3	Day 6	Day 9	Day 31
FVC (L)	4.79	1.16	1.24	1.67	3.44
FEV_1 (L)	3.91	0.90	0.90	1.43	2.91
FEV_1 (%)	82	78	88	86	85
FRC (L)	3.59	1.59	2.23	2.15	2.52
RV (L)	1.86	1.24	2.20	1.71	1.11
TLC (L)	7.39	2.26	3.37	3.43	4.54
DLCO (ml/min/mm Hg)	42.7		13.0	13.8	24.3
Pa_{O_2} (mm Hg) ($F_{I_{O_2}}$ =			54	57	74
0.21)		47	43	40	37
Pa_{CO_2}, mm Hg		41	7.43	7.41	7.46
pH, arterial		7.41			

[a] These values follow the development of acute, pulmonary edema, which was recognized during cesarean section being performed to deliver twins from a 32-year-old woman with indolent labor. Mechanical ventilation was discontinued after 8 hours with resolution of dyspnea by 24 hours and no significant radiologic clearing by 72 hours postpartum. Rapid radiologic resolution occurred thereafter, and the patient had no pulmonary symptoms.

(Table 4.7). Serious consideration must now be given to the entrance of soluble mediators rather than fragments of trophoblast and decidual tissue, which would account for the noncardiac pulmonary edema and acute lung injury syndrome seen during premature or complicated labor—commonly and probably erroneously attributed to the tocolytic agents.

Elderly Patients

It is difficult to distinguish between the effects of disease and the changes that result from aging in humans, particularly the deterioration due to environmental contamination. This discussion describes and emphasizes anatomic and functional variables as well as host defense mechanisms and immunosenescence of the respiratory systems of the elderly and indicates implications that predispose to pneumonia.

Structural Changes

Structural changes with age may occur in both the thorax and the lung.

Thoracic Cage

The rib cage stiffens progressively with advancing years and becomes fixed at a higher volume. The shape of the chest changes as dorsal kyphosis develops owing to degeneration of the intervertebral discs and thoracic spine. This forward curvature is associated with upward rotation of the ribs and upward displacement of the sternum, resulting in an increase in the anteroposterior diameter. Normally, the ratio of anteroposterior to lateral dimensions is approximately 0.75. When this ratio reaches about 0.9, a barrel deformity, so characteristic of old age, is recognizable. This configuration was thought at one time to represent a distinct pulmonary disease of the elderly and was referred to as senile emphysema. The physiologic changes and functional capacity of these patients, however, are no different from those of individuals of the same age without barrel deformities; hence the term senile emphysema should be abandoned. The structural deformation of the chest does, however, interfere with pulmonary function.

Lung

The lung also undergoes changes. Morphologically, they consist in dilatation of the airspaces, a decrease in the number and thickness of elastic fibers surrounding them, and an increase in the size and number of alveolar pores. When the walls of respiratory bronchioles and alveolar ducts or alveoli degenerate as well, pathologists describe the alterations as those of emphysema rather than old age.

In a series of 138 routine autopsies performed at an urban general hospital in the United States,[69] both destruction and dilatation of airspaces were found in 68% of men and 24%of women beyond the third decade of life. These observations are illustrated by age groups in Figure 4.16. The data clearly demonstrate a sex difference in the incidence of the criteria for the pathologic diagnosis of emphysema and further suggest that in men beyond the sixth decade of life this incidence does not increase. It should not be inferred from these studies that 68% of men beyond the third decade have clinically significant emphysema, only that parenchymal destruction after that age progresses to an extent that fulfills the pathologic standards for this diagnosis. The incidence appears to be so high in men beyond the fifth decade that, from a practical standpoint, the physician must assume the presence of these pathologic changes in all elderly men. It is not true of women (Fig. 4.16).

Supporting Structure of the Lung

Some of the important derangements in pulmonary function that occur with aging result from variations in the mechanical properties of the lung. These alterations have, as would be expected, a morphologic counterpart consisting in changes in the pulmonary supporting structure, the connective tissue. This acellular tissue, which gives the lung its form and structure, is composed of mucopolysaccharides and fibrous proteins (collagen, elastin, reticulin).

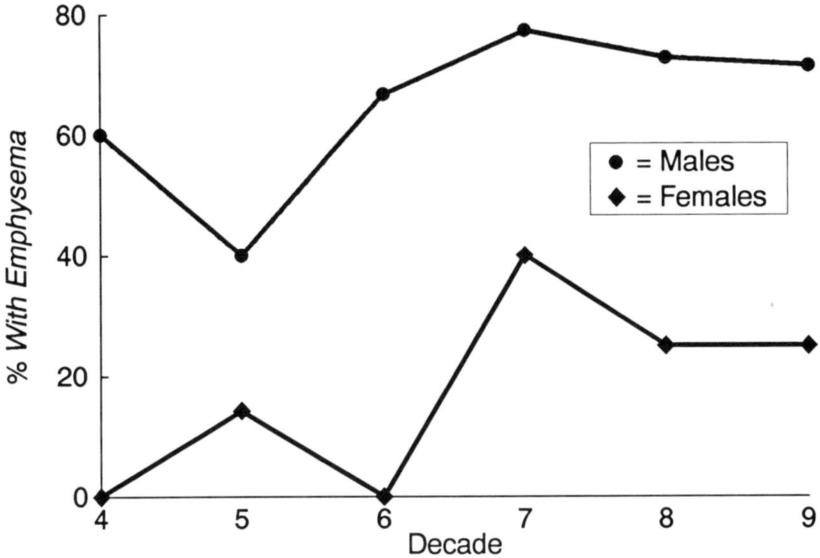

FIGURE 4.16. Incidence of pathologic diagnoses of emphysema (dilatation of air spaces associated with destruction of the walls of respiratory bronchioles, alveolar ducts, or alveoli) at routine autopsy. (Data from Thurlbeck.[69])

The content of mucopolysaccharides does not appear to change with age. Collagen, which constitutes approximately 30% of total body protein and up to 25% of the dry weight of lung, is distributed with elastin as a meshwork that serves as a supporting structure. Its fibers have a high Young's modulus and defy stretching, a property that probably prevents pulmonary overdistension. In the young lung the fibers are only sparsely interconnected by cross-links and can therefore be easily deformed by forces directed on them laterally. As age progresses, although the concentration of collagen in the lung does not change, the fibers become more closely bound to one another, and lateral deformation of the lung becomes more limited by preventing the transmission of displacing forces from one fiber to another. This progressive aggregation of collagen accounts, in large measure, for the increasing stiffness of the lung with age and the effect of this rigidity on pulmonary function.

The consequences of age on reticulin, another important component of connective tissue, have not been directly measured. Yet the questionable assumption has been offered that because of their close chemical similarity the changes that have been observed in collagen apply also to reticulin.

Elastin, the protein of which elastic fibers are composed, makes up about 8% of the solid structure of the lung. Unlike collagen, it is not rigid; rather, it is highly extensible, a property thought to account for elastic pulmonary recoil during exhalation. Curiously enough, the concentration of elastin in the lungs of both men and women increases with the approach of senscence despite concomitant progressive decrease in the elastic retractive force of the lung. This seemingly paradoxical concurrence may be the result of distortion in the geometric distribution of elastic fibers, hindering their function, even though their numbers are increased.

Vascular Bed

The vascular bed within the lung also undergoes progressive alterations with age from the third decade on. Elastic fibers in the media of the pulmonary vessels are generally replaced by fibrous tissue, thereby reducing the extensibility of the pulmonary trunk of an elderly person by approximately one-half when compared with that of a young subject. As age advances, the arterial tree changes from a highly distensible system of low resistance to one of reduced elasticity and increased resistance. These modifications are functionally similar to those that occur in the surrounding lung.

Summary

The structural remodeling in the lung associated with age consists in the following: (1) Dilatation of the airspaces distal to the terminal bronchioles and an increase in the number and size of alveolar pores beyond the sixth decade in approximately 72% of men and 22% of women. These alterations fulfill the pathologic criteria for the diagnosis of emphysema. (2) There is no change in the concentration of collagen, but there is aggregation of its fibers, which tends to stiffen the lung. (3) There are similar alterations in the pulmonary vascular bed. (4) The lung becomes rigid despite an increase in elastin, which may fail in its retractive function because of geometric distortion.

Functional Changes

Mechanics

The resting pulmonary volume, that is, the volume of gas contained in the lung at the end of a normal quiet expiration, is designed as the functional residual capacity (FRC). It is determined by the algebraic sum of two opposing factors: the elastic recoil of the lung and the elastic recoil of the chest wall. These forces within the lung tend to effect collapse and reduce its volume, whereas those of the thorax are directed toward expansion. The independent consequence of each can be seen when the chest of a cadaver is opened: The lungs collapse, and the thorax springs out. In the normal young subject, these opposing actions are such that the FRC is approximately 50% of the total lung capacity. As age advances, the elastic pulmonary recoil is reduced, and the progressively more rigid chest becomes fixed at a higher volume. The result is an amplified expansion of the lung, both at the end of normal, quiet exhalation (FRC) and after a full expiration (residual volume).

The reason for the loss of pulmonary elasticity with age is not known, but it may be due to the structural changes discussed in the preceding section. According to Laplace's law, the pressure within a sphere is directly proportional to the tension at its surface but inversely related to its radius of curvature. Because the airspaces become dilated with age, this pressure, and therefore the elastic recoil, would be expected to decrease. Pulmonary surfactant, by its effect on surface tension, is an important determinant of the elasticity of the lung, but its formation and activity do not change with age.

Opinions differ concerning the consequence of aging on the resistance to flow in the airways, but the best evidence indicates that it does not change. This point distinguishes normal elderly individuals from patients with symptomatic pulmonary emphysema, in whom an increase in airway resistance is a cardinal feature.

An important and often overlooked change with age is a decrease in the strength of the muscles of respiration. The maximal pressure exerted by elderly persons at the end of a normal exhalation is 50% that of young subjects and at the end of inspiration 61%. Under resting conditions this impairment of strength is insignificant, but in older postoperative patients it can become of practical import by sharply limiting the force of the cough, which is so essential to the prevention of atelectasis and pulmonary infection.

Static Lung Volume

Pulmonary volumes have been measured at different ages in many studies. The largest series included 135 individuals equally distributed between the third and ninth decades.[70] The changes in lung volume with senescence are illustrated by data chosen from subjects included in this investigation who had no symptoms or signs of pulmonary disease: The body shrinks with age; and between the third and ninth decades the height decreased by 6%, weight by 23%, and body surface area by 14%. Because pulmonary volume is a function of body size, the data are most meaningful when expressed as volume per square meter of surface area. The results so calculated, but charted as percent change, are shown in Figure 4.17.

The absolute level of total lung capacity decreases with age but, when expressed in relation to surface area, it does not change; what does vary, however, is the distribution of this total volume between subdivisions. Residual volume and functional residual capacity increase up to the sixth decade, by 90% and 60%, respectively; the vital capacity is reduced perforce. The resting tidal volume does not alter with age; hence both inspiratory and expiratory reserves are progressively diminished up to the seventh decade. The increase in residual volume, similar to the change

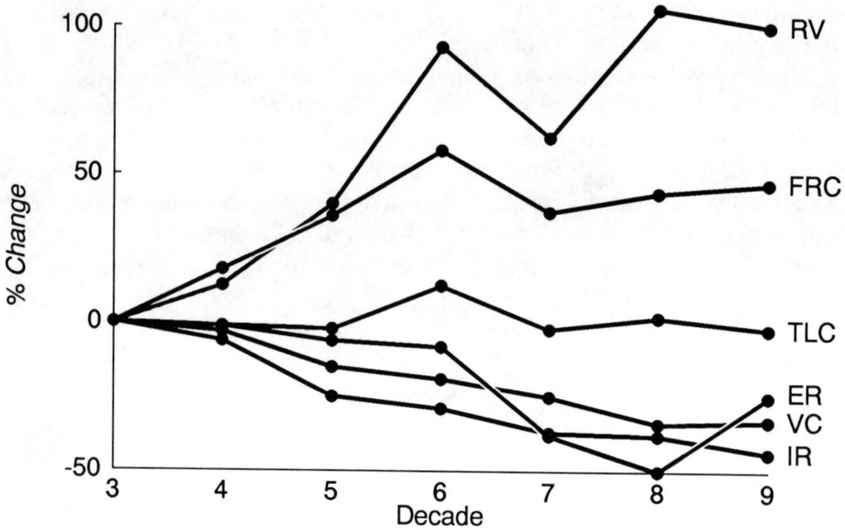

FIGURE 4.17. Percent change in static lung volumes in normal subjects at various ages compared to values found during the third decade of life. All data are expressed as volume per square meter of body surface area. RV = residual volume; FRC = functional residual capacity; TLC = total lung capacity; ER = expiratory reserve; VC = vital capacity; IR = inspiratory reserve. (Data from Norris et al.[70])

found in pulmonary emphysema, represents the primary variable for which there is adequate explanation. The suppression of the other subdivisions must result from the encroachment of residual volume, as total lung capacity does not vary. From a functional standpoint, it means that the capacity of the lungs as a ventilator of the blood and their function as a bellows are diminished with age, whereas the immovable fraction of gas, the residual volume, which causes contamination of each breath, is increased. At rest and during mild exercise, this change makes little difference because the limits are not taxed; but under conditions of stress, when large ventilatory volumes are required, these alterations can become critical. Additional impingement, as may be caused by postoperative atelectasis or pneumonia, can impose new and potentially lethal limits on an already restricted system. The high mortality rate from postoperative pulmonary complications in elderly patients is a manifestation of this loss of ventilatory reserve.

Dynamic Lung Volumes

The lung volumes described in the preceding section indicate the dimensions of the gas compartments of the lung: They are static measurements that do not necessarily reflect the capacity of the system for dynamic function. Ventilatory volumes, on the other hand, convey this function by introducing the dimension of time and describing thereby the dynamic limits of the system.

The resting tidal volume does not change with age or respiratory frequency. Deadspace ventilation, however, increases. Alveolar ventilation [(tidal volume × frequency) − (deadspace × frequency)] diminishes, but it does so in parallel with decreased oxygen requirements, keeping the relation between alveolar ventilation and metabolism constant throughout adult life.[71]

The maximal breathing capacity (MBC), also called maximal voluntary ventilation, is defined as the maximal volume of gas that can be breathed per minute by ventilatory effort. Age differences in MBC calculated for the same subjects shown in Figure 4.17, also expressed as liters per minute per square meter of body surface, show that the greatest fall in MBC occurred between the third and sixth decades, beyond which it decreased by only another 10% to a value in the seventies and eighties equal to 50% of that during the third decade of life. In this study, the reduction in MBC with age was due to the fact that elderly people breathed more slowly during the test while keeping their tidal volumes equal to those of the younger subjects. This difference in performance probably results from the combined effects of rigidity of the thoracic cage, loss of muscular strength and velocity of contraction, inability to perform sustained work, and decreased coordination.[71]

Gas Exchange

The functional changes in the respiratory system with aging are not confined to the static volumes and ventilatory capacities but include all aspects of gas exchange between the lung and the blood. The net effect of aging on gas exchange is manifested by a slight fall in arterial oxygen tension, which results largely from an inequality in the distribution of inspired gas in the lung in relation to the distribution of blood flow.

In addition to derangements in ventilation-perfusion relations in the elderly, there is a decrease in the diffusing capacity of the lung. The decline of diffusing capacity with age has been interpreted as the result of a decrease in the effective pulmonary capillary area due to diminution in cardiac output.

The changes in the relations of ventilation to perfusion and in diffusing capacity of the lung with aging result in a slight fall in arterial oxygen pressure and hemoglobin saturation. Typical results are shown in Figure 4.18, drawn from the data of one study.[72] The fall in oxygen tension does not represent a serious defect, even during the eighth decade; the predicted value of 70 mm Hg is equivalent to that found in normal young people residing at an altitude of 5000 feet. Although the absolute level of

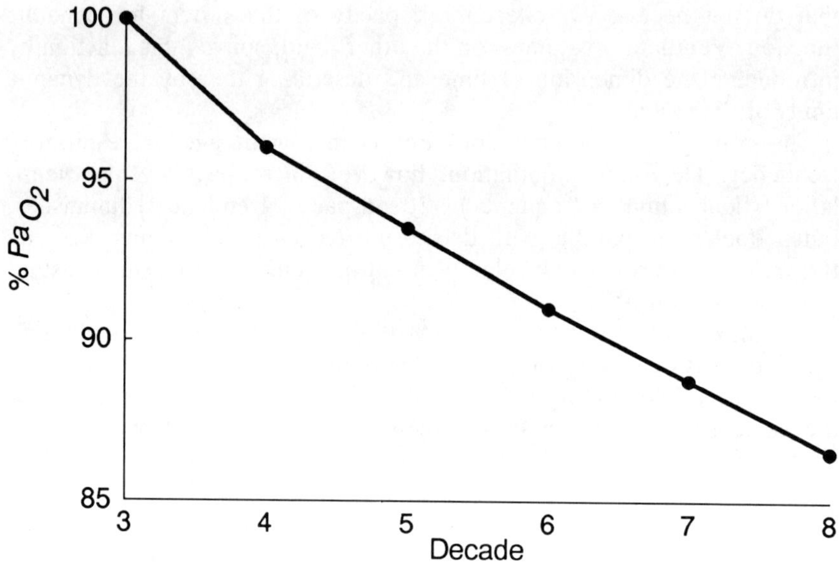

FIGURE 4.18. Percent change in arterial partial pressure of oxygen (Pa_{O_2}) with age in normal subjects. For calculation of absolute values, 90 mm Hg can be assumed to be normal during the third decade. (Data from Robinson.[72])

PO_2 is not critically low, the fact that it is reduced because of disordered pulmonary function indicates again a restriction imposed by age, which can manifest as more severe hypoxia if further limitations are placed on the system by postoperative pain, depressant drugs, the development of pulmonary atelectasis, infection, or other stress. The partial pressure of carbon dioxide, the pH, and the bicarbonate content of arterial blood are all unchanged by advancing age.

Regulation of Respiration

The fact that the relation between alveolar ventilation and metabolism remains constant throughout life indicates that the stability of the ventilatory control system is maintained. However, the ventilatory responses to hypoxia and hypercapnia decrease in the elderly owing primarily to alterations in central mechanisms that control efferent outflow to the respiratory muscles.

The common occurrence of Cheyne-Stokes breathing in elderly subjects during sleep may represent a subtle derangement of ventilatory control. Some loss of integrative function is also suggested by the observation that the administration of small doses of morphine to elderly subjects may produce Cheyne-Stokes breathing in the wakeful state. It occurs despite the fact that a single dose of morphine produces no more ventilatory depression in elderly subjects than it does in the young.[71]

Host-Defense Mechanisms

Upper Airway

A decrease in the acuity of perception and reflex activity has long been thought to accompany the aging process. Laryngeal closure due to chemical mucosal irritation (Kratschmer reflex) was found to be profoundly impaired in the elderly with nearly a sixfold increase in threshold from the third to the ninth decade of life.[73] The decrease in such protective activity has been proposed as an explanation for an increased incidence of silent aspiration in the elderly and the reported increased incidence of bronchopneumonia.[73] In addition, impaired mucociliary clearance has been reported in the elderly in part because of a loss of ciliated cells.

Cell-Mediated Immunity

Decreased cell-mediated immunity with aging has been well documented. There is a decrease in delayed hypersensitivity as determined by skin testing to both old (immunologic memory) and new antigens. The aged T cells show a wide spectrum of activity, as illustrated by a variably impaired proliferative response in part related to decreased interleukin-2 (IL-2) secretion and to decreased expression of IL-2 receptor.[74] Other abnormalities detected include decreased numbers of T lymphocytes, both CD4+ and CD8+ cells, as well as excessive T-suppressor-cell activity.[75] Studies have failed to detect abnormalities in macrophage function in the elderly, a major component of successful immunosurveillance.

Humoral Immunity

The ability of the bone marrow to generate B cells does not diminish with aging, although immunoglobulin levels do decrease. Immunization with pneumococcal capsular antigens and influenza vaccine demonstrates a blunted antibody response in the elderly. This defect in antibody production appears to be due to altered T-lymphocyte function.[74]

Cellular Immunity

Studies of neutrophil function in the elderly have suggested decreases in chemotactic response, phagocytic activity, and superoxide anion production.[74]

Summary

Although these changes of immunologic attrition appear mild, the attack ratio for pneumonia increases with age as does the severity. These observations are thought to be related to senescence of the immune system, increasing susceptibility. The anatomic changes and decreased functional reserve of the respiratory system is responsible for the age-related increase in severity resulting in increased hospitalization and mortality associated with pneumonia. Finally, the importance of comorbidity and enhanced microaspiration is thought to be responsible for changes from a predominantly gram-positive to gram-negative oropharyngeal flora and the predilection for developing nosocomial pneumonia.

Hypersensitivity Pneumonitis

Hypersensitivity pneumonitis, also known as allergic alveolitis, is not an infectious entity but represents an inflammatory response of the lung due to chronic exposure to inorganic, or more commonly organic, antigen (Table 4.8). Different antigens have given rise to a variety of specific occupational terminology (i.e., farmers' lung and pigeon breeders' disease). It has been classically described in relation to occupational exposure; but though it is environmental, it is not necessarily related to the workplace and is being increasingly appreciated to also be a consequence of nonoccupational exposure. The etiologic agents are diverse; more than 50 sources of antigen have been described, including bacteria, fungi, protozoa, animal or avian proteins, plants, and chemicals, but the clinical manifestations and pulmonary pathology are uniform.[76] The evolution of BAL has greatly enhanced early diagnosis and our understanding of the pathogenesis.

Factors that influence hypersensitivity pneumonitis are the physical characteristics of the agent and the dose inhaled. The antigen must be particulate in nature, small enough to reach the terminal airways (1–3 μm); and there must be prolonged, repeated exposure. Such high antigen dosage presumably accounts for the association with occupational exposure rather than the occasional environmental contact, though

TABLE 4.8. Causes of hypersensitivity pneumonia.

Antigen	Exposure	Syndrome
Thermoactinomyces vulgaris	Moldy hay	Farmers' lung
Aureobasidium pullulans	Air conditioner	Ventilation pneumonitis
Micropolyspora faeni	Water	Humidifier lung
Aspergillus clavatus	Moldy barley	Malt workers' lung
Thermophilic actinomycetes	Mushroom compost	Mushroom workers' lung
Thermoactinomyces sacchari	Moldy sugar cane	Bagassosis
Mucor stolonifer	Paprika dust	Paprika splitters' lung
Cryptostroma corticale	Maple wood bark	Maple bark strippers' lung
Penicillium caseii	Moldy cheese	Cheese washers' lung
Penicillium frequentans	Moldy cork	Suberosis
Avian proteins	Avian excreta and shedding	Bird fanciers' (pigeon breeders') lung
Toluene diisocyanate	Polyurethane foam	TDI pneumonitis
Phthalic anhydride	Heated epoxy resin	Epoxy resin lung
Sitophilus granarius	Wheat weevils	Millers' lung

exposure variables have been poorly documented. Host factors, although poorly defined, are important in the pathogenesis of hypersensitivity pneumonitis, as only a small percentage (<10%) of those exposed (attack rate) develop the disease. Interestingly, cigarette smoking appears to exert a protective effect against this disorder, with associated low serum precipitin values. The mechanism of this protective effect of tobacco smoke remains unclear. The BAL fluid contains the specific precipitins for the causal antigens, as does the serum. Humoral diagnostic techniques, however, are limited, as serum precipitins to suspect antigen may be present in 50% of exposed but asymptomatic patients or absent in patients with overt disease.

When established hypersensitivity pneumonitis exists, BAL reveals a typical lymphocyte alveolitis with a striking lymphocyte predominance in a hypercellular fluid.[77] The lymphocyte numbers are higher in symptomatic patients than in exposed workers who are asymptomatic. Remission as a result of avoidance or of treatment is associated with a decrease in the number of lymphocytes. Phenotypic studies have shown that it is a T lymphocytosis, with the B cells representing a small percentage of the total amount. The predominant T-cell subset is CD8+ cells (suppressor-cytotoxic subset) though the total number of CD4+ (helper/inducer) cells is increased and there is a decrease in the CD4+/CD8+ ratio. The profile returns to normal with remission after removal from exposure. It has been suggested that the cells recovered by lavage from individuals with hypersensitivity pneumonitis have functional abnormalities compatible with an ongoing immune response, but which cells are toxic and which cells are protective is not clear. The role of suppressor T cells in the clinical expression of hypersensitivity pneumonitis has been emphasized and is related to the concept of functional immune regulatory imbalance with a loss of functional suppression of disease activity.

Finally, with acute exposure to antigen, an increase in BAL neutrophils and eosinophils (without eosinophilia) is seen, and this recruitment has been attributed to an antigen-directed early inflammatory response. Large numbers of mast cells are found as well, and their release of vasoactive mediators may be of significance with respect to morbid chronic fibrotic reactions. Continued exposure in some individuals does not necessarily lead to progressive deterioration, whereas others may show a progressive decline in pulmonary function despite antigen avoidance. It has been shown that only the intensity of the alveolitis, not its composition, distinguishes normal farmers from patients with farmer's lung.[78] No correlation was observed between BAL mast cell yield and clinical or laboratory evaluation of pulmonary function. The number of alveolar macrophages in hypersensitivity pneumonitis is normal. It has been concluded from these findings that this disease involves immune complex and cell-mediated tissue injury acting in combination with nonimmunologic factors in reaction to inhaled antigens.

References

1. Fang G-D, Fine M, Orloff J, et al: New and emerging etiologies for community-acquired pneumonia with implications for therapy: a prospective multicenter study of 359 cases. Medicine (Baltimore) 1990;69:307–316.
2. Gwaltney JM Jr, Sande MA, Austrian R, Hendly JO: Spread of Steptococcus pneumoniae in families. II. Relation of transfer of S. pneumoniae to incidence of colds and serum antibody. J Infect Dis 1975;132:62–68.
3. Shackelford PG, Feigin RD: Periodicity of susceptibility to pneumococcal infection: influence of light and adrenocortical secretions. Science 1973;182:285–287.
4. Pachon J, Prados MD, Capote F, et al: Severe community-acquired pneumonia: etiology, prognosis, and treatment. Am Rev Respir Dis 1990;142:369–373.
5. Brown RB, Sands M, Ryczak M: Community-acquired pneumonia caused by mixed aerobic bacteria. Chest 1986;90:810–814.
6. Woodhead MA, Arrowsmith J, Chamberlain-Webber R, et al: The value of routine microbial investigation in community-acquired pneumonia. Respir Med 1991;85:313–317.
7. Dreyfuss D, Djedaini K, Weber P, et al: Prospective study of nosocomial pneumonia and of patient and circuit colonization during mechanical ventilation with circuit changes every 48 hours versus no change. Am Rev Respir Dis 1991;143:738–743.
8. Hanson LC, Weber DJ, Rutalla WA: Risk factors for nosocomial pneumonia in the elderly. Am J Med 1992;92:161–166.
9. Atherton ST, White DJ: Stomach as source of bacteria colonizing respiratory tract during artificial ventilation. Lancet 1978;2:968–969.
10. Driks MR, Craven DE, Celli BR, et al: Nosocomial pneumonia in intubated patients given sucralfate as compared with antacids or histamine type 2 blockers: the role of gastric colonization. N Engl J Med 1987;317:1376–1382.
11. Andrews CP, Coalson JJ, Johanson WG: Diagnosis of nosocomial bacterial pneumonia in acute diffuse lung injury. Chest 1981;80:254–258.
12. Aerdts SJA, Van Dalen R, Clasener HAL, et al: Antibiotic prophylaxis of respiratory tract infection in mechanically ventilated patients: a prospective, blinded, randomized trial of the effect of a novel regimen. Chest 1991;100:783–791.
13. Gastinne H, Wolff M, Delatour F, et al: A controlled trial in intensive care units of selective decontamination of the digestive tract with nonabsorbable antibiotics. N Engl J Med 1992;326:594–599.
14. Garibaldi RA, Britt MR, Coleman ML, et al: Risk factors for post-operative pneumonia. Am J Med 1981;70:677–680.
15. Tisi GM: Pre-operative evaluation of pulmonary function: validity, indications and benefits. Am Rev Respir Dis 1979;119:293–310.
16. Lawrence VA, Page CP, Harris GD: Pre-operative spirometry before abdominal operations: a critical appraisal of its predictive value. Arch Intern Med 1989;149:280–285.
17. Ford GT, Whitelaw WA, Rosenal TW, et al: Diaphragm function after abdominal surgery in humans. Am Rev Respir Dis 1983;127:431–436.

18. Nunn JF, Coleman AJ, Sachithanandan T, et al: Hypoxaemia and atelectasis produced by forced expiration. Br J Anaesth 1965;37:3–12.
19. Bendixen HH, Hedley-White J, Laver MB: Impaired oxygenation in surgical patients during general anesthesia with controlled ventilation: a concept of atelectasis. N Engl J Med 1963;269:991–996.
20. Henderson Y: The physiology of atelectasis. JAMA 1929;93:96–98.
21. O'Donohue WJ Jr: National survey of the usage of lung expansion modalities for the prevention and treatment of post-operative atelectasis following abdominal and thoracic surgery. Chest 1985;87:76–80.
22. Bodey GP, Powell RD Jr, Hersh EM, et al: Pulmonary complications of acute leukemia. Cancer 1966;19:781–793.
23. Tryka AF, Godleski JJ, Fanta HH: Leukemic cell lysis pneumopathy: a complication of treated myeloblastic leukemia. Cancer 1982;50:2763–2770.
24. Hildebrand FL Jr, Rosenow EC II, Haberman TM, Tazelaar HD: Pulmonary complications of leukemia. Chest 1990;98:1233–1239.
25. Saito H, Anaissie EJ, Morice RC, et al: Bronchoalveolar lavage in the diagnosis of pulmonary infiltrates in patients with acute leukemia. Chest 1988;94:745–749.
26. Witte RJ, Gurney JW, Robbins RA, et al: Diffuse pulmonary alveolar hemorrhage after bone marrow transplantation: radiographic findings in 39 patients. AJR 1991;157:461–464.
27. Ettinger NA, Trulock EP: Pulmonary considerations of organ transplantation. Part 2. Am Rev Respir Dis 1991;144:213–223.
28. Barnes PF, Bloch AB, Davidson PT, Snider DE Jr: Tuberculosis in patients with human immunodeficiency virus infection. N Engl J Med 1991;324:1644–1650.
29. Horsburgh CR Jr: Mycobacterium avium complex infection in the acquired immunodeficiency syndrome. N Engl J Med 1991;324:1332–1338.
30. El-Sadr W, Simberkoff MS: Survival and prognostic factors in severe Pneumocystis carinii pneumonia requiring mechanical ventilation. Am Rev Respir Dis 1988;137:1264–1267.
31. Bennet CL, Garfinkle JB, Greenfield S, et al: The relation between hospital experience and in-hospital mortality for patients with AIDS-related PCP. JAMA 1989;261:2975–2979.
32. Wachter RM, Russi MB, Bloch DA, et al: Pneumocystis carinii pneumonia and respiratory failure in AIDS: improved outcomes and increased use of intensive care units. Am Rev Respir Dis 1991;143:251–256.
33. Sankary RM, Turner J, Lipavsky A, et al: Alveolar-capillary block in patients with AIDS and Pneumocystis carinii pneumonia. Am Rev Respir Dis 1988;137:443–449.
34. Smith DE, Wyatt J, McLuckie A, Gazzard B: Severe exercise hypoxemia with normal or near normal x-rays: a feature of Pneumocystis carinii infection. Lancet 1988;2:1049–1051.
35. Kagawa FT, Kirsch CM, Yenokida GG, Levine ML: Serum lactate dehydrogenase activity in patients with AIDS and Pneumocystis carinii pneumonia. Chest 1988;94:1031–1033.
36. Kreuger JJ, Sayre VA, Karetzky M: Bronchoalveolar lavage-induced pneumothorax. Chest 1988;94:440–441.

37. Krueger JJ, Sayre VA, Karetzky, M: Infectious interstitial emphysema in AIDS. N J Med 1987;84:489–491.
38. Aronin PA, Mahaley MS Jr, Rudnick SA, et al: Prediction of BCNU pulmonary toxicity in patients with malignant gliomas: an assessment of risk factors. N Engl J Med 1980;303:183–188.
39. Martin WJ II, Rosenow EC III: Amiodarone pulmonary toxicity: recognition and pathogenesis. Part 2. Chest 1988;93:1243–1248.
40. White DA, Rankin JA, Stover DE, et al: Methotrexate pneumonitis: bronchoalveolar lavage findings suggest an immunologic disorder. Am Rev Respir Dis 1989;139:18–21.
41. Castellino RA, Glatstein E, Turbow MM, et al: Latent radiation injury of lungs or heart activated by steroid withdrawal. Ann Intern Med 1974;80:593–599.
42. Gross NJ: Pulmonary effects of radiation therapy. Ann Intern Med 1977;86:81–92.
43. Gibson PG, Bryant DH, Morgan GW: Radiation-induced lung injury: a hypersensitivity pneumonitis? Ann Intern Med 1988;109:288–291.
44. Keane TJ, Van Dyk J, Rider WD: Idiopathic interstitial pneumonia in bone marrow transplantation: the relationship with total body irradiation. Int J Radiat Oncol Biol Phys 1981;7:1365–1370.
45. Clark CJ, Reid WH, Gilmour WH, Campbell D: Mortality probability in victims of fire trauma: revised equation to include inhalation injury. BMJ 1986;292:1303–1305.
46. Clark CJ, Campbell D, Reid WH: Blood carboxyhaemoglobin and cyanide levels in fire survivors. Lancet 1981;1:1332–1335.
47. Baud FJ, Barriot P, Toffis V, et al: Elevated blood cyanide concentrations in victims of smoke inhalation. N Engl J Med 1991;325:1761–1766.
48. Helpern M, Rho Y-M: Deaths from narcotism in New York City: incidence, circumstances, and post morteum findings. NY State J Med 1966;66:2391–2408.
49. Clemmesen C, Lassen NA: Treatment of circulatory shock in narcotic poisoning. Dan Med Bull 1963;10:100–103.
50. Wendt VE, Puro HE, Shapiro J, et al: Angiothrombotic pulmonary hypertension in addicts: "blue velvet" addiction. JAMA 1964;188:755–757.
51. Ettinger NA, Albin RJ: A review of the respiratory effects of smoking cocaine. Am J Med 1989;87:664–668.
52. Murray RJ, Albin RJ, Mergner W, Criner GJ: Diffuse alveolar hemorrhage temporarily related to cocaine smoking. Chest 1988;93:427–429.
53. Taylor RF, Bernard GR: Airway complications from freebasing cocaine. Chest 1989;95:476–477.
54. Mendelson CL: The aspiration of stomach contents into the lungs during obstetric anesthesia. Am J Obstet Gynecol 1946;52:191–204.
55. Amberson JB Jr: Aspiration pneumonia. Int Clin 1937;22:126–138.
56. Gardner AMN: Aspiration of food and vomit. Q J Med 1958;27:227–245.
57. Teabeaut JR II: Aspiration of gastric contents: an experimental study. Am J Pathol 1952;28:51–67.
58. Colebatch HJH, Halmagyi DFJ: Reflex airway reaction to fluid aspiration. J Appl Physiol 1962;17:787–794.

59. Berry REL, Sanslow CA: Clinical manifestations and treatment of congestive atelectasis. Arch Surg 1963;87:169–183.
60. Awe WC, Fletcher WS, Jacob SW: The pathophysiology of aspiration pneumonitis. Surgery 1966;60:232–239.
61. Cameron JL, Mitchell WH, Zuidema GD: Aspiration pneumonia: clinical outcome following documented aspiration. Arch Surg 1973;106:49–52.
62. Bartlett JG, Gorbach SL, Finegold SM: The bacteriology of aspiration pneumonia. Am J Med 1974;56:202–207.
63. Finland M: Pneumonia and pneumococcal infections with special reference to pneumococcal pneumonia. Am Rev Respir Dis 1979;120:481–502.
64. Cugell DW, Frank NR, Gaensler EA, Badger TL: Pulmonary function in pregnancy. 1. Serial observations in normal women. Am Rev Tuberc 1953;67:1–30.
65. Milne JA, Howie AD, Pack AI: Dyspnea during normal pregnancy. Br J Obstet Gynaecol 1978;85:260–263.
66. Gaensler EA, Patton WE, Verstraeten JM, Badger TL: Pulmonary function in pregnancy. III. Serial observations in patients with pulmonary insufficiency. Am Rev Tuberc 1953;67:55–73.
67. Taylor G, Pryse-Davies J: The prophylactic use of antacids in prevention of the acid-pulmonary-aspiration syndrome (Mendelson's syndrome). •Lancet 1966;1:288–291.
68. Edwards G, Morton HJV, Pak EA, Wylie WD: Death associated with anaesthesia: a report on 1000 cases. Anesthesia 1956;11:194–220.
69. Thurlbeck WM: The incidence of pulmonary emphysema: with observations on the relative incidence and spatial distribution of various types of emphysema. Am Rev Respir Dis 1963;87:206–215.
70. Norris AH, Shick NW, Landowne M, Falzone JH Jr: Pulmonary function studies: age differences in lung volumes and bellows function. J Gerontol 1956;11:379–387.
71. Tenney SM: Ventilatory control in old age. In Cander L, Moyer JH (eds): Aging of the lung. Orlauds, FL: Grune & Stratton, 1964, pp. 143–151.
72. Robinson S: Experimental studies on physical fitness in relation to age. Arbeitsphysiologie 1938;19:251–323.
73. Pontoppidan H, Beecher HK: Progressive loss of protective reflexes in the airway with the advance of age. JAMA 1960;174:2209–2213.
74. Simons RJ, Reynold HY: Altered immune status in the elderly. Sem Respir Infect 1990;5:251–259.
75. Verghese A, Berk SL: Bacterial pneumonia in the elderly. Medicine (Baltimore) 1983;62:271–285.
76. Arellano JLP, Sanchez RS, Encinas IP, et al: Pathogenesis of hypersensitivity pneumonitis. Allergol Immunopathol 1989;17:225–232.
77. Shellito JE: Hypersensitivity pneumonitis. Semin Respir Med 1991;12:196–203.
78. Laviolette M, Cormier Y, Loiseau A, et al: Bronchoalveolar mast cells in normal farmers and subjects with farmers lung: diagnostic, prognostic and physiologic significance. Am Rev Respir Dis 1991;144:855–860.

5
Historical, Physical, and Laboratory Clues to the Diagnosis of Pneumonia

BURKE A. CUNHA

Pneumonia may be defined as an infectious process involving the lungs. It may be acute, subacute, or chronic, and it may be due to a wide variety of infectious agents including bacteria, viruses, and fungi, with bacterial pneumonias the lungs are the primary site of organ involvement, but with viral and atypical bacterial pathogens extrapulmonary manifestations are common. Tuberculosis and fungal disease may be limited to the lung or, if the infection is disseminated, result in extrapulmonary manifestations involving multiple organs. The clinical problem is to differentiate the treatable pneumonias from untreatable infectious processes and non-infectious conditions mimicking pneumonia. Because the bacterial and atypical pneumonias are the most common and readily treatable with antimicrobial therapy, the diagnostic approach is directed at ruling out or identifying specific bacterial pathogens.

Patients present with a variety of signs and symptoms, so the syndromic approach to diagnosis is the most sensible, the best, and sometimes the only way to arrive at a reasonable working differential diagnosis. Careful analysis of the history combined with pertinent physical findings help to narrow diagnostic possibilities and suggest specific etiologies for the patient's pulmonary complaints.[1–4] It is the chest roentgenogram, however, that defines the process as pulmonary and suggests broad diagnostic categories in which to classify the pulmonary process. Therefore the chest roentgenogram is helpful for differentiating a typical pneumonia from an atypical pneumonia but is not usually helpful for arriving at a specific etiologic diagnosis. It is even more helpful for eliminating whole categories from diagnostic consideration. This purpose is the real strength of the plain film, which reveals what the process is not rather than what it is in most cases. For example, a diffuse honeycomb pattern on a chest film suggests that the process is not infectious but does not reveal what the initial pulmonary process was that resulted in end-stage pulmonary disease manifested by "honeycombing" on the plain chest film.[5–8]

The critical factor in syndromic diagnosis is combining nonspecific findings, whether they are laboratory findings or chest film abnormalities, so as to increase diagnostic specificity. Always look for uncommon but specific findings that immediately point to a specific diagnosis. For example, the finding of hypophosphatemia in a patient with an atypical pneumonia presentation immediately suggests the possibility of legionnaires' disease.

This approach works even by combining nonspecific findings with long differential diagnoses if one can "bunch" and "clump" diagnostic data with mental dexterity and adroitness. For example, the differential diagnosis for pleural effusion is considerable, as is the differential diagnosis for hilar nodal involvement. When a pulmonary infiltrate is found in conjunction with a pleural effusion and hilar adenopathy, the differential diagnosis is quickly limited to a relatively few disease entities by combining these three findings, which when taken by themselves would have not provided the answer. The search for diagnostic clues, preferably specifically but also nonspecifically in groups, directs the astute clinician to arrive quickly, with minimal information, at a fairly precise diagnosis that permits early empiric antimicrobial therapy.[9,10] For this reason, the chapter contains many tables of differential diagnostic features to assist the clinician in finding diagnostic information that can be combined to assist in the diagnosis of the patient with pneumonia.

The use of diagnostic "pearls" represents another important aspect of medical education and diagnostic decision making. Aphorisms help decide between two conditions that are similar or provide information to allow a specific diagnosis. This information is helpful adjunctively when combined with conflicting or difficult diagnostic dilemmas suggested by the history, physical examination, and chest film. For example, if the differential diagnosis is between Wegener's granulomatosis and Churg-Strauss allergic granulomatosis, the presence of eosinophilia, if due to the pulmonary process, immediately eliminates Wegener's granulomatosis as a diagnostic possibility. Similarly, eosinophilia is not part of pulmonary or disseminated tuberculosis; and in the absence of other causes of eosinophilia, this finding alone goes strongly against the diagnosis of *Mycobacterium tuberculosis* in any of its myriad manifestations.[1,11]

It is also not often appreciated that a patient presents with a nonspecific syndrome complex that nevertheless has the "diagnostic flavor" of certain diseases. For example, an elderly emaciated man with a pulmonary infiltrate and pulmonary symptoms that have persisted for weeks immediately suggests a chronic pulmonary process, which may be tuberculous, neoplastic, or fungal. Just as importantly, it immediately eliminates nearly all common bacterial and viral pathogens. This "feeling" that patients give you immediately suggests the appropriate diagnostic approach that may be refined with additional laboratory tests.[9,10]

Although the focus of this chapter is on arriving at a syndromic diagnosis on which to base early empiric therapy, which is important because it is of the greatest benefit to the patient, it should not be forgotten that the aim of the diagnostic workup is to arrive at a specific etiologic diagnosis.[2,3] A definitive diagnosis should be sought in all cases but is not always available in a timely fashion and in some cases, is not possible at all. The clinician, however, should endeavor to make every effort to arrive at a specific etiologic diagnosis. It may be done by blood cultures or by recovery of a specific pathogen from pleural fluid or tissue samples. Techniques vary from a variety of staining techniques to culture of the organism or serologic methods. Because definitive diagnosis, except for the common bacterial pneumonias, is often delayed or not possible, every effort must be directed to use the syndromic diagnostic approach to efficiently and effectively devise a diagnostic and therapeutic approach to the patient's pulmonary problems.[12–14]

Clues from the History

It has long been said that "the history is the diagnosis." This Oslerian aphorism remains true today and is helpful in many patients with non-infectious and infectious pulmonary disorders.[1] The historical clues to pneumonia begin with questioning the patient about exposure to sick people or special environmental conditions. More important diagnostic information is available by analyzing underlying diseases, the age of the individual, and any associated condition that may suggest the predisposition to specific pulmonary pathogens.[2,5] For example, pneumonia in children and young adults is likely to be due to *Mycoplasma*, one of the respiratory viruses, or *Chlamydia pneumoniae*, but it must be appreciated that bacterial pneumonias also are not uncommon in this age group. Similarly, elderly patients may have viral pneumonias but, excluding viral influenza, are more likely to have bacterial or atypical pneumonias. Alcoholics are predisposed to infection by the pneumococcus, *Klebsiella*, and *M. tuberculosis*, and to aspiration pneumonia. Individuals coming from chronic care facilities with pneumonias are likely to have *Streptococcus pneumoniae*, *Hemophilus influenzae*, or *Klebsiella* as a cause for their infectious pneumonia, other factors aside.[15] Patients with human immunodeficiency virus (HIV) presenting initially almost invariably have *Pneumocystis carinii* pneumonia (PCP), but on subsequent admissions may have a relapse of PCP or a variety of other pathogens including *Mycobacterium avium-intracellulare*, *Salmonella*, or *Legionella*.[2,12] Infections in leukopenic compromised hosts are determined by the profoundness and duration of the leukopenia. Early after chemotherapy, most infections tend to be nonpulmonary and due to aerobic gram-negative bacilli (e.g., *Pseudomonas aeruginosa*). After more than 2 weeks of profound leukopenia, the possibility of disseminated fungal diseases (e.g., *Aspergillus*) increases with time. These patients do not have gram-positive infections except as related to intravenous access devices, and gram-positive pneumonias in these patients are distinctly uncommon.[1,2]

These patients also may have a variety of noninfectious pulmonary problems, including leukoagglutination reactions involving the lungs, radiation pneumonitis, or a variety of drug-induced pulmonary diseases secondary to chemotherapeutic agents.[16] By examining the data in this way, one uses historical information to suggest specific diagnostic possibilities or, at the very least, broad diagnostic categories.

Symptoms are less specific in general and therefore provide less useful information. Combining nonspecific symptom clues with other information, however, enhances their value. For example, dyspnea is a common symptom of a wide variety of pulmonary diseases, but severely progressive dyspnea that develops over a week or more suggests PCP.[2] Once again the rapidity of the time course combined with the relatively nonspecific symptoms of dyspnea helps eliminate a variety of pulmonary disorders that may produce dyspnea more slowly (e.g., a variety of interstitial lung diseases).[11,12] Viral pneumonias may also some produce some dyspnea over a week, but again there should be other associated symptoms (e.g., fevers or myalgias) that would point toward a viral etiology. Similarly, severe bacterial pneumonias would not present solely with dyspnea after a week or more of acute shortness of breath in the absence of any other symptoms.[17] In contrast, if one is fortunate enough to have a patient with symptoms that do not ordinarily accompany most pneumonias, the uncommon but specific finding is of great diagnostic significance. For example, if an adult patient presents with an ill-defined pulmonary infiltrate and abdominal pain, *Legionella* is the most likely diagnostic possibility. Once again we have combined a typical pneumonia presentation on the chest film with an extrapulmonary finding to rapidly limit diagnostic possibilities.[9] Analogously, ear pain in a patient with pneumonia suggests pneumococcus, group A streptococci, *H. influenzae*, *Branhamella catarrhalis*, or *Mycoplasma* pneumonia, and the finding of the less common but more specific bullous myringitis immediately points to *Mycoplasma* as the cause of the patient's problems.[10] Similarly, a sore throat due to pharyngitis in a patient with pneumonia eliminates immediately pneumococcus and *H. influenzae* from diagnostic consideration, as these organisms are not associated with pharyngitis but commonly colonize the oropharynx.[18]

Underlying medical diseases also suggest specific putative pathogens. The diagnostic approach here is to recognize that the underlying condition is associated with a specific host defense defect, which in turn predisposes to a limited number of possible pathogens.[1,2] A patient with pneumonia and asplenia should have *S. pneumoniae*, *H. influenzae*, or *Neisseria meningitidis* pneumonia.[19] Patients with silicosis or pneumoconiosis are predisposed to *M. tuberculosis*; similarly, patients with *M. tuberculosis* or silicosis, which results in scarred and fibrosed lungs, may in turn predispose to adenocarcinoma; rarely, the two may even coexist. The most important part of the diagnostic approach is to appreciate the value of the method of looking for findings with high diagnostic specificity and in combining nonspecific findings to increase diagnostic accuracy.[9,10] Clues from the history are presented in Table 5.1.

Clues from the Physical Diagnosis

Physical diagnosis is most helpful for determining if the patient has consolidation or pleural effusion. Other physical diagnostic findings are helpful in specific situations (e.g., apical dullness suggesting tuberculosis, chest wall sinuses suggesting actinomycosis or bronchogenic carcinoma, or the relatively "quiet lungs" on auscultation typical of the viral pneumonias). Except for pleural effusion and consolidation, the most important physical findings are generally not helpful for diagnosing specific causes of pulmonary disease.[20] The physical examination is somewhat more helpful by providing extrapulmonary findings that may provide clues to the cause of the pulmonary process. In a patient with an atypical pneumonia and

TABLE 5.1. Pneumonia: historical clues.

Clues	With lung infiltrates suggest
Environmental clues	
Soil/plant contact	Legionnaires' disease Histoplasmosis Blastomycosis Sporotrichosis
Zoonotic clues	
Bird contact	Psittacosis Blastomycosis Histoplasmosis Cryptococcosis Q fever
Cat contact	Tularemia Q fever
Rabbit contact	Tularemia
Dog contact	*Dirofilaria immitis*
Host clues	
Age	
Children/young adults	*Mycoplasma* *C. pneumoniae* Viral pneumonias
Elderly	*Streptococcus pneumoniae* *Hemophilus influenzae* *Klebsiella* Legionnaires' disease Viral influenza Aspiration pneumonia/anaerobic abscess *M. tuberculosis*

TABLE 5.1. *Continued*

Clues	With lung infiltrates suggest
Special populations	
Alcoholics	*S. pneumoniae*
	Klebsiella
	M. tuberculosis
	Aspiration pneumonias/anaerobic abscess
Chronic care facilities	*S. pneumoniae*
	H. influenzae
	Klebsiella
	M. tuberculosis
	C. pneumoniae
IV drug abusers	*Staphylococcus aureus*
	Septic pulmonary embolism
	Pseudomonas aeruginosa
	Pneumocystis carinii[a]
	M. tuberculosis/M. avium-intracellulare
HIV	PCP
	M. tuberculosis
	M. avium-intracellulare
	Salmonella
	Legionella
	CMV
	Histoplasmosis
	S. pneumoniae
	Klebsiella
	H. influenzae
Leukopenia (prolonged and profound)	*Aspergillus*
	Mucormycosis
	Cryptococcosis
	Pseudomonas
Organ transplant	Cytomegalovirus
	Herpes simplex virus
	Aspergillus
	Cryptococcosis
	PCP
Foreign travel	*M. tuberculosis*
	Q fever
	Melioidosis
	Paragonamiasis
Symptom clues	
Cough (nonproductive)	*Mycoplasma*
	Legionella
	Q fever
	C. pneumoniae
	Tularemia
	Viral pneumonia
Chest pain (pleuritic)	Bacteremic pneumonia
	Viral influenza
Dyspnea (severe)	Viral pneumonia
	PCP
	Severe bacteremic pneumonia

(*continued*)

TABLE 5.1. *Continued*

Clues	With lung infiltrates suggest
Night sweats	*M. tuberculosis*
	Histoplasmosis
Abdominal pain	*Legionella*
Ear pain	*Mycoplasma*
	S. pneumoniae
	H. influenzae
	B. catarrhalis
Sore throat	*Mycoplasma*
	C. pneumoniae
	Viral influenza
	Group A streptococci
	Adenovirus
Hoarseness	
Acute	Viral influenza
	C. pneumoniae
Chronic	*M. tuberculosis*
Diarrhea	*Mycoplasma*
	Legionella
Headache (severe)	Psittacosis
	Q fever
Mental confusion	*Legionella*
	Mycoplasma
Abdominal pain	Legionnaires' disease
Muscle aches (severe)	Cocci
	Viral influenza
	Mycoplasma
	Psittacosis
Nosebleed	Psittacosis
Underlying condition/disease	
Asplenia	*S. pneumoniae*
	H. influenzae
	N. meningitidis
Uremia	*M. tuberculosis*
COPD	*S. pneumoniae*
	H. influenzae
	Klebsiella
	B. catarrhalis
Pulmonary alveolar proteinosis	*Nocardia*
	Cryptococcosis
Silicosis/coal mining	*M. tuberculosis*
Sarcoidosis	*M. tuberculosis*
Lymphoma/malignancy	*M. tuberculosis*
Blood transfusion	PCP
Chickenpox exposure	Varicella
Corticosteroid therapy	*M. tuberculosis*
	Aspergillosis
Urinary tract infection	*E. coli*
Periodontal disease	Actinomycosis
	Aspiration pneumonia/anaerobic abscess

TABLE 5.2. Pneumonia: physical diagnosis clues.

System clues	With pneumonia suggests
HEENT	
Horder's spots	Psittacosis
Seborrheic dermatitis (severe)	PCP
Conjunctivitis	Adenovirus
Otitis/bullous myringitis	*Mycoplasma*
Pharyngitis	*Mycoplasma* *Chlamydia pneumoniae* Viral infection Adenovirus
Nose ulcer	Histoplasmosis
Tongue ulcer	Histoplasmosis
Oral ulcers (severe)	PCP Histoplasmosis
Hairy leukoplakia	PCP
Perioral ulcerations/conjunctivitis (Steven-Johnson syndrome)	*Mycoplasma*
Chest	
Erythema multiforme	*Mycoplasma*
Chest wall sinuses	Actinomycosis *M. tuberculosis* Sporotrichosis
Seborrheic dermatitis (severe)	PCP
Abdomen	
Hepatosplenomegaly	*M. tuberculosis* Histoplasmosis Q fever Psittacosis
Extremities	
Erythema multiforme	*Mycoplasma*
Folliculitis (severe)	PCP
Erythema nodosum	Coccidioidomycosis Histoplasmosis Blastomycosis *M. tuberculosis* Group A streptococci
Ecthyma gangrenosum	*Pseudomonas* *Serratia*
Skin ulcers	Blastomycosis Sporotrichosis Tularemia Histoplasmosis
Vesicular lesions	Varicella
Obscure phlebitis	Psittacosis

HEENT = head, eyes, ears, nose, and throat.

macular facial spots, the diagnosis of psittacosis is highly likely. Conjunctivitis in the neonate with pneumonia immediately suggests *Chlamydia*, where as conjunctivitis in an adult points to adenoviral pneumonia.[2,4] Certain associations are nearly pathognomonic and, although unusual, are virtually diagnostic when found (e.g., tongue ulcers for disseminated histoplasmosis and hairy leukoplakia in HIV patients with PCP pneumonia).

Unfortunately, all findings are not present in every case, and one must be constantly alert to seize on the diagnostic significance of uncommon but specific findings.[9] For example, an atypical pneumonia plus erythema multiforme on the skin is virtually diagnostic of *Mycoplasma* pneumonia, as no other pneumonia is associated with this skin manifestation.[21] The clinician must be cautious when associating erythema multiforme with a pneumonia, as the patient could be receiving an antibiotic (e.g., trimethoprim-sulfamethoxazole) for the pneumonia or an unrelated urinary tract infection that could result in a drug reaction manifested by erythema multiforme.[1] Once again, never analyze findings in a vacuum, but always apply them in the proper clinical context and preferably in concert with other findings to avoid diagnostic errors.[9,10] Clues from the physical diagnosis are presented in Table 5.2.

Clues from the Chest Film

It is not commonly appreciated that the behavior of the infiltrate on the chest film is as important to the diagnosis as its general appearance. Rapidly developing pulmonary infiltrates suggest limited processes that are capable of producing such roentgenographic abnormalities.[6,8] Gram-negative bacillary pneumonias, *Staphylococcus aureus* infection, aspiration pneumonia, and legionnaires' disease characterize infectious possibilities, whereas congestive heart failure and adult respiratory distress syndrome (ARDS) are the most common noninfectious entities that appear rapidly. Similarly, infiltrates that rapidly resolve are almost never infectious and suggest left ventricular failure, localized pulmonary edema, and acute eosinophilic pneumonias or pulmonary drug reactions.[1,4]

The predominant location of the infiltrate on the chest film or lobar predisposition has important diagnostic significance.[7,8] Symmetric peripheral infiltrates suggest a noninfectious etiology (e.g., pulmonary drug reactions). Unilateral pulmonary infiltrates suggest bacterial pneumonias, actinomycosis, nocardiosis, Q fever, or *Crytococcus neoformans*. Noninfectious asymmetric pulmonary infiltrates suggest such entities as adenocarcinoma, large-cell anaplastic carcinoma, vasculitis, systemic lupus erythematous (SLE), or Loeffler syndrome.[16] In contrast, perihilar infiltrates suggest viral pneumonias, fungal disease, pertussis, or PCP, as well as a wide variety of noninfectious processes.[22–25]

Focal infiltrates are a difficult diagnostic problem but usually represent a bacterial process rather than a noninfectious one. Most of the noninfectious causes of pulmonary infiltration are generalized processes and tend not to be focal (e.g., chemical pneumonitis, pulmonary drug reactions). Radiation pneumonitis, however, tends to be focal and confined to the radiation fields; similarly, pulmonary embolus and infarction as well as localized pulmonary edema or bronchogenic carcinomas may present with localized or focal infiltrates.[25,26] In general, diffuse infiltrates are noninfectious but may be a manifestation of any of the viral pneumonias or PCP.

Lastly, the speed of resolution of an infiltrate provides important diagnostic information regarding the cause of the pulmonary infiltrate. Among the infections, tuberculosis and lung abscesses are the commonest examples in this category.[27] Noninfectious conditions are more commonly responsible for slowly resolving infiltrates (e.g., chronic pulmonary drug reactions, Wegener's granulomatosis, repeated aspiration).[26] An infiltrate that resolves slowly or not at all suggests a postobstructive pneumonia or underlying carcinoma. However, do not forget the entity known as "delayed resolution of pneumococcal pneumonia," in which pulmonary abnormalities may persist on the chest roentgenogram for up to 14 weeks after initial diagnosis (Table 5.3).

Certain diseases, infectious or noninfectious, have a predilection for certain areas of the lung. This information may be used diagnostically in a general sense but is useful only when combined with other historical, physical, or laboratory features. In general, the upper lung zone involvement is characteristic of tuberculosis, histoplasmosis, and coccidioidomycosis.[27–30] Anaerobic aspiration pneumonia due to mechanical causes is commonest in the upper lung fields, as is *Proteus* and *Klebsiella* among the bacterial pneumonias. It should be appreciated that any bacterial pneumonia may

TABLE 5.3. Pneumonia: clues from the chest film—infiltrates.

Infectious agents	Noninfectious agents
Rapidly progressive infiltrates	
Legionnaires' disease	Congestive heart failure
Aspiration pneumonia	Noncardiac pulmonary edema
S. aureus	ARDS
Gram-negative pneumonia	Systemic lupus erythematosus (SLE)
Peripheral infiltrates	
Actinomycosis	Loeffler syndrome
Nocardiosis	Pulmonary drug reactions
	Adenocarcinoma
	Large-cell anaplastic carcinoma
	Vasculitis
	SLE
	Fat emboli

(*continued*)

TABLE 5.3. *Continued*

Infectious agents	Noninfectious agents
Perihilar infiltrates	
Viral pneumonias	Squamous cell carcinoma
Pertussis	Small-cell anaplastic (oat cell) carcinoma
PCP	
Histoplasmosis	Silicosis
Cryptococcosis	Congestive heart failure
Coccidioidomycosis	Pulmonary alveolar proteinosis
Chlamydia trachomatis	Sarcoidosis
Focal infiltrates	
Bacterial pneumonia	Bronchogenic carcinoma
	Chemical pneumonitis
	Pseudolymphomas
	Localized pulmonary edema
	Pulmonary infarct
	Pulmonary drug reactions
	Radiation pneumonitis
Diffuse infiltrates	
PCP	Pulmonary edema
Viral pneumonias	Noncardiac pulmonary edema
	Chemical pneumonitis
	Radiation pneumonitis
	Cancer with lymphangitic spread
	Pulmonary fibrosis
	Pulmonary alveolar proteinosis
	Wegener's granulomatosis
	Bilateral massive aspiration
	SLE
	Uremia
	Drug reactions
	ARDS
	Sarcoidosis
Rapidly resolving infiltrates	
None	Pulmonary edema
	"Vanishing tumor" (localized pulmonary edema)
	Acute pulmonary drug reactions
	Acute eosinophilic pneumonias
Slowly resolving infiltrates	
Abscesses	Repeated aspiration
Inadequate/inappropriate therapy	Pulmonary emboli
Legionnaires' disease	Postobstructive pneumonias/carcinoma
Tuberculosis	Bronchoalveolar carcinoma
S. pneumoniae	Lymphomas
PCP	Chronic pulmonary drug reactions
	Bronchopulmonary aspergillosis
	Wegener's granulomatosis

involve the upper lungs, but *Klebsiella* is found in the upper lobes more commonly than group A streptococcal pneumonia or *B. catarrhalis* pneumonia, for example.[2,4] Noninfectious disorders with an upper lung zone preference include eosinophilic granulomas, psittacosis, and Loeffler syndrome. Midlung zones are affected by infectious bacterial pneumonias (e.g., *S. pneumoniae*, *H. influenzae*) or a wide variety of noninfectious conditions (e.g., sarcoidosis, hypersensitivity pneumonitis, lymphomas). Infectious diseases have a predilection for the lower zones of the lung; pneumococcus and *H. influenzae* have a predilection for the right lower

TABLE 5.4. Pneumonia: chest film clues—lung zone predilection.

Infectious agents	Noninfectious agents
Upper lung zone	
Tuberculosis	Eosinophilic granulomas
Histoplasmosis	Silicosis
Coccidioidomycosis	Bronchial adenoma
Atypical tuberculosis	Loeffler syndrome
Klebsiella	Extrinsic allergic alveolitis
Proteus	Sarcoidosis
Aerobic aspiration pneumonia/abscess	Radiation pneumonitis
	Ankylosing spondylitis
Mid-lung zone	
S. pneumoniae	Metastatic carcinoma
H. influenzae	Bronchial adenomas
	Eosinophilic granulomas
	Lymphomas
	Idiopathic pulmonary hemosiderosis
	Goodpasture syndrome
	Sarcoidosis
	Extrinsic allergic alveolitis
	Silicosis
	Hypersensitivity pneumonitis
Lower lung zone	
Cryptococcosis	Idiopathic hemosiderosis
Sporotrichosis	Metastases
Mycoplasma	Goodpasture syndrome
Melioidosis	Drug-induced pulmonary disease
H. influenzae	Extrinsic allergic alveolitis
S. pneumoniae	Arteriovenous malformation
Group A streptococci	Pulmonary infarct
Tularemia	Rheumatoid nodules
Q fever	Wegener's granulomatosis
Psittacosis	Fibrosing alveolitis
Legionella	
C. pneumoniae	
Amebiasis	
E. coli	
Hydatid cysts	

lobe, for example.[31] Noninfectious lower lung processes include Goodpasture syndrome, drug-induced pulmonary disease, hypersensitivity pneumonitis, pulmonary infarcts, and metastatic disease.[25,26] Again, care must be taken to avoid trying to diagnose the problem based on these isolated, nonspecific findings alone. Always try to combine such nonspecific findings with other nonroentgenographic clues (Table 5.4).

Cavitary lesions, when present, are important diagnostic clues. Relatively few pulmonary diseases, infectious or noninfectious, result in cavities. When cavities are present they are usually thick-walled. The finding of a thin-walled cavity quickly limits differential diagnostic possibilities to sporotrichosis, coccidioidomycosis, paragonamiasis, or atypical tuberculosis, among the infectious etiologies.[4] It should be remembered that most of the thick-walled cavitary lesions, over time, develop into thin-walled lesions. If the process is subacute versus chronic, argue against the noninfectious etiology.[6,7] Thick-walled cavitary lesions that are noninfectious are usually due to squamous cell carcinoma, Wegener's granulomatosis, rheumatoid nodules, lymphoma, metastatic carcinoma, or bronchoalveolar carcinoma.[25,26] The clinician should combine the cavitary lesion with the presence of other features of the chest film; for example, rapidly progressive infiltrates with cavitary lesions favor the diagnosis of a bacterial pneumonia or anaerobic pneumonitis versus a granulomatous or noninfectious pneumonia (Table 5.5).

TABLE 5.5. Pneumonia: clues from chest film—cavitary lesions.

Infectious agents	Noninfectious agents
Thick-walled lesions	
Staphylococcus aureus	Squamous cell carcinoma
Klebsiella	Pulmonary infarction
Escherichia coli	Silicosis
Pseudomonas	Wegener's granulomatosis
Tuberculosis	Rheumatoid nodules
Histoplasmosis	Lymphoma
Blastomycosis	Sarcoidosis
Aspergillus	Metastatic carcinoma
Melioidosis	Metastatic sarcoma
Anaerobic lung abscess	Bronchioalveolar carcinoma
Septic pulmonary emboli	Melanoma
Nocardia	
Thin-walled lesions[a]	
Sporotrichosis	Wegener's granulomatosis
Coccidioidomycosis	
Paragonamiasis	
Atypical tuberculosis	

[a] Many thick-walled cavitary lesions become thin-walled over time.

Hilar adenopathy alone is not confused with pneumonia; but when it is found in concert with a pulmonary infiltrate it is helpful for limiting diagnostic possibilities. Hilar adenopathy may be viewed as unilateral or bilateral in terms of differential diagnosis. *Mycoplasma* and viruses are unusual causes of hilar adenopathy, and when hilar adenopathy occurs it is only in children.[32–34] In adults, hilar adenopathy suggests tuberculosis, fungus infection, or, if the patient has an atypical pneumonia, tularemia. Noninfectious etiologies are more common causes of both unilateral or bilateral hilar adenopathy (e.g., bronchogenic carcinoma, lymphomas, SLE).[12] Bilateral hilar adenopathy is most strongly associated with sarcoidosis but is also a feature of lymphomas. Once again, associated clues may provide the key to the differential diagosis. For example, if a patient presents with bilateral hilar adenopathy, a pulmonary infiltrate, and pleural effusion, the diagnosis of lymphoma is favored over sarcoidosis, as pleural effusions are uncommon with sarcoidosis.[5,6] Similarly, if there is a clear channel between the hilar nodes and the cardiac shadow, the diagnosis of sarcoidosis is enhanced. The same thing is true of right paratracheal adenopathy in concert with symmetric bilateral hilar adenopathy, suggesting the diagnosis of sarcoidosis.[8] Calcification of the hilar nodes, except for silicosis, is usually due to tuberculosis or histoplasmosis. Be careful not to confuse calcifications in adjacent structures as being in the hilar nodes (e.g., a calcified aortic aneurysm[7,8] (Table 5.6).

Pleural effusions occurring alone do not indicate pneumonia; but when present in conjunction with an ipsilateral pulmonary infiltrate, they provide an important diagnostic clue to the etiology of the pulmonary process. Pleural effusions may be classified according to their size,

TABLE 5.6. Pneumonia: clues from the chest film—hilar adenopathy.

Infectious agents	Noninfectious agents
Bilateral hilar adenopathy	
Fungi	Sarcoidosis
Tularemia	Bronchogenic carcinoma
Tuberculosis	Lymphomas
Mycoplasma	Leukemias
Viral pneumonias	Silicosis
	Systemic lupus erythematosus
Unilateral hilar adenopathy	
Tuberculosis	Bronchogenic carcinoma
Fungi	Metastases
Tularemia	Lymphomas
Mycoplasma	Atypical measles
Calcified hilar nodes	
Tuberculosis	Silicosis
Histoplasmosis	

rapidity of accumulation or reaccumulation, and their bilaterality.[35,36] Unilateral pleural effusion on an infectious basis suggests *H. influenzae* or *S. pneumoniae* as the most likely bacterial pathogen. Among the granulomatous diseases, primary tuberculosis is the most common cause of unilateral pleural effusion.[1,4] Noninfectious causes of pleural effusion include a wide variety of disorders; but most commonly unilateral pleural effusions are due to congestive heart failure, pancreatitis, malignancy, or pulmonary infarction. Bilateral pleural effusions are never infectious, even if associated with pulmonary infiltrates.[36] The most common cause of bilateral pleural effusion by far is congestive heart failure. Unilateral or bilateral pleural effusions without pulmonary infiltrates suggest a subdiaphragmatic collection, or abscess. A good example of an abdominal cause for pleural effusion in concert with a pulmonary infiltrate is pancreatitis-induced ARDS. The size of a pleural effusion is also somewhat helpful in the differential diagnosis. Moderate pleural effusions are characteristic of *H. influenzae*, tularemia and primary tuberculosis, whereas a large pleural effusion that is infectious immediately points to group A streptococci.[8,10] Among the noninfectious causes, a large pleural effusion or a rapidly recurring pleural effusion immediately points to a neoplastic etiology. Small to moderate effusions are due to a wide variety of noninfectious conditions (e.g., pulmonary infarction, pancreatitis, SLE, congestive heart failure nephrosis, cirrhosis, or ascites).[35] Combining the pleural effusion with other findings to increase diagnostic accuracy again emphasizes the principle of "bunching" information to increase diagnostic accuracy. Pleural effusion occurs with cardiomegaly virtually only with primary tuberculosis or with associated tuberculous pericarditis. Almost all other etiologies are noninfectious. Pleural effusion with hilar enlargement, argues against the fungal etiology, and favors tuberculosis.[27,30] Among the noninfectious etiologies, bronchogenic carcinomas and lymphomas head the list. Focal infiltrates suggest a bacterial process, although, again, neoplastic disorders and pulmonary embolism may present in this fashion. The diagnostic clues from pleural effusions are presented in Table 5.7.

Chest nodules by themselves usually represent granulomatous disease or malignancy. When found in association with a pulmonary infiltrate, however, they suggest a wider range of diagnostic possibilities.[12] Pulmonary nodules may be classified as solitary or multiple, diffuse, localized, or cavitating. Multiple nodules in a patient with atypical pneumonia suggest *Legionella micdadei* or Q fever. The only viral pneumonia with nodular densities is adenoviral pneumonia.[1,36] The ovoid densities are not truly nodules and are therefore not considered in this differential diagnostic list. Septic pulmonary emboli are characterized by temperatures of more than 102°F and an identifiable distant source in the pelvis or arm in a patient with a history of intravenous drug abuse. Most other infectious multiple pulmonary nodules are caused by subacute or chronic diseases due to the higher bacteria, *M. tuberculosis*, or fungi. Noninfectious causes

TABLE 5.7. Pneumonia: chest film clues—pleural effusion.

Infectious agents	Noninfectious agents
Unilateral pleural effusion	
S. pneumoniae	Chronic heart failure
Klebsiella	Neoplasms
H. influenzae	Metastases
Tularemia	Meig syndrome
Mycoplasma	Postthoracotomy
Primary tuberculosis	Postmyocardial infarction syndrome (Dressler syndrome)
	SLE
	Pancreatitis/ARDS
	Pulmonary infarction
	Subphrenic collection/abscess
Bilateral pleural effusion	
None	Congenital heart failure
	Cirrhosis/ascites
	Pancreatitis
	Subdiaphramatic abscess
	Pulmonary infarction
	Metastases
	SLE
	Postmyocardial infarct syndrome
	Nephrosis
	Hypothyroidism
	Drug-induced pulmonary disease
	Meig syndrome
Size of pleural effusion	
None or small effusion	Small to moderate effusion
Streptococcus pneumoniae	Pancreatitis
Mycoplasma	Pulmonary infarct
Legionella	Meig syndrome
	Drugs
Moderate	Nitrofurantoin
H. influenzae	Methysergide
Tularemia	Drug-induced SLE
Primary tuberculosis	SLE
	Rheumatoid nodules
	Cirrhosis or ascites
	Congestive heart failure
	Nephrosis
Large	Large
Group A streptococci	Malignancy
Pleural effusion with cardiomegaly	
Viral infection (only with CHF)	Congestive heart failure
	Pulmonary embolism
Primary tuberculosis	Neoplasms
	Rheumatoid nodule
	Postpericardiotomy syndrome
	SLE

(continued)

TABLE 5.7. *Continued*

Infectious agents	Noninfectious agents
Pleural effusion with hilar enlargement	
Primary tuberculosis	Pulmonary embolism
Pertussis	Bronchogenic carcinoma
	Lymphomas
	Metastases
Pleural effusion with focal infiltrates	
Pneumonia/empyema	Pulmonary embolism
Primary tuberculosis	Neoplasms
H. influenzae	Bronchogenic cardinoma
S. pneumoniae	Lymphomas
Group A streptococci	
Mycoplasma	
Tularemia	

SLE = systemic lupus erythematosus; ARDS = adult respiratory distress syndrome; CHF = congestive heart failure.

include such diverse entities are metastatic carcinoma, Wegener's granulomatosis, rheumatoid nodules, ateriovenous malformations, and nonsepticpulmonary emboli.[23,25] Diffuse fine nodules are suggested by eosinophilic granulomas, sarcoidosis, or hypersensitivity pneumonitis. Among the noninfectious causes of cavitary nodules are squamous cell carcinoma and bronchoalveolar carcinoma, which are often confused with anaerobic lung abscesses. Similarly, cavitation is a feature of Wegener's granulomatosis, and sometimes this entity can be confused with infectious causes. Wegener's granulomatosis is frequently associated with hemoptysis, which is less common in the infectious conditions it mimics.[12] The patient with septic pulmonary emboli is seriously ill and has an underlying recognizable source of the emboli. Patients with *Nocardia* do not commonly present with hemoptysis, nor do those with cryptococcosis.[16] Tuberculosis with fibrocaseous disease do not present predominantly with nodules as do those with Wegener's granulomatosis. In this way, by combining other features with a chest roentgenogram, one can quickly eliminate possibilities. The differential diagnosis of nodules in the chest film is presented in Table 5.8.

There are a variety of other findings on the chest film that limit the diagnostic possibilities if not suggest a specific etiology. For example, the "bulging fissures sign" indicates volume expansion and is most commonly associated with *Klebsiella* pneumonia. However, any infectious or noninfectious process that can result in lobar expansion may produce the same sign.[8,12] Therefore do not forget other infectious etiologies or bronchoalveolar carcinoma as a cause for this roentgenographic finding. Moreover, spontaneous pneumothorax is usually associated with bullous lung diseases; and do not fail to consider eosinophilic granuloma,

TABLE 5.8. Pneumonia: chest film clues—nodules.

Infectious agents	Noninfectious agents
Solitary pulmonary nodule	
Tuberculosis	Bronchogenic cancer
Histoplasmosis	Metastasis (kidney, colon, ovary, testis, Wilms' tumor, sarcoma
Coccidioidomycosis	Lymphoma
Cryptococcosis	Plasmacytoma
Nocardia	Rheumatoid nodules
Dirofilaria	Wegener's granulomatosis
Abscess	Arteriovenous malformation
	Pulmonary infarct
	Hamartoma
	Hematoma
	Bronchial adenomas
	Sarcoidosis
Multiple pulmonary nodules	
Legionella micdadei	Wegener's granulomatosis
Septic pulmonary emboli	Caplan syndrome
Abscesses	Metastasis (kidney, colon, ovary, testes, melanoma)
Histoplasmosis	Lymphoma
Coccidioidomycosis	Arteriovenous malformation
Cryptococcosis	Pseudolymphoma
Nocardia	Pulmonary infarction
Tuberculosis	Rheumatoid nodules
Q fever	Silicosis
Hydatid cyst	Atypical measles
Paragonamiasis	
Adenovirus	
Diffuse fine nodules	
Viral pneumonia	Hypersensitivity pneumonitis
Miliary tuberculosis	Eosinophilic granuloma
	Sarcoidosis
Cavitating nodules	
Septic pulmonary emboli	Squamous cell carcinoma
Nocardia	Bronchoalveolar cell carcinoma
Cryptococcosis	Melanoma
Coccidioidomycosis	Osteosarcoma
Aspergillosis	Lymphoma
Abscesses	Wegener's granulomatosis
	Rheumatoid nodules

metastatic osteogenic sarcoma, or beryliosis as a cause of spontaneous pneumothorax in the appropriate clinical setting.[7,8] Similarly, legionnaires' disease and PCP have been associated with spontaneous pneumothorax, albeit uncommonly, although one would never diagnose legionnaires' disease or PCP on this basis alone. It is always inadvisable to diagnose "in a vacuum" basing one's impressions solely on the chest film. Rather, one should always endeavor to synthesize the diagnostic clues as an aid in diagnosis.[10]

Laboratory Clues

Basic laboratory tests provide useful adjunctive indirect clues to the pulmonary process. A complete blood count (CBC) is commonly obtained on all patients with pneumonia, and one should specifically look for leukopenia, eosinophilia, basophilia, or thrombocytopenia. Any of these findings provides useful diagnostic information when no extrapulmonary process is responsible for the abnormality. For example, eosinophilia in concert with a pulmonary infiltrate always suggests a noninfectious etiology with the exception of helminthic migration through the pulmonary vasculature or a fungal pneumonia, most commonly coccidiodomycosis.[2,37] Basophilia is associated only with varicella pneumonia among all of the infectious diseases but suggests the possibility of carcinoma or lymphoma when the etiology of the pulmonary infiltrate is obscure. Monocytosis suggests tuberculosis, lymphoma, SLE, or carcinoma.[4] Leukopenia in an acutely ill patient suggests a viral process, usually viral influenza, overwhelming pneumococcal or streptococcal sepsis, disseminated histoplasmosis, or tuberculosis; it is also an indirect indicator of PCP in a patient with HIV.[27] Liver function tests should be obtained on all patients with pneumonias because abnormalities of liver function immediately suggest an atypical pathogen in a patient with acute pneumonia or miliary tuberculosis or lymphoma in a patient with a subacute or chronic illness.[1,21] Laboratory tests from routine blood work are presented in Table 5.9.

Blood cultures should be performed on all patients with pneumonias, as they may provide a retrospective specific bacterial diagnosis. Blood cultures should always be preposed when the patient is first seen—before antimicrobial therapy is started. Positive blood culture results must be interpreted in the appropriate clinical context, as is true with all laboratory tests, but it may be the only way to make the diagnosis in a patient incapable of producing sputum. Blood culture positivity relates to the timing of the blood culture sample (i.e., in relation to the onset of the infectious pneumonia). Blood culture positivity is directly related to the *volume* of blood obtained rather than the number of specimens. Blood culture positivity also is related to the pathogen causing the pneumonia; that is, certain pathogens have a high bacteremic potential (e.g., *S. pneumoniae*, *H. influenzae*), whereas others are rarely recovered from blood cultures (e.g., *Serratia* or *Acinetobacter*).[2,4] If a sputum specimen is unobtainable, the diagnosis may be mode retrospectively by testing the patient for urinary antigens to *Hemophilus*, pneumococcus, or *Legionella*. It should be remembered that antigen urea is slow to develop and may be

TABLE 5.9. Pneumonia: laboratory clues from serum tests.

Abnormality	Infectious associations
Leukopenia	Viral influenza PCP Miliary tuberculosis *Streptococcus pneumoniae* *Staphylococcus* Histoplasmosis (disseminated)
Eosinophilia	Coccidioidomycosis Helminths
Basophilia	Varicella
Monocytosis	Tuberculosis Lymphoma SLE Carcinoma
Thrombocytopenia	Sarcoidosis SLE Lymphoma Miliary tuberculosis Histoplasmosis (disseminated) Influenza ARDS PCP (HIV) Drug-induced
Hypergammaglobulinemia	Sarcoidosis PCP (HIV)
Abormal liver function tests	Psittacosis Miliary tuberculosis Legionnaires' disease Q fever

negative initially, but once the process is initiated it persists over long periods. Therefore be careful not to misinterpret an initial negative urinary antigen test as evidence against a particular pathogen. The test should be considered negative only if it remains negative weeks into the infectious process. Similarly, serum serologic tests, which are useful for epidemiologic purposes or a retrospective serologic diagnosis, should be negative initially during the acute pneumonia but become positive weeks or months later. Once again, be careful not to ascribe acute pulmonary infiltrates to a positive *Legionella* or *Mycoplasma* serology, especially in low titer, as the positive test usually indicates previous exposure rather than acute disease.[1,2,4]

Sputum, when available, provides the most immediate and useful clue to the diagnosis of community-acquired bacterial pneumonia. For a sputum sample to be correctly interpreted, it must be properly collected, represent

TABLE 5.10. Pneumonia: diagnostic clues from sputum.

Sputum findings	Infectious agents
Foul smell	Oral anaerobes (aspiration)
Creamy yellow or salmon color	*Staphylococcus aureus*
Currant-jelly color	Pneumococcus
	Klebsiella
Raspberry-syrup color	Pneumonic plague
Red color (pseudohemoptysis)	*Serratia*
Blood-streaked (hemoptysis)	*Klebsiella*
	Viral influenza
	Meningococcus
	Pneumonic plague
No PMNs	Q fever
PMNs	Bacterial pneumonia
Eosinophils	Helminths (pulmonary migration phase)
Mononuclear cells	*Legionella*
	Mycoplasma
Mixed flora	Aspiration pneumonia

the lower respiratory tract flora, and be void of oropharyngeal contamination. Such contamination is evidenced on microscopic examination of the sputum by finding epithelial squamous cells in the specimen. This specimen should be disregarded and the culture results ignored. The gross examination of the sputum in terms of its color, consistency, and odor provide an initial impression. Purulent, fixed sputum favors a bacterial etiology, whereas thin or mucoid sputum suggests an atypical pneumonia or a malignant process. Blood-flecked sputum suggests most commonly pneumococcus or *Klebsiella*. The finding of purulence correlates well with the presence of polymorphonuclear neutrophils (PMNs) in the microscopic examination of the sputum. In general, the more purulent the sputum, the higher the PMN count, a condition that favors a bacterial etiology.[12] Atypical pneumonias, in general, with the occasional exception of *Legionella*, present with a mononuclear cell predominance, although usually in low numbers[31,38] (Table 5.10).

Gram stain of the sputum provides specific information as to the cause of the bacterial pneumonia. Gram-stained sputum may be misleading in a patient with chronic obstructive pulmonary disease (COPD) or anaerobic pneumonitis, where the results of the sputum Gram stain and culture show mixed or normal flora and provide no useful diagnostic information. A properly collected sputum sample that shows a predominant organism is the most useful. The type of organism (i.e., bacilli versus cocci) and the configuration of the organism provide specific diagnostic information. Gram-positive cocci in the smear may represent streptococci, pneumococci, or staphylococci. Overly decolorized streptococci may even resemble

TABLE 5.11. Pneumonia: diagnostic clues from sputum (Gram stain).

Finding	Organism	Comments
Gram positive		
Diplococci	*Streptococcus pneumoniae*	Coffee bean configuration (lancet-shaped)
Cocci (grape-like clusters)	*Staphylococcus aureus*	May be seen together with short chains or pairs
Cocci (short chains or pairs)	Group A streptococci	Length ≃ virulence Smaller than streptococci
Comma-shaped	*Nocardia*	Sometimes appear like "Chinese letters" on Gram stain
Gram negative		
Coccobacillary (pleomorphic)	*Hemophilus influenzae*	Encapsulated
Bacilli	*Klebsiella*	Plump and encapsulated
Diplococci	*Neisseria meningitidis* *Branhamella catarrhalis*	Kidney-bean-shaped

H. influenzae, *Branhamella*, or *Acinetobacter*.[22] The configuration of organisms among gram-positive organisms is most useful. Gram-positive cocci in pairs may represent pneumococci, streptococci, or an early staphylococcal infection. However, if grape-like clusters are present, even if in small number, *S. aureus* can be reliably diagnosed. If the Gram stain shows predominantly diplococci with occasional short chains, the diagnosis of *S. pneumoniae* can be made with confidence. A Gram stain showing many short chains of small cocci, even if some are present in pairs, points immediately to a group A streptococcal etiology. Gram-negative bacillary enteric organisms cannot be differentiated by Gram stain,[2,4] although the trained observer can differentiate *Pseudomonas* from *Klebsiella* from *H. influenzae*. An experienced microscopist can also easily distinguish the oral pigmented *Bacteroides* found in aspiration pneumonia/anaerobic lung abscesses from other aerobic gram-negative bacilli by Gram stain alone. The presence of gram-negative diplobacilli immediately suggests the diagnosis of *Neisseria meningitidis* or *B. catarrhalis*. Sputum Gram stain findings are presented in Table 5.11.

Although the presence of a pleural effusion adds another dimension to the chest film differential diagnosis, analysis of the fluid provides more definitive information and further limits diagnostic possibilities. The gross appearance of the pleural effusion fluid is usually helpful and in some cases can be diagnostic (e.g., hydatid cyst fluid, mesothelioma, chylous effusion). Much emphasis is usually given to differentiating transudates from exudates, but this information generally adds little diagnostic help to the case. There are only three causes of transudates: heart failure, nephrosis, and cirrhosis.[1,36] These conditions should be clinically obvious and not require lactate dehydrogenase (LDH) ratio analysis to make

TABLE 5.12. Pneumonia: diagnostic clues from pleural fluid.

Findings	Infectious agents	Noninfectious agents
Bloody	Tuberculosis Tularemia	Mesotheliomas Pulmonary infarct Carcinoma Metastases
Whitish	Empyema Hydatid cysts	Chylous effusion
Brownish	Empyema Amebic cysts	Parapneumonic effusion
Yellow-green	—	Rheumatoid arthritis
pH $\leqslant$ 7.3	Tuberculosis Rheumatoid arthritis	Bronchogenic carcinoma (rarely)
↓ Glucose	Tuberculosis Bacteria Fungi *Mycoplasma*	Carcinoma Rheumatoid nodules SLE Lymphomas Esophageal rupture
↑ Protein	Tuberculosis	Carcinoma Rheumatoid arthritis
↑ Amylase	None	Pancreatitis/pseudocyst Adenocarcinoma Esophageal rupture
Extracellular debris	Abscesses Anaerobic empyema	Rheumatoid arthritis
PMNs	Bacteria Early tuberculosis	Idiopathic pleural effusion Pancreatitis Abdominal abscess CHF
Lymphocytes	Tuberculosis	Carcinoma
Eosinophils	Fungi Helminths	Lymphomas Mesotheliomas Pleural effusion Pneumothorax Pulmonary drug regimens Idiopathic effusions

the diagnosis from pleural effusion fluid. Virtually all other causes are exudative in nature and do not require further tests to document what should be obvious. There are some exceptions, but in general differentiation of a exudate from a transudate is not helpful.

Microscopic examination of the pleural fluid is somewhat helpful. PMN predominance usually suggests early tuberculosis or a bacterial pneumonia but is also found with idiopathic pleural effusions, pancreatitis, and abdominal abscesses. PMNs are found in low numbers in effusions due to congestive heart failure. Lymphocytic predominance suggests tuberculosis or carcinoma, whereas eosinophils point to fungi or a variety of noninfectious causes.

Usually neglected but of great diagnostic importance is the pH of the fluid. A pH of less than 7.3 usually points to tuberculosis or rheumatoid arthritis but rarely is associated with bronchogenic carcinomas.[36] A low glucose level points to a bacterial, tuberculous, or fungal etiology among the infectious causes but is also associated with carcinoma, rheumatoid nodules, SLE, or lymphomas. An elevated pleural fluid protein level suggests rheumatoid arthritis, carcinoma, or tuberculosis.

Once again, the findings should be combined to increase diagnostic specificity, and therefore finding decreased glucose and increased protein in a patient with a pleural fluid pH of less than 7.3 strongly favors the diagnosis of tuberculosis. Extracellular debris is characteristic of rheumatoid arthritis, as is a yellow-greenish fluid. A grossly bloody fluid suggests malignancy or pulmonary infarction and argues against the diagnosis of tuberculosis.[1,25] Among the atypical pneumonias, bloody pleural effusion is associated only with tularemia. A serosanguineous pleural effusion suggests tuberculosis, group A streptococci, or malignancy.[2,3] Clues that can be obtained pleural fluid are outlined in Table 5.12.

Synthesis of Diagnostic Clues

The clinician uses whatever historical physical chest film or laboratory clues that are available in combination to rule in or exclude a bacterial or atypical pneumonia. The diagnostic approach is directed at identifying a treatable disease so empiric therapy may be begun as soon as possible. A definitive diagnosis of collagen vascular diseases and malignant disorders is secondary because they usually do not present an immediate threat to the patient's health on presentation. Using the syndromic approach and differential diagnosis, each disease usually presents with a particular profile.

It is not coincidental that diseases occur in some individuals with certain underlying diseases or host defense defects; it is the age, underlying disease, and host defect that predisposes the patient to specific pathogen groups. Furthermore, pathogens pathophysiologically cause disease in a stereotyped fashion, and therefore they "behave" in a predictable fashion most of the time. For example, the pneumococcus prefers the lower lobe and does not cavitate. Therefore if there is a lower lobe segmental or lobar defect that is cavitating, one can confidently state that the process is not due to pneumococcus, remembering that the chest film is more useful in a negative sense, to exclude diagnostic possibilities, than it is to make a specific etiologic diagnosis. If a patient with a lower lobe process also has an increased bilirubin level, the only bacterial pneumonia that routinely

TABLE 5.13. Pneumonia: common bacteria—differential diagnosis.

Organism	Historical host factors	Sputum	Chest film	Pleural effusion	Cavitation	Comments
S. pneumoniae	Elderly; COPD/CHF; alcoholism; asplenia	Encapsulated; may be blood-tinged; gram-pos. diplococci	RLL preference; multilobe involvement common; occasional bronchopneumonia pattern	Usually none but may be small unilateral effusion; empyema uncommon	None	In ETOH may have associated ABE or meningitis; ↑ bilirubin; bacteremia common
H. influenzae	Elderly; chronic care facilities/nursing home patients; children ≤6 years old; COPD	Encapsulated pleomorphic gram-neg. bacilli	RLL common, but any lobe possible; occasional bronchopneumonia pattern	Common (⅓) small to moderate sized; empyema uncommon	None	Both encapsulated and unencapsulated strains pathogenic; bacteremia common
Group A streptococci	Postviral influenza uncommon, history of pharyngitis in 2/3	Gram-pos. cocci in chains	Lower lobe preference	Large (hydrothorax) effusion often obscuring infiltrate; empyema not uncommon	None	Pleuritic chest pain common early feature; pleural effusion fluid is serosanguineous; bacteremia occasionally
S. aureus	Usually in the postinfluenza setting; children; IV drug	Gram-pos. cocci in clusters; may be blood-tinged	No lobar predilection; multilobar involvement common	Effusion uncommon; empyema common	Early common feature; thick-walled cavitation; pneumatoceles in children	Severe hypoxemia/cyanosis; patient clinically very "sick"; bacteremia common

Klebsiella	ETOH; chronic care facility/ nursing home patients; postviral influenza	Encapsulated plump pleomorphic gram-neg. bacilli; may be blood-tinged	Upper lobe preference; "bulging fissure sign"	Effusion uncommon; empyema common	Common thick-walled cavities	Chronic *Klebsiella* may mimic reactivation tuberculosis; bacteremia occasionally
B. catarrhalis	COPD; elderly	Gram-neg. diplococci	Lower lobe preference	None	None	Uncommon in normal hosts; resembles *H. influenzae*, *Acinetobacter*, or *N. meningitidis* on sputum Gram stain; bacteremia uncommon
E. coli	Elderly; recent urinary tract manipulation, prostatitis	Unencapsulated gram-neg. bacilli	Lower lobe preference; bronchopneumonia pattern common	Effusion uncommon; empyema not uncommon	Uncommon	Usually from antecedent or concomitant *E. coli* urinary tract infection; bacteremia common

COPD = chronic obstructive pulmonary disease; CHF = congestive heart failure; ETOH = alcohol abuse; RLL = right lower lobe; ABE = acute bacterial endocarditis.

does that is pneumococcus, not *H. influenzae* or *B. catarrhalis*. Similarly, if a patient presents with an ill-defined lower lobe infiltrate and has diarrhea, the likelihood of *Mycoplasma* or *Legionella* is enhanced. Approaching diseases in this way gives pathogens certain "profiles" that are a compilation of diagnostic clues ascribable to an organism or process.[9,10] This information for the common community-acquired bacterial pneumonias is presented in Table 5.13.

The atypical pneumonias are usually differentiated from the typical bacterial pneumonias by their less acute onset, except for *Mycoplasma* and legionnaires' disease, and by their extrapulmonary findings. All of the pathogens responsible for the atypical pneumonias cause systemic diseases that have predominant pulmonary manifestations; however, the clue to diagnosing an atypical pneumonia resides in combining the extrapulmonary features.

The chest film is most helpful for differentiating an atypical from a typical bacterial process. In general, bacterial pneumonias usually produce segmental or lobar infiltrates unless the process is a bronchopneumonia.[1,2] If the process is diffuse and ill-defined, an atypical etiology is favored. It must be kept in mind that atypical pneumonias may present with segmental or lobar infiltrations that closely resemble a bacterial pneumonia, (most characteristic of psittacosis and legionnaires' disease). Being careful never to diagnose in a vacuum solely on the basis of the chest film, the clinician should endeavor to use the extrapulmonary findings that are present with the atypical pneumonias to readily differentiate them from the bacterial pneumonias as well as from each other. A pulse temperature deficit in a patient with an ill-defined lower lobe infiltrate immediately suggests legionnaires' disease, psittacosis, or Q fever, and definitely excludes *Mycoplasma* pneumonia, tularemia, or *C. pneumoniae*.[26] Liver function abnormalities are not characteristic of typical bacterial pneumonias and immediately suggest an atypical pathogen. Elevated liver function test results argue against the diagnosis of *Mycoplasma* pneumonia, tularemia, and *C. pneumoniae*. Elevated cold agglutinins (≥1:64) strongly suggest at *Mycoplasma* etiology for the patient's symptoms. Acute hoarseness usually suggests a viral pneumonia; but among the atypical pneumonias, it is a common feature of *Chlamydia pneumoniae* infection in young adults.[26] The diagnostic features of the atypical pneumonias are presented in Table 5.14.

The subacute or chronic pneumonias are a problem unto themselves. Most of these disorders are not infectious, but the common infectious etiologies include tuberculosis and the fungal pneumonias. Tuberculosis and histoplasmosis have nearly the same clinical spectrum of disease. Crytococcosis, sporotrichosis, and blastomycosis can usually be readily differentiated from tuberculosis or histoplasmosis. Reactivation tuberculosis is manifested by apical disease with or without fibrocavitary involvement of the upper lobes. Histoplasmosis may present in a similar

TABLE 5.14. Diagnostic features of atypical pneumonias.

Manifestations	Mycoplasma pneumonia	Legionnaires' disease	Psittacosis	Q fever	Tularemia	Chlamydia pneumoniae
Symptoms						
Mental confusion	−	+	±	−	−	−
Headache	±	+	+	+	−	−
Meningismus	−	−	+	−	−	−
Myalgias	+	+	+	+	−	−
Ear pain	±	−	−	−	−	±
Pleuritic pain	±	+	±	±	−	−
Abdominal pain	−	+	−	−	−	−
Diarrhea	±	+	±	±	−	−
Hoarseness	−	−	−	−	−	+
Signs						
Rash	± (erythema multiforme)	−	± (Horder's spots)	−	−	−
Raynaud's phenomenon	±	−	−	−	−	−
Nonexudative pharyngitis	+	+	−	−	−	+
Hemoptysis	−	±	±	±	−	−
Lobar consolidation	−	±	±	±	±	−
Cardiac involvement	±	±	±	±	−	−
Splenomegaly	−	−	+	−	−	−
Relative bradycardia	−	+	+	+	−	−
Chest film findings						
Infiltrate	Patchy	Patchy/ consolidation	Patchy/ consolidation	Multiple rounded pleura-based opacities	Ovoid, bodies	Single circumscribed infiltrate
Bilateral hilar adenopathy	−	−	−	−	+	−
Pleural effusion	± (small)	±	±	−	+ (bloody)	±
Laboratory findings						
WBC count	Elevated	Elevated	Normal	Normal	Normal	Normal
Hypophosphatemia	−	+	−	−	−	−
Increase in SGOT/SGPT	−	+	+	+	−	−
Cold agglutinins	+	−	−	−	−	−
Microscopic hematuria	−	+	−	−	−	−

Source: Adapted from Cunha.[21]

TABLE 5.15. Pneumonias: clinical spectrum of histoplasmosis.

Hematologic signs
Thrombocytopenia
Anemia
Leukopenia
Pancytopenia
Splenomegaly
Generalized adenopathy
Eosinophilia
Dermatologic signs
Erythema nodosum
Skin ulcers
Gastrointestinal signs
Granulomatous hepatitis
Intestinal ulceration
Pulmonary signs
"Thick-walled" cavities
Apical infiltrates
Coin lesions
Hilar adenopathy
"Buckshot" calcifications
Miliary calcifications
"Marching cavities"
Mediastinal fibrosis
Obstruction of pulmonary/artery vein[a]
Obstruction of superior vena cava[a]
Cardiac
Endocarditis
Pericarditis
Ear, nose, and throat signs
Nose ulcers
Lip ulcers
Gum ulcers
Mouth ulcers
Tongue ulcers
Laryngeal ulcers
Neurologic signs
Chronic meningitis
Other signs
Addison's disease

Source: Adapted from Cunha BA: Histoplasmosis. Infect Dis Pract 1986;9:1–8.

[a] Secondary to lymph node compression/mediastinal fibrosis.

fashion. Acute primary tuberculous pneumonia is associated with a pleural effusion, but it is not a feature of reactivation tuberculosis. Histoplasmosis in the commonest fungal disease likely to be encountered and may present in disseminated form in HIV patients and compromised hosts. Once again, the diagnostic approach involves looking for specific features (e.g., tongue ulcers, which suggest the diagnosis of histoplasmosis, or a constellation of nonspecific findings that when combined may provide as nearly specific information).[28–30] For example, a patient with pulmonary infiltrates and erythema nodosum may have tuberculosis or histoplasmosis. However, if eosinophils are present in the periphery, the diagnosis of histoplasmosis is favored because eosinophilia is not a feature of tuberculosis.[1] In this way, the diagnostic workup can be directed until a specific diagnosis is made. The many manifestations of histoplasmosis are presented in Tables 5.15 and 5.16.

TABLE 5.16. Infectious granulomatous pneumonias.

Findings	Histoplasmosis	Tuberculosis	Blastomycosis
Fever			
Double quotidian fever	−	±	−
Laboratory tests			
Pancytopenia	+[a]	+	−
Hypergammaglobulinemia	−	−	−
Leukemoid reaction	−	+	−
Chest roentgenogram			
Miliary calcification	+	±	−
Hilar adenopathy	+	−	−
Pleural effusion	−	+	−
Abdominal roentgenogram			
Liver/spleen calcification	+	−	−
Organ involvement			
Meningitis	+[a]	+	−
Oropharyngeal ulcers	+[a]	±	−
Pulmonary infiltrates	+	+	±
Endocarditis	+	−	−
Addison's disease	+[a]	+	−
Granulomatous hepatitis	+	+	±
Splenomegaly	+[a]	±	±
Generalized adenopathy	+	±	−
Intestinal ulcers	+[a]	±	−
Bone/joint lesions		+	+
Glomerulonephritis	−	−	−
Epididymoorchitis	−	+	+
Granulomatous prostatitis	+	−	+
Skin ulcers	+[a]	±	+
Erythema nodosum	+	+	±

Source: Adapted from Cunha BA: Histoplasmosis. Infect Dis Pract 1986;9:1–8.
[a] Only in disseminated histoplasmosis.

The diagnosis of nosocomial pneumonia in the febrile leukopenic compromised host, organ transplant patient, and HIV-positive patient depend on demonstrating the putative pathogen in tissue. General principles apply to these as well as other patients, but a specific diagnosis depends on a definitive test or demonstration of the organism in tissue.[39,40] One can predict, in general, the group of pathogens likely to infect an organ transplant patient early versus later but cannot differentiate among pathogens in each category. For example, cytomegalovirus (CMV) and HIV commonly coexist with PCP pneumonia in organ transplant patients. Only lung biopsy can differentiate these two disease entities, which present in a similar fashion and frequently coexist.[2,4] In the leukopenic compromised host, only generalities can be made, but these principles are nontheless useful for the initial approach to the patient. Early, after induction chemotherapy, aerobic gram-negative pathogens predominate. The longer that intravenous access devices remain, the more likely is intravenous line sepsis to occur due to gram-positive organisms or fungi. The longer the neutropenia persists, the more likely it is that a disseminated fungal mycoses will supervene. Definitive diagnosis of disseminated fungal disease depends on demonstrating tissue invasion, not superficial recovery of, the organism from mucosal surfaces.[1,3] Similarly, the HIV patient initially may present with PCP if diffuse infiltrates are present. However, focal infiltrates suggest a bacterial etiology that may be due to common pathogens or intracellular organisms (e.g., *Salmonella*, *Legionella*). HIV patients presenting with recurrent pulmonary infiltrates require a definitive diagnostic procedure, as it may be due to a variety of opportunistic pathogens as well as noninfectious diseases (e.g., Kaposi sarcoma of the lung).

In addition to clues from the history, physical examination, chest film, and laboratory tests, the clinician needs other diagnostic caveats to help with the differential diagnosis of community-acquired pneumonias. This aphorismic approach utilizing diagnostic "pearls" frequently is the way to solve complex clinical problems. Aphorisms provide bits of clinical wisdom that are helpful in telling what the diagnosis is not or in differentiating between two similar disease entities. Pneumonia aphorisms and diagnostic pulmonary pearls should be applied to the case in addition to, not instead of, the aforementioned diagnostic process.

Pneumonia Aphorisms

1. Recurrent pneumonias may be due to immunodeficiencies (antibody deficiency, complement deficiency, cell-mediated deficiency, or phagocyte disorders).

2. Hypereosinophilic immunoglobulin E (IgE) syndrome or Job syndrome is associated with recurrent pneumonitis.

3. Patients prone to recurrent pneumonia may have an underlying disorder. Do not forget to consider seizure disorder, alcoholism, intravenous drug abuse, diabetes, sickle cell anemia, renal failure, esophageal diverticulum, or tracheoesophageal fistula.

4. Kartagener syndrome is suggested by the combination of pneumonia, recurrent sinusitis, and otitis plus situs inversus.

5. Pulmonary sequestration is a development abnormality involving lung sequestered from bronchi, predisposing to recurrent pneumonia.

6. Myeloma or chronic lymphatic leukemia with pneumonia is usually due to *Hemophilus influenzae*, *Streptococcus pneumoniae*, or *Staphylococcus aureus* because of defects in patient's the B lymphocytes.

7. Selective IgA deficiency is a rare cause of recurrent pneumonias. Recurrent sinopulmonary infections are uncommon; and although IgA deficiency is the most common immunodeficiency, it is usually asymptomatic.

8. The usual pathogens in chronic granulomatous disease are *S. aureus* and occasionally gram-negative aerobic bacilli. Remember that infections with coagulase-negative organisms, streptococci, *H. influenzae*, or pneumococci are rare. Look for associated hepatosplenomegaly and lymphadenopathy.

9. The conditions associated with recurrent pneumonias include chest abnormalities: bronchogenic carcinomas, silicosis, kyphoscoliosis, previous pulmonary surgery, previous pulmonary tuberculosis, asthma, chronic bronchitis, or congestive heart failure.

10. Systemic diseases associated with recurrent pneumonias include alcoholism, diabetest, chronic lymphocytic leukemia, lymphoma, myeloma, sickle cell disease, cerebrovascular accident, neutropenia, systemic steroid treatment, hypogammaglobulinemia, and systemic lupus erythematosus (SLE).

11. Aspiration pneumonia rarely requires more than penicillin therapy, as most aspirated oral anaerobes are sensistive to most antibiotics. However, if "pigmented" oral *Bacteroides* is present in large numbers, or if *S. aureus* is present, the β-lactamases produced by these organisms inactivate penicillin, and treatment with a β-lactamase-resistant drug (e.g., clindamycin) is required.

12. Invasive *Aspergillus* infections (e.g., *Aspergillus* pneumonia) are associated with negative or low-titer *Aspergillus* precipitins in the peripheral blood. High levels of *Aspergillus* precipitins are associated with bronchopulmonary aspergillosis, which is a noninfectious immunologic reaction to the fungus.

13. Nasal cultures are worthless for the diagnosis of pneumonia, except in the case of febrile, leukopenic compromised hosts where surveillance nasal cultures positive for *Aspergillus* predict subsequent invasive or disseminated *Aspergillus* infection.

14. *Candida* pneumonia probably does not exist. Similarly *Torulopsis glabrata* pneumonias are also exceedingly rare or do not exist at all.

15. Be careful not miss the diagnosis of PCP pneumonia with a near-normal chest roentgyenogram. The patient's severe and progressive dyspnea suggesting PCP can be verified by finding a greatly reduced carbon monoxide diffusing capacity and a positive gallium scan of the lungs.

16. Cytomegalovirus (CMV) pneumonia is virtually never found in normal hosts. In immunocompromised hosts it is most commonly associated with PCP.

17. In renal transplant patients, common community-acquired organism (e.g., *S. pneumoniae*, *H. influenzae*, *S. aureus*) are important pathogens up to day 30 after transplantation and after day 120, but not during the intervening 30–120 days.

18. Viral and fungal pathogens are most common 30–120 days after renal transplant, when cell-mediated immunity is maximally depressed. Pathogens include CMV, *Nocardia*, and *Aspergillus*.

19. *Legionella* pneumonia may be community-acquired and has the same presentation when nosocomially acquired. Look for the organism in the hospital's water supply.

20. Pneumonia in a patient with herpes labialis is pneumococcal until proved otherwise. Herpes labialis occurs in up to 30% of patients with pneumococcal pneumonia.

21. Pneumococcal pneumonia may be associated with leukopenia or leukocytosis. Be wary of a patient presenting with right upper quadrant pain and isolated elevation of the bilirubin level. Indirect hyperbilirubinemia may be a clue to pneumococcal pneumonia or represent Dubin-Johnson syndrome in a patient with a pneumonia due to another etiology.

22. Asplenic individuals may present with fulminant shock and sepsis disseminated intravascular coagulation (DIC) due to overwhelming pneumococcal infection, which rarely can produce the same picture in apparently "normal" individuals.

23. Pneumococcal empyema is unusual today, and pleural effusion is uncommon.

24. Complete histologic resolution is the rule with pneumococcal pneumonia; however, delayed resolution of pneumococcal pneumonia may take up to 14 weeks.

25. Pneumococcal bacteremia is particularly associated with cirrhosis, hypergammaglobulinemia, and asplenism.

26. The pneumococcal vaccine does not protect everyone who is immunized. Serotypes in the pneumococcal vaccine do not represent all organisms responsible for pneumococcal pneumonria. Furthermore, compromised hosts have impaired antibody responses that frequently result in inadequate or no protection.

27. More than 60% of patients with group A streptococcal pneumonia have an antecedent history of pharyngitis, but only 20% of these patients have positive throat cultures for the organism.

28. With group A streptococcal pneumonia, the higher the pleural fluid white blood cell count is over 20,000 cells/mm^3, the more likely is empyema.

29. The longer the chains of streptococci in Gram-stained sputum, the more pathogenic and virulent is the organism.

30. Group A streptococcal pneumonia is characterized in virtually all cases by large pleural effusions. Persistent pleuritic chest pain heralds empyema.

31. Group B streptococcal pneumonia occurs only in neonates and is the most common manifestation of early-onset group B streptococcal infection. The chest film appearance mimics that of pneumococcal pneumonia, but cyanosis is a clue to the group B streptococcal etiology.

32. Staphylococcal pneumonia follows not only viral influenza infection but may follow measles or other minor upper or lower respiratory infections.

33. Pneumothorax commonly is associated with staphylococcal pneumonia, but pneumatoceles are found primarily in children and not adults.

34. After viral influenza, *S. aureus* is the most common pathogen, but pneumococcus, *H. influenzae*, and *Klebsiella* should also be considered.

35. Staphylococcal pneumonia is characterized by widely scattered pulmonary infiltrates, but pneumatoceles and consolidation are unusual. Multiple abscesses that cavitate occur in approximately 25% of cases.

36. *Nocardia* species are obligate aerobes, are weakly acid-fast, and produce branching filaments. In contrast, *Actinomyces* are anaerobic, are non-acid-fast, and have sulfa granules.

37. Aspiration pneumonia that occurs after a week or more of hospitalization should be treated as a nosocomial pneumonia because "hospital" flora are aspirated. For this reason, specific antianaerobic coverage should not be added to the regimen.

38. *Acinetobacter* pneumonia is nearly always nosocomial, and its treatment includes respiratory support equipment. Be wary because *Acinetobacter* is a common nosocomial colonizer of the wounds, skin, and sputum.

39. *Serratia* pneumonia is uncommon; and when it does occur, it does not cavitate.

40. Community-acquired *Acinetobacter* pneumonia is rare but is as sociated with positive blood cultures, whereas nosocomial *Acinetobacter* infection is never associated with bacteremia.

41. Chronic *Klebsiella* pneumonia resembles tuberculosis. However, chronic *Klebsiella* pneumonia is associated with thin-walled cavities, unlike *Mycobacterium* tuberculosis, which is associated with thick-walled cavities.

In addition, the sputum shows gram-negative encapsulated bacilli with *Klebsiella* pneumonia and not with pulmonary tuberculosis.

42. *Proteus* pneumonia is the only nosocomial pneumonia with a predisposition for the upper lobes.

43. *Pseudomonas* pneumonia is always nosocomial except in patients with cystic fibrosis.

44. Virtually all *Proteus* pneumonias originate from the urinary tract. On roentgenogram, *Proteus* pneumonia resembles *Klebsiella* pneumonia, except that cavitation is unusual. In a patient with an antecedent history of urinary tract infection, *Escherichia coli* and *Proteus* pneumonias are the most likely diagnostic possibilities.

45. Hemoptysis associated with a nosocomial pneumonia suggests *Serratia marcescens* pneumonia. It may be differentiated from true hemoptysis of testing the sputum for hemoglobin. Pseudohemoptysis is related to prodigiosin, which gives the red color to sputum.

46. A "pertussoid cough" in a young infant with peripheral eosinophilia suggests *Chlamydia* rather than *Bordetella* pertussis.

47. In a child with pneumonia, more than 60% lymphocytes on the peripheral smear suggests pertussis. The "shaggy heart sign" may be seen on chest roentgenogram.

48. The only pneumonias associated with epistaxis are psittacosis and pertussis. Subconjunctival hemorrhage in the pneumonia patient immediately suggests pertussis.

49. Meningococcal pneumonia occurs primarily in closed military recruit populations and is usually due to group Y serotypes. The usual presentation is that of a diffuse bronchopneumonia, and bacteremia occurs in fewer than 10% of patients.

50. The only pneumonia presenting with a low serum phosphorus level in the absence of other causes of hypophosphatemia is that due to *Legionella*.

51. Ovoid densities on the chest film suggest *Legionella micdadei*, tularemia, or adenoviral pneumonia.

52. With primary tuberculous pneumonia with a large effusion, the PPD test is often negative. Primary tuberculosis, which occurs most of ten in the very young and the very old, is characterized by a lower lobe infiltrate and a pleural effusion.

53. False-positive tuberculin skin tests may be attributed to technical difficulties, nonspecific pertubations and immunity such as from recent acute viral infections (e.g., measles, Ebstein-Barr virus, CMV), steroid therapy, dehydration, malnutrition, hypothyroidism, and old age. Viral immunization, sarcoidosis, immunosuppressive therapy, radiotherapy, and lymphoreticular malignancies may also be responsible for a negative skin test.

54. Be careful not to miss tuberculosis (TB) with a negative PPD if the patient has primary TB with a large tuberculous effusion, miliary TB, far-

advanced TB, or very early TB. The patient can also have TB and be rendered anergic by a superimposed disease (e.g., HIV infection).

55. Cold agglutinin titers seen in *Mycoplasma* infection peak during the second and third weeks of illness. Cold agglutinins are IgM antibodies that bind to the big I antigen on the erythrocyte.

56. A lobar infiltrate with consolidation in the absence of pleuritic chest pain suggests psittacosis. Splenomegaly occurs in 10–70% of patients with psittacosis. Splenomegaly in a patient with pneumonia suggests psittacosis or Q fever.

57. Respiratory syncytial virus (RSV) causes tracheobronchitis in adults but pneumonia in children.

58. Measles pneumonia predominantly involves the lower lobes, and the disease parallels the cutaneous manifestations. Measles pneumonia may be fatal in severely immunocompromised hosts and in the very young and the malnourished patient.

59. *Staphylococcus aureus*, pneumococcus, and *H. influenzae* are the most common pathogens in postmeasles pneumonia.

60. Ebstein-Barr virus (EBV) mononucleosis rarely presents with interstitial infiltrates. Hilar adenopathy, paratracheal node enlargement, and pleural effusions have been reported. Patients with EBV mononucleosis do not get secondary bacterial pneumonias.

61. The patient with pneumonia and skin petechial hemorrhages or purpura, not in shock or in DIC, suggests adenvirus as a cause.

62. The physical examination in viral influenza pneumonia patients is unremarkable, as is the chest film. Rales and rhonchi in these patients suggest superimposed bacterial pneumonia.

63. Secondary bacterial pneumonia in a patient with viral influenza usually occurs about a week after the beginning of the influenza illness when the patient is clinicallyimproving. There is a recrudescence of fever, and the chest film shows a segmental or lobar defect.

64. Uncomplicated asthma is not associated with pulmonary infiltrates or fever.

65. Aspergillomas have been associated with chronic cavitary pulmonary diseases including tuberculosis, histoplasmosis, sarcoidosis, and ankylosing spondylitis. *Aspergillus* precipitins are positive in 80% or more of patients. The chest film usually reveals a soft-tissue density surrounding by a crescent of air that delineates the fungus ball in the cavity.

66. Invasive pulmonary aspergillosis occurs only in severely immunocompromised hosts (e.g., patients with leukemia or lymphoma, those on chemotherapy, renal transplant patiens). Do not forget that invasive aspergillosis is also associated with prolonged treatment with antibiotics and therapy with corticosteroids.

67. The diagnosis of all invasive fungal infections of the lung requires biopsy proof of tissue invasion. Mere recovery of an organism from a

protected brush or bronchoalveolar lavage (BAL) specimen does not prove its pathogenicity in the lung.

68. Blastomycosis does not involve the gastrointestinal tract or the central nervous system. Calcification is not a feature of blastomycosis.

69. Crytococcal pneumonia sometimes is characterized by blood-streaked sputum and pleuritic chest pain. Cryptococcal pneumonia occurs almost always in immunosuppressed individuals. Sputum cultures are usually negative with cryptococcal pneumonia. If skin lesions are present, they should be biopsied, as the organism is present in large numbers in these lesions.

70. In a patient with pneumonia and meningitis, do not fail to consider cryptococci, tuberculosis, *Toxoplasma*, CMV, *Nocardia*, legionnaires' disease, or *Mycoplasma* meningoencephalitis.

71. Herpes simplex meningitis is rarely if ever associated with herpes pneumonitis.

72. The patient with malaria may have noncardiac pulmonary edema or adult respiratory distress syndrome (ARDS), but pulmonary infiltrates are not due to secondary pneumonia.

73. An elevated right hemidiaphragm in association with pulmonary infiltrates suggests amebiasis or echinococcosis. Neither of these diseases is associated with peripheral eosinophilia.

74. Except with congenitally acquired disease, toxoplasmosis never causes pneumonia by itself in adults. Toxoplasmosis is a common co-pathogen in patients with HIV. Lung infiltrates due to *Toxoplasma* are difficult to differentiate from those due to other pathogens. LUNG Biopsy is needed for a definitive diagnosis.

75. Eosinophilia is uncommon with dog heartworm (Dirofilaria immitis). The chest film shows one or more coin lesions, but most patients are asymptomatic. Some have chest pain, cough, fever, or hemoptysis.

76. In a patient with hemoptysis from Southeast Asia, tuberculosis, melioidosis, or paragonamiasis should be considered. Be careful not to forget that paragonamiasis frequently coexists with pulmonary tuberculosis.

77. Bacterial pneumonia can activate quiescent tuberculosis, a common phenomenon in elderly patients. Therefore if an elderly patient is recovering from a bacterial pneumonia and subsequently becomes worse and develops a new pulmonary infiltrate, consider reactivated tuberculosis in the differential diagnosis.

References

1. Wilson JD, Braunwald E, Isselbacher KJ, et al (eds): Harrison's Principles of Internal Medicine, 12th ed. New York: McGraw-Hill, 1991.
2. Gorbach SL, Bartlett JG, Blacklow NR (eds): Infectious Diseases. Philadelphia: Saunders, 1992.

3. Braude AI (ed): Infectious Diseases and Medical Microbiology, 2nd ed. Philadelphia: Saunders, 1986.
4. Mandell GL, Gordon-Douglas R Jr, Bennett JE (eds): Principles and Practice of Infectious Diseases, 3rd ed. New York: Churchill Livingstone, 1985.
5. Chapman S, Nakielny R: Aids to Radiological Differential Diagnosis, 2nd ed. London: Baillière Tindall, 1990.
6. Burgener FA, Kormano M: Differential Diagnosis in Conventional Radiology, 2nd ed. New York: Thieme, 1991.
7. Lippington GA, Jamplis RW: A Diagnostic Approach to Chest Diseases, 2nd ed. Baltimore: Williams & Wilkins, 1977.
8. Reed JC: Chest Radiology, 3rd ed. St. Louis: Mosby-Year Book, 1991.
9. Cunha BA: Pneumonias acquired from others. I and II. Postgrad Med 1987;82:126–156.
10. Cunha BA, Strampfer MJ: Pearls and pitfalls. In: Brandstetter RD (ed): Pulmonary Medicine. Oradell, NJ: Medical Economics, 1989.
11. Seaton A, Seaton D, Leitch AG: Crofton & Douglas's Respiratory Diseases, 4th ed. Oxford: Blackwell, 1989.
12. Brandstetter RD (ed): Pulmonary Medicine. Oradell, NJ: Medical Economics, 1989.
13. Pennington JE (ed): Respiratory Infections: Diagnosis and Management. New York: Raven Press, 1983.
14. Jacobs RF (ed): Pediatric pulmonary infections. Semin Respir Infect 1987;2(3):145–187.
15. Murphey SA: Host defenses in the respiratory tract. In Levison ME (ed): The Pneumonias. Boston: John Wright-PSG, 1984.
16. Golish JA, Curtis PS: Unusual pneumonias. In Brandstetter RD (ed): Pulmonary Medicine. Oradell, NJ: Medical Economics, 1989.
17. Gleckman RA: Pneumonia: update on diagnosis and treatment. J Geriatr 1991;46:49–50, 55–56.
18. Palmar LB: Bacterial colonization: pathogenesis and clinical significance. Clin Chest Med 1987;8:455–466.
19. Hoeprich PD, Jordan MC: Infectious Diseases, 4th ed. Philadelphia: Lippincott, 1989.
20. Sapira JD: The Art and Science of Bedside Diagnosis. Baltimore: Urban & Schwarzenberg, 1990.
21. Cunha BA: Atypical pneumonias. Postgrad Med 1991;90:89–101.
22. Wollschlager CM, Khan FA, Khan A: Utility of radiography and clinical features in the diagnosis of community acquired pneumonia. Clin Chest Med 1987;8:393.
23. Matthay RA (ed): Pulmonary manifestations of systemic disease. Clin Chest Med 1989;10:469–818.
24. Hunnighake GW, Fauci AS: Pulmonary involvement in collagen vascular diseases. Am Rev Respir Dis 1979;119:471.
25. Leatherman JW (ed): Noninfectious pulmonary infitrates. Semin Respir Infect 1988;3:179–274.
26. Brandstetter RD, Hausen HS, Desvarieux H: Noninfectious pulmonary disorders radiographically mimicking infection. Infect Dis Pract 1991;15:1–8.
27. Marino PL: Complications of pneumonia. In Levison ME (ed): The Pneumonias. Boston, John Wright-PSG, 1984.

28. Davies SF (ed): Fungal diseases. Semin Respir Infect 1986;1(1):1–65.
29. Davies SF: Fungal diseases. Semin Respir Infect 1990;5(2):91–154.
30. Sarosi GA, Davies SF (eds): Fungal Diseases of the Lung. Orlando, FL: Grune & Stratton, 1986.
31. Raju L, Khan F: Bacterial pneumonias. In Brandstetter RD (ed): Pulmonary Medicine. Oradell, NJ: Medical Economics, 1989.
32. Snepar R: Adenovirus. In Levison ME (ed): The Pneumonias: Boston: John Wright-PSG, 1984.
33. Poporad GA: Influenza. In Levison ME (ed): the Pneumonias. Boston: John Wright-PSG, 1984.
34. Cate TR, Ruben FL (eds): Viral pneumonias. Semin Respir Infect 1987;2(2):84–144.
35. Sahn SA (ed): Infections of the pleural space. Semin Respir Infect 1988;3(4):289–394.
36. Lowell JR: Pleural Effusions. Baltimore: University Park Press, 1977.
37. Weller PF: Parasitic pneumonias. In Pennington JE (ed): Respiratory Infections: Diagnosis and Management. New York: Raven Press, 1983.
38. Sarosi GA (ed): Community-acquired pneumonia. Semin Respir Infect 1989;4(1):1–72.
39. Toews GB: Nosocomial pneumonias. Clin Chest Med 1987;8:467–480.
40. Pennington JE (ed): Hospital-acquired pneumonias. Semin Respir Infect 1987;2(1):1–81.

6
Pneumonia: Diagnostic Techniques

ROBERT D. BRANDSTETTER

Diagnosis of a lower respiratory tract infection can be simple, as in a young immunocompetent individual, or difficult, as in patients who have underlying cardiopulmonary or systemic illness. Although our antimicrobial pharmacology today effectively eliminates a broad spectrum of offending organisms, it remains desirable to identify the causative organism so specific therapy can be offered. Knowledge of the infectious organism also has epidemiologic considerations.

Pneumonia is defined separately from other infections of the lower respiratory tract, such as tracheitis, tracheobronchitis, bronchitis, bronchiolitis, bronchiectasis, lung abscess, and empyema. The criteria for pneumonia involve various clinical, radiographic, and laboratory evidence of infection (Table 6.1).

It is usual, acceptable practice to proceed from noninvasive to invasive techniques for the diagnosis of pneumonia. According to the nature of the infection, diagnosis may be reasonably assumed by direct sputum examination and culture, or it may depend on open lung biopsy (Table 6.2). Between these two extremes lies an impressive spectrum of diagnostic modalities: nasotracheal suction, transtracheal aspiration, bronchoscopy with various sleeved catheters, percutaneous lung aspiration, thoracocentesis, blood cultures, and serologic studies. It is not uncommon to utilize one or all of these examinations in the process of establishing a diagnosis.

Expectorated Sputum

The first diagnostic test that should be performed when evaluating a patient with suspected pneumonia is the examination of expectorated sputum (Table 6.3). In the event a patient cannot perform a deep cough, efforts should be made to induce a cough by inhalation of a bronchial irritant such as propylene glycol. Although there are considerable limitations to the diagnostic value of an examination of the sputum (Table 6.4), it is the simplest, most cost-effective technique available.

TABLE 6.1. Diagnosis of pneumonia.

For the diagnosis of pneumonia, one of the two following criteria must be met.

1. Crackles or dullness to percussion upon physical examination of the chest *and* any of the following:
   - Change in nature of sputum or new onset of sputum
   - Positive blood culture
   - Isolation of organism from pleural space or parenchyma (bronchoscopy with plugged telescoping catheter specimen brush, transpercutaneous lung aspiration, open lung biopsy)
2. Chest radiographic examination with new or progressive infiltrate, consolidation, cavitation, or pleural effusion *and* any of the following:
   - Change in nature of sputum or new onset of sputum
   - Positive blood culture
   - Isolation of organism from pleural space or parenchyma (bronchoscopy with plugged telescoping catheter specimen brush, transpercutaneous lung aspirate, open lung biopsy)
   - Isolation of virus or detection of viral antigen in respiratory secretions
   - Diagnostic single antibody titer (IgM) or fourfold increase in paired serum samples (IgG) for pthogen
   - Histopathologic evidence of pneumonia

Source: CDC definitions for nosocomial infections. Am Rev Respir Dis 1989;139:1058–1059. With permission.

TABLE 6.2. Laboratory procedures for diagnosis of pneumonia.

- Expectorated sputum
- Nasotrachael suction
- Transtracheal aspiration
- Bronchoscopy
  - Bronchial washings
  - Bronchoalveolar lavage
  - Plugged telescoping catheter brush
  - Transbronchial needle aspiration
  - Transbronchial biopsy
- Transthoracic needle aspiration
- Thoracocentesis
- Open lung biopsy
- Blood culture

A sputum sample should be considered meaningful for examination if it is grossly purulent and if fewer than 10 squamous epithelial cells or more than 25 leukocytes per low-powered microscopic field are seen. Under such conditions the cultured specimen more closely resembles transtracheal aspirates than contaminated saliva.[1]

Although limitations exist regarding the interpretation of the Gram stain for "typical bacteria" (excluding such species as *Mycoplasma* and

TABLE 6.3. Laboratory stains useful for diagnosis of pneumonia.

Stain	Organism
Gram stain	"Typical" aerobic and anaerobic bacteria
Acid-fast stain (Ziehl-Neelsen) or fluorochrome stain	Mycobacteria
Grocott's modified Gomori methenamine silver stain	*Pneumocystis carinii*
Direct immunofluorescence (DFA)	*Legionella* sp. *Bordetella pertussis*
Potassium hydroxide (KOH) with phase contrast Gomori methenamine silver stain (GMS)	Fungal sp.
Cytologic preparation	Cytomegalovirus (owl's eye)
Gram stain or modified carbol fuchsin stain	*Nocardia*

TABLE 6.4. Limitations to the interpretation of expectorated sputum.

Contamination of upper airway with nonpathogen flora
Colonization of upper airway with potential pathogens
Previous antibiotic therapy
Deficiencies in specimen processing

Legionella), certain microbes found in expectorated sputum should make one suspect strongly the pathogenicity of that organism. *Mycobacterium* species and *Pneumocystis carinii* organisms, when appropriately stained (Table 6.4), may be found in expectorated sputum and indicate disease.

Nasotracheal Suction

Sputum may be obtained from patients who are either uncooperative or unable to cough by passing a soft suction catheter through the nose and into the trachea. Limitations when interpreting the specimen are the same as those for expectorated sputum, with the additional concern of vocal cord trauma from the catheter.

Transtracheal Aspiration

Transtracheal aspiration was developed in an effort to avoid contamination of the upper airway.[2,3] The technique involves placing a 14-gauge needle-catheter into the cricothyroid membrane. A sample of tracheal secretions is then obtained by aspiration.

The main advantage of this procedure is the high sensitivity of culture results. Only 1% false-negative cultures have been reported in a large series of nearly 400 patients,[3] and the same excellent results were found in the diagnosis of anaerobic infections.[4]

False-positive results, however, in the setting of colonization of the tracheobronchial tree (coexisting bronchitis) has limited the usefulness of this procedure for the diagnosis of pneumonia.[5] Accordingly, the procedure should not be performed when chronic underlying lung disease is present, and concern exists about contamination by nonpathogenic organisms.

The popularity of transtracheal aspiration has also decreased because of its associated complications. Hemoptysis, subcutaneous emphysema, arrhythmias, and death have rarely been reported.[6–8] Furthermore, the procedure is contraindicated in uncooperative patients and in the setting of a coagulation disorder.

Bronchoscopy With Plugged Telescoping Catheter Brush

Should expectorated sputum not be of benefit in establishing which organism is responsible for the infection, transtracheal aspiration and bronchoscopy are the subsequent procedures of choice. Most pulmonologists prefer bronchoscopy.

Flexible fiberoptic bronchoscopy allows direct visualization of the airways in the process of diagnosing and treating certain respiratory disorders. As in the circumstance of nasotracheal suction, organisms in the posterior oropharynx are dragged down into the tracheobronchial tree with the bronchoscope. In addition, as was found with transtracheal aspiration, where colonization may give false-positive results upon culturing a specimen, the bronchoscope is also subject to this limiting feature.

In 1979 a technique was introduced to eliminate the problem of contaminating the upper airways by nonpathogenic bacteria.[9] A sterile sample brush within a telescoping double catheter, occluded by a distal polyethylene glycol plug (BFW brush, Medi-Tech Corp, Watertown, MA) is utilized. Upon reaching the site to be sampled, the protected brush catheter is inserted through the inner suction channel of the scope and advanced under direct visualization several centimeters beyond the end of the bronchoscope. The inner telescoping cannula containing the specimen sampling brush is then advanced 2 cm, jettisoning the protective polyethylene glycol plug, and specimens are obtained by advancing the brush into secretions. The brush is then retracted into the inner cannula, and the entire unit is removed from the bronchoscope.

Quantitative cultures of the specimen are prepared in order to distinguish pathogens from nonpathogens. Respiratory pathogens are usually present in concentrations of at least 10^3 colony-forming units (cfu)/ml due to the fact that the initial specimen is diluted 100–1000 times in Ringer's lactate solution.

A number of studies have shown the benefit of this procedure,[10] whose use has been extended to patients who are intubated and undergoing mechanical ventilation.[11] Although other studies have shown false-positive rates,[12,13] the methodology of the studies were questioned, leaving the protected brush technique as a sensitive procedure for identifying the etiology of a pneumonia.[14,15]

Bronchoscopy is a safe technique when performed with the patient monitored and receiving supplemental oxygen.[16,17] Complications include fever, dysrhythmias, and minor hemorrhage. Laryngospasm and cough are minimized by instillation of lidocaine, although reduction in the yield of cultures may be expected with such a technique.[18]

Bronchial Washings

Bronchial washings are of little value, not being much better than expectorated sputum for diagnosing the cause for pneumonia. Isotonic saline is injected down the suction channel of the scope into the bronchus. Secretions are then aspirated into a sterile trap. As with expectorated sputum, finding *Mycobacterium* or *Pneumocystis* should alert the physician to the pathogenesis of the pneumonia.

Bronchoalveolar Lavage

Bronchoalveolar lavage (BAL) is a particularly useful technique when a sample from the alveolus is to be obtained. BAL involves wedging the bronchoscope into a distal bronchus, followed by instillation of 100–200 ml of isotonic saline. At least 50% of the total infusion should be returned by suction.[19]

The BAL technique is most beneficial for diagnosing opportunistic lung disease, in particular *Pneumocystis carinii*.[20] When transbronchial biopsy is used in addition to BAL, the diagnostic yield increases.[21] BAL is also of value in the diagnosis of cytomegalovirus, *Mycobacterium*, and fungal infections of the lung.

Bronchoalveolar lavage is a safe procedure, with complications that include fever, minor hemorrhage, and exacerbation of respiratory failure.[8] Serious complications are rare, and no deaths have been reported. Accordingly, BAL is an effective technique for the diagnosis of respiratory infections in the immunosuppressed patient.

Transbronchial Needle Aspiration

Transbronchial needle aspiration was introduced originally for the diagnosis of malignancy in subcarinal and mediastinal nodes.[8] Using the same technique, with the addition of a double-lumen catheter with a protective polyethylene glycol plug (Microvasive, Milford, MA), this procedure was found to be as reliable as the protected brush.[22] The ability of the needle to penetrate the bronchial wall and directly aspirate infected lung parenchyma thus limits contamination by the upper airway and bronchial flora.

Transbronchial Biopsy

The last procedure performed by flexible fiberoptic bronchoscopy for diagnosing pneumonia is transbronchial biopsy. A forceps is introduced through the bronchoscope channel into the lung parenchyma. The patient is instructed to exhale, at which time a specimen is taken.

The diagnostic yield appears to be enhanced with diffuse rather than localized infiltrates[23] and in combination with BAL.[21] The lung infections diagnosed include viruses (cytomegalovirus, herpes simplex), fungi (*Candida*, *Cryptococcus*, *Aspergillus*), mycobacteria, and *Pneumocystis carinii*.[24] Gram-positive, gram-negative, and nocardial infections may also be identified with transbronchial biopsy.[24]

Transbronchial biopsy is associated with complications ranging from pneumothorax, to fever, to fatal hemorrhage.[25] Additional complications may be expected in the setting of hypoxia, thrombocytopenia, coagulation abnormalities, and azotemia and in patients who are mechanically ventilated.

Transthoracic Needle Aspiration

Transthoracic needle aspiration (TNA) was originally introduced for the diagnosis of masses and peripheral nodules. Over the past several years it has regained interest as a procedure for diagnosing pulmonary infections.[26] Various techniques have been described, all being performed under either fluoroscopic or computed tomographic guidance. The procedure may incorporate any one of the following techniques: insertion and withdrawal under continuous suction, negative pressure during several back-and-forth movements, or insertion with suction only during withdrawal.[27] Needle sizes range from 18 to 25 gauge, and the needles are inserted only during suspended respiration. By this direct percutaneous route of sampling the lung parenchyma, the problem of upper airway contamination is thus avoided.

The TNA technique appears to be of particular benefit for peripheral infiltrates and infiltrates in immunocompromised patients.[28,29] Multiple pathogens may be diagnosed, including opportunistic fungi, *Nocardia*, *Mycobacterium*, *Legionella*, and *Pneumocystis carinii*. After discounting obvious skin organisms, a positive culture obtained by TNA can be considered diagnostic of the etiologic agent of pneumonia.[8]

A continuous problem with TNA, however, is the frequency of false-negative cultures. Small sampling area, inability to localize the pneumonic area precisely, small inoculum volume, and skill of the operator have been suggested as reasons for failure to identify the causative organism.[30]

Complications of TNA are significant and include pneumothorax and life-threatening hemoptysis.[28] Compared with previously reported studies, however, the use of an ultrathin needle (24–25 gauge) produces significantly fewer complications while sustaining an excellent diagnostic yield.[31]

There are definite contraindications to TNA, including patients undergoing mechanical ventilation and those with suspected vascular lesions or pulmonary hypertension. In addition, patients with bullous emphysema or a coagulopathy should not be considered for this procedure.

Thoracocentesis

Pleural effusions accompany infectious parenchymal disease in as many as 30% of patients with the pneumonic processes. Removing pleural fluid for diagnostic measures is a simple procedure, where a 18- to 21-gauge needle is inserted through the skin and into the pleural space. As little as 2 ml of fluid can provide the information necessary to diagnose a parapneumonic effusion or an empyema.

Gram stain of the specimen obtained can provide a rapid diagnosis of bacterial pneumonia, with treatment initiated pending culture results. An infection may be suspected, again pending cultures when there is a low pleural fluid pH ($\leq$7.3) or low pleural fluid glucose ($\leq$30 mg/dl).[32]

Thoracocentesis is a safe procedure when supplemental oxygen is administered[33] and the patients is cooperative with no coagulation abnormalities. Hypoxia, pneumothorax, and hemorrhage (hemothorax) are the most frequently encountered complications. In difficult cases where pleural fluid is loculated, thoracocentesis can be performed with ultrasound guidance.

Open Lung Biopsy

Open lung biopsy is reserved for patients in whom a diagnosis has not been reached using less invasive procedures. Most often the patient is immunosuppressed. A 3- to 4-cm piece of lung tissue obtained by open lung biopsy provides the microbiologist with the least contaminated specimen.

Pulmonary infiltrates in immunosuppressed patients are caused not only by infectious organisms but by underlying disease, drug-induced disease, or other new or unrelated conditions. A number of excellent studies have demonstrated the high diagnostic yield of open lung biopsy, with results available within 3 hours in nearly 50% of the patients.[34,35] Opportunistic lung infection with *Pneumocystis carinii*, cytomegalovirus, or *Mycobacterium avium intracellulare* are frequently diagnosed by this procedure.

In carefully selected patients, the complications of open lung biopsy are low compared with other invasive procedures. Pneumothorax, hemorrhage, fever, and rarely death have been reported.[24]

Blood Culture

When blood cultures are positive, they provide exact diagnosis of a bacteremic pneumonia. Positive results, however, are uncommon. With pneumococcal pneumonia, blood cultures are positive in 8–50% of hospitalized patients.[36] In patients with the adult respiratory distress syndrome, bacteremia was present in only 27% of patients with lung infection.[37] Anaerobic pneumonias have even a lower rate of associated positive blood cultures.

Special Tests for Diagnosis of Pneumonia

Table 6.5 outlines some of the special tests that are available for diagnosis of pneumonia. The techniques include the analysis of either respiratory secretions or serum. The tests are of limited value, however, because of their specific nature, lack of availability, and expense.

Skin Testing for Fungal Pneumonia

Skin testing for the diagnosis of fungal diseases is seldom useful. A positive skin test (histoplasmosis, coccidioidomycosis) does not establish a causal relation for a given clinical condition unless the previously negative skin test status of the individual is known. Conversely, with disseminated illness, a negative skin test is the rule; hence a nonreactive skin test does not rule out clinically significant histoplasmosis or coccidioidomycosis. Skin testing should not be performed for diagnosis in individual patients but should be reserved for epidemiologic investigations. At the present time, good skin test antigen exists for histoplasmosis and coccidioidomycosis but not for blastomycosis.

TABLE 6.5. Special tests useful for diagnosis of pneumonia.

Examination	Organism
Bacterial antigen assay	
Countercurrent immunoelectrophoresis	Group B streptococci
Coagglutination	*N. meningitidis*
Latex particle	*H. influenzae* B antigen
	Pneumococcal antigen
Monoclonal antibody-antigen	Cytomegalovirus
Antibody assay	
Specific antibodies	Respiratory syncytial virus
	Influenza A and B virus
	Parainfluenza virus
	Mycoplasa pneumoniae
	Chlamydia psittaci
	Coxiella burnetii
Immunofluorescence technique	
Indirect immunofluorescence antibodies (1:128 titer or fourfold or greater change)	*Legionella* sp.
Immunofluorescence	Respiratory syncytial virus
	Parainfluenza (types 1–3)
	Influenza A and B virus
	Adenovirus
	Cytomegalovirus
Enzyme-linked immunosorbent assay	Respiratory syncytial virus

Serologic Testing for Fungal Pneumonia

Serologic testing remains a viable method for the diagnosis of the endemic mycoses, but in general these tests take several weeks to become positive. By the time the positive results are known, most patients have recovered. With acute fulminating infections, where an answer would be especially useful, the tests usually are negative.

References

1. Murray PR, Washington JA: Microscopic and bacteriologic analysis of expectorated sputum. Mayo Clin Proc 1975;50:339–344.
2. Irwin RS, Garrity FH, Erickson AD, et al: Sampling lower respiratory tract secretions in primary lung abscess: a comparison of the accuracy of four methods. Chest 1981;79:559–565.
3. Bartlett JG: Diagnostic accuracy of transtracheal aspiration bacteriologic studies. Am Rev Respir Dis 1977;115:777–782.
4. Bartlett JG, Rosenblatt JE, Finegold SM: Percutaneous transtracheal aspiration in the diagnosis of anaerobic pulmonary infection. Ann Intern Med 1973;79:535–540.

5. Bjerkestrand G, Digranes A, Schreiner A: Bacteriological findings in transtracheal aspirates from patients with chronic bronchitis and bronchiectasis. Scand J Respir Dis 1975;56:201–207.
6. Pratter MR, Irwin RS: Transtracheal aspiration guidelines for safety. Chest 1979;76:518–520.
7. Spencer DC, Beaty HN: Complications of transtracheal aspiration. N Engl J Med 1972;286:304–306.
8. Busk MF, Rosenow EC, Wilson WR: Invasive procedures in the diagnosis of pneumonia. Semin Respir Infect 1988;3:113–122.
9. Wimberly N, Faling LJ, Bartlett JG: A fiberoptic bronchoscopy technique to obtain uncontaminated lower airway secretions for bacterial culture. Am Rev Respir Dis 1979;119:337–343.
10. Pollock HM, Hawkins EL, Bonner JR, et al: Diagnosis of bacterial pulmonary infections with quantitative protected cultures obtained during bronchoscopy. J Clin Microsc 1983;17:255–259.
11. Chastre J, Viau F, Brun P, et al: Prospective evaluation of the protected specimen brush for diagnosis of pulmonary infections in ventilated patients. Am Rev Respir Dis 1984;130:924–929.
12. Fletcher EC, Mohr JA, Levin DC, et al: Bronchoscopic diagnosis of pulmonary infections: comparison of protected-specimen brush and cytology brush with lung aspirates. West J Med 1983;138:364–370.
13. Halperin SA, Suratt PM, Gwaltney JM, et al: Bacterial cultures of the lower respiratory tract in normal volunteers with and without experimental rhinovirus infection using a plugged device catheter system. Am Rev Respir Dis 1982;125:678–680.
14. Bamberger DM: Diagnosis of nosocomial pneumonia. Semin Respir Infect 1988;3:140–147.
15. Roig J, Aguilar X, Ruiz J, et al: Comparative study of Legionella pneumophila and other nosocomial-acquired pneumonias. Chest 1991;99:344–350.
16. Brandstetter RD: Flexible fiberoptic bronchoscopy in the intensive care unit. J Intens Care Med 1989;4:248–264.
17. Karetzky MA, Garvey JW, Brandstetter RD: Effect of fiberoptic bronchoscopy on arterial oxygen tension. NY State J Med 1974;74:62–63.
18. Tobin MJ: Diagnosis of pneumonia: techniques and problems. Clin Chest Med 1987;8:513–527.
19. Martin WJ, Smith TF, Brutinel WM, et al: Role of bronchoalveolar lavage in the assessment of opportunistic infections: utility and complications. Mayo Clin Proc 1987;62:549–557.
20. Stover DE, Zaman MB, Hajdu SI, et al: Bronchoalveolar lavage in the diagnosis of diffuse pulmonary infiltrates in the immunosuppressed host. Ann Intern Med 1984;101:1–7.
21. Broaddus C, Dake MD, Stulbarg MS, et al: Bronchoalveolar lavage and transbronchial biopsy for the diagnosis of pulmonary infections in the acquired immunodeficiency syndrome. Ann Intern Med 1985;102:749–752.
22. Lorch DG, John JF, Tomlinson JR, et al: Protected transbronchial needle aspiration and protected specimen brush in the diagnosis of pneumonia. Am Rev Respir Dis 1987;136:565–569.
23. Feldman NT, Pennington JE, Ehrie MG: Transbronchial lung biopsy in the compromised host. JAMA 1977;238:1377–1379.

24. Matthay RA, Moritz ED: Invasive procedures for diagnosing pulmonary infection: a critical review. Clin Chest Med 1981;2:3–18.
25. Brandstetter RD, Croce SA, Schiaffino E, et al: Flexible fiberoptic bronchoscopy in the hospitalized elderly. NY State J Med 1984;84:546–548.
26. Torres A, Jimenez P, de la Bellacasa JP, et al: Diagnostic value of nonfluoroscopic percutaneous lung needle aspiration in patients with pneumonia. Chest 1990;98:840–844.
27. Bartlett JG: Diagnosis of bacterial infections of the lung. Clin Chest Med 1987;8:119–134.
28. Bartlett JG: Invasive diagnostic techniques in respiratory infections. In Pennington JE (ed): Respiratory Infections: Diagnosis and Management. New York: Raven Press, 1983, pp. 55–77.
29. Castellino RA, Blank N: Etiologic diagonsis of focal pulmonary infection in immunocompromised patients by fluoroscopically guided percutaneous needle aspiration. Radiology 1979;132:563–567.
30. Palmer DL, Davidson M, Luck R: Needle aspiration of the lung in complex pneumonias. Chest 1980;78:16–21.
31. Zavala DC, Scohell JE: Ultra thin needle aspiration of the lung in infectious and malignant disease. Am Rev Respir Dis 1981;123:125–131.
32. Light RW, MacGregor MI, Ball WC Jr, Luchsinger PC: Diagnostic significance of pleural fluid pH and PCO_2. Chest 1973;64:591–596.
33. Brandstetter ED, Cohen RP: Hypoxemia after thoracentesis: a predictable and treatable observation. JAMA 1979;242:1060–1061.
34. Toledo-Pereyra LH, DeMeester TR, Kinealy A, et al: The benefits of open lung biopsy in patients with previous nondiagnostic transbronchial lung biopsy: a guide to appropriate therapy. Chest 1980;77:647–650.
35. Cockerill FR, Wilson WR, Carpenter HA, et al: Open lung biopsy in immunocompromised patients. Arch Intern Med 1985;145:1398–1404.
36. Bartlett JG: Bacteriological diagnosis of pulmonary infections. In Sackner MA (ed): Diagnostic Techniques in Pulmonary Disease. Part II. New York: Marcel Dekker, 1981, pp. 707–745.
37. Seidenfeld JJ, Pohl DF, Bell RC, et al: Incidence, site, and outcome of infections in patients with adult respiratory distress syndrome. Am Respir Dis 1986;134:12–16.

7
Presentation of Pneumonia

MONROE KARETZKY

Clinical Presentation

Dyspnea

The sensation of shortness of breath—dyspnea, or breathlessness—characterized by tachypnea and variable degrees of hypoxemia and hypocapnea is a characteristic clinical phenomenon of pneumonia and occurs even in the absence of pleuritic pain or fever. The alveolar hyperventilation reflected by the hypocapnia has been found to persist in patients with lobar pneumonia even after arterial hypoxemia is eliminated with oxygen therapy. A process of elimination can be observed in the long-standing efforts to attribute the sensation of breathlessness to objective criteria. Classic breath-holding studies have shown dyspnea to be alleviated by a rebreathing maneuver or with inspiration of oxygen and carbon dioxide gas mixtures that resulted in no improvement in either arterial hypoxemia or the associated respiratory acidosis. Thus linkage to chemoreceptor activity has been largely unsuccessful.

Almost all of the afferent impulses arising from airway and intrapulmonary receptors are carried in the vagus nerves. Classic studies in dogs have reported that the tachypnea of lobar pneumonia was entirely dependent on intact vagi. Subsequently, stretch receptors of vagal afferents were shown to be of significance but not critical. More recent studies with differential block suggest that the lung receptors that are excited are those innervated by nonmyelinated vagal afferents.[1] These J receptors lie in the interstitial space of the lung at the alveolar level. The inflammatory mediators presumably act to depolarize these chemically sensitive non-myelinated nerve endings. It has been suggested that J-receptor stimulation alone or in conjunction with the stimulation of irritant receptors is responsible for the tachypnea of pneumonia. Others, meanwhile, have suggested the importance of mechanoreceptors in the thoracic wall, including joint receptors, tendon organs, and muscle spindles.

Muscle spindles, especially prominent in the intercostal muscles in contrast to the diaphragm, are found within the special intrafusal fibers that are arranged in parallel with the main, extrafusal muscle fibers. The annulospiral receptor would be stretched (and stimulated) if shortening of the extrafusal fiber was impeded so it did not match the intrafusal muscle fiber shortening; enhancement of afferent impulses would then induce further extrafusal fiber contraction (length servo).[2] The contractile extrafusal fibers of a muscle receive the integrated output of the respiratory centers through alpha motoneurons, whereas the gamma motoneurons innervate the intrafusal fibers within the muscle spindles (fusiform system). Misalignment between these intra- and extrafusal systems was therefore suggested as a neuroanatomic mechanism of dyspnea.

Finally, the ongoing search was diverted from classic anatomic and physiologic concepts of cause and effect as both neurophysiologists and respiratory physiologists turned to concepts of the systems engineer. This diversion allowed a concept of appropriateness of response as perceived by the "respiratory center," be it volume or rate of gas flow or thoracopulmonary expansion (respiratory psychophysics) that has continuously gained support and remains at the forefront in current models of the pathogenesis of dyspnea. A unifying concept of the mechanism of detection of both resistive and elastic loads proposed a role for several responsible receptors: probably joint receptors and the muscle spindle to detect volume change, and the Golgi tendon organ to detect tension and resulting airflow. The methodology involves parameters of magnitude scaling and threshold discrimination of perceived effort as psychophysical measurement techniques for assessing the magnitude of "length-tension inappropriateness."[3,4]

The restrictive lung disease of pneumonia is therefore characterized by tachypnea and hyperventilation attributed to inappropriately increased drive with an increased sense of effort from mechanical changes in the lungs and altered afferent length-tension signals. It is further mediated by enhanced pulmonary reflexes from inflammatory changes in the lung parenchyma. There is also a mechanism of adaptation of respiratory control mechanisms to the increased elastic load in order to minimize the work of breathing. It has been suggested that dyspnea is probably not due to respiratory muscle fatigue in pneumonia, though fatigue may increase the intensity of dyspnea.

In conclusion, no specific peripheral site (dyspnea receptor) is uniquely essential for load detection or perception, but integrated afferent pathways and sites of dyspnogenesis exist that may include the cerebral cortex and central motor command.[5] There is now considerable evidence that discharges from intramuscular receptors project to the cerebral cortex. It is also apparent that much of this confusion as to the mechanism of breathlessness arises from the qualitative description of the sensation and the inability to quantitate accurately what in fact may be different sensations.

Cough

Cough is both a diagnostic sign and symptom of most pulmonary diseases and an indicator of the adequacy of an important pulmonary defense mechanism. It has also been the basis for a lucrative and controversial field of pharmacology: the efforts to suppress a sometimes annoying and debilitating symptom when its functional value is either inapparent or insufficient to tolerate its associated discomfort. More than 600 formulations of cough remedies are on sale in the United States, many on an over-the-counter basis; this class of drugs is the fifth most frequently prescribed.[6]

Cough is characterized by a preliminary deep inspiration, facilitated by glottal dilation, that is highly variable in magnitude but generally not exceeding 50% of vital capacity. This phase is followed by a forced expiration against a closed glottis for the initial 0.2–0.3 second. This period of closure is considered functionally to enhance the effectiveness of the cough but is thought to vary in an unknown manner in the presence of disease and in the elderly. The explosive phase of coughing is no less effective if the glottis remains open, however, and patients with tracheostomies can produce an efficient cough provided there is normal respiratory muscle strength.[7] The intrathoracic and intraabdominal pressures are elevated to 50–100 mm Hg, achieving expiratory flow rates exceeding 6–7 L/second. This step is again facilitated by active glottal participation, in this phase dilation. The air is explosively emitted at speeds up to 12 meters/second, causing vibration of the upper airways and accounting for the sound that accompanies the cough. The sound is influenced by the violence of the oscillations resulting from forces as high as 300 mm Hg and achieving speeds over 200 meters/second; the compliance of the tissues which is influenced by the degree of inflammation and the nature and quantity of secretions.

The stimuli to the respiratory tract that cause coughing also cause reflex bronchoconstriction in the periphery that may last a minute or more. As the glottis opens, intraluminal pressure within the airways rapidly falls; pleural pressure remains high, however, setting the conditions for dynamic compression of central airways, which accounts for most of the volume change in the airways. Thus the efforts of coughing are superimposed on constricted airways, resulting in greater velocity and therefore turbulence of gas flow, loosening particles attached to mucosal surfaces. It also serves to stabilize the airway walls, enhancing the strength of the cough and minimizing dynamic collapse. In the presence of respiratory muscle disease or expiratory muscle weakness, the maximum expiratory flow rate is decreased owing to the reduced dynamic airway compression. The clearance of mucus is then impaired because of the decreased linear velocity of airflow and shearing force, thereby predisposing to atelectasis and pneumonia.

The neural interactions are intricate, with the mediation of axon reflexes along branches of the sensory end-organs that release neuropeptides, such as substance P and other neuropeptokinins. The motor pathway also releases neuropeptides, such as vasoactive intestinal peptide, a smooth muscle relaxant. Thus the bronchomotor response to cough stimuli is a complex balance of constrictor and dilator influences. The observation has been reported that inhaled β-adrenergic drugs may be efficacious in the treatment of cough, but their action may be elaborate, affecting epithelium, mast cells, or airway vascular beds rather than just simply relaxing airway smooth muscle.[8]

The high air velocity necessary to shear mucus from the airway walls can be achieved only down to the sixth or seventh generation of bronchi. Its effectiveness is further dependent on the viscosity and other physical properties of the mucus. The degree of adhesion of the mucus to the airway epithelium is thought to be influenced by both its lipid components and the degree of hydration. Moreover, the underlying periciliary fluid layer may greatly facilitate mobilization. The actual thickness of the mucous layer is also important. It appears essential that an increased amount of mucus (hypersecretion) is present for cough to be an effective clearance mechanism. Cough is not thought to play a role in clearing normal secretions. The lack of detailed information about the significance of the viscoelastic properties of mucus leaves our attempts to facilitate cough and alter the properties of secretions not only empiric but highly speculative.

Involuntary coughing is an entirely vagal phenomenon related to inflammatory or mechanical abnormalities in the upper airways. A variety of chemical and mechanical irritants can cause coughing. Coughing cannot be induced from the smaller airways and alveoli. Teleologically, it can be reasoned that cough at this level would be ineffective because gas could not be made to move fast enough. Although the larynx is observed to be more sensitive to cough stimuli than the tracheobronchial tree, analysis of the cough mechanisms of the latter is simpler because the sensory innervation of the tracheobronchial tree is not as complex as that of the larynx (Table 7.1).

The cough receptors are variously identified as myelinated irritant and nonmyelinated nerve terminals within the bronchial epithelium. The rapidly adapting receptors are concentrated on the walls of the larger airways and are sensitive to topical anesthesia. They have vagal myelinated fibers; and if vagal conduction is blocked, the cough reflex is inhibited. These receptors decrease with age and loss of the cough reflex. The afferent pathways for the cough reflex pass up the vagal nerve fibers to the medulla oblongata, where they relay in or near the nucleus of the tractus solitarius. From here on, where they connect to the brainstem respiratory complex is unknown; but this "cough center" is presumably the site of action of some antitussive drugs such as codeine. The central

TABLE 7.1. Afferent nerves associated with cough reflex.

Sensory nerve characteristics	Location
Myelinated receptors	
Irritant—mechanical, chemical	Mucosal surface of larynx, extra- and intrathoracic airways
Stretch	
Rapidly adapting: intraepithelial—mechanical	Mucosal surface of proximal extra- and intrathoracic tracheobronchial tree
Slowly adapting: smooth muscle—length change	Smooth muscle of proximal extra- and intrathoracic bronchial tree
Nonmyelinated receptor	
C-fiber—chemical	
Bronchial	Mucosal surface of larynx, proximal extra- and intrathoracic airways
Pulmonary (J receptors)	Peripheral airways; also inhibition

nervous system (CNS) control of coughing is characterized by the ability to voluntarily initiate coughing. Thus patients with brainstem damage, although lacking a cough reflex, can still voluntarily induce coughing to clear the upper airways. Hypoxia, if severe enough, can inhibit the cough reflex through a central rather than a peripheral action via the chemoreceptors.

Pulmonary C-fiber receptors, also called J receptors, can inhibit the cough reflex. For nearly all lung conditions associated with coughing (e.g., airway inflammation, responses to allergens, infections) the magnitude of the cough reflex depends on this interaction. Similarly, therapeutic efficacy of various antitussive drugs may also depend on their selective action on the reflexes. Thus a drug that stimulates C fibers might be antitussive.

There are several mechanisms proposed for enhancement of the cough reflex following infection. The most apparent is a result of epithelial denudation, exposing afferent nerve endings and thereby enhancing their accessibility to mechanical or chemical stimuli. The infection itself results in the release of inflammatory mediators, which also may serve to sensitize sensory receptors directly and by enhancing epithelial permeability. A similar mechanism of "up-regulation" due to an increase in bradykinin has been suggested for the cough associated with the administration of angiotensin-converting enzyme inhibitors.[9] With pneumonia or early pulmonary edema, irritant receptors may be stimulated as airways become distorted by pressure from surrounding fluid-filled alveoli. It has been further suggested that when there is consolidation of a large mass of lung, as with lobar pneumonia, the cough may be due to the nonexpansibility of that part of the lung, with distortion of the trachea and main bronchi triggering cough receptors.

Both mucous glycoprotein and serum transudate are present in normal bronchial secretions, but the concentration of glycoprotein mucus is greater than that of serum transudate. A normal tracheobronchial tree responds to infection by increasing the concentration of both mucus glycoprotein and serum transudate in almost similar amounts. In addition, there is a shift in the type of mucous glycoprotein to a more sialylated and sulfated form. The danger of successful mucolytic treatment, given systemically or by aerosol administration (which perhaps fortunately has not yet been clearly achieved), is that destruction of the viscoelastic properties of mucus would prevent its effective clearance by cough. On the contrary, it may be argued that after finding low viscoelasticity during the assessment of physicochemical properties of mucus agents that promote restructuring or cross-linking would be more appropriate. Under such conditions, a mucospissic agent should then be given to optimize cough efficacy. Moreover, the rheologic characteristics favoring mobilization of mucus by the shearing force of a cough do not appear to be the same as those that enhance mucociliary clearance, further complicating the design and choice of mucolytic agents and expectorants.

Fever

Thermogenesis and Pyrogens

Body temperature is normally rigidly maintained within a narrow range of 97°–99°F, made possible by the existence of elaborate regulatory mechanisms that control an apparatus geared to the efficient containment or dissipation of the heat that results from the body's metabolic and biologic processes. The febrile response of pneumonia, characteristic of infection, is just one of a variety of immunologic, inflammatory, and malignant processes capable of disrupting this homeostatic state. Thus temperature elevation (or depression), though a nonspecific manifestation, has been an enduring clinical prerequisite for the diagnosis of pneumonia.

Pyrogens, exogenous or endogenous, are substances that alter the setpoint of the thermoregulatory processes governed by a controller in the region of the rostral preoptic portion of the hypothalamus. Neural influences, however, are not limited to a specific anatomic site. A circadian and other thermal biorhythms exist, as illustrated by body temperature alterations associated with the sleep–wake, menstrual, and activity cycles. The clinical significance of the thermal diurnal rhythm lies in its exaggeration or elimination as a result of infection.

Contemporary thinking is that, except for the continuous fevers of pneumonia or CNS damage, evaluation of the febrile pattern is without value. The classic febrile patterns remain in the medical students' core curriculum, however, along with the associated manifestations of "night sweats" and leukocytosis. The medical students' dilemma of discerning the meaning and correlation of restrained, quotidian, double quotidian, tertian, quartan, biphasic, intermittent, diurnal reversal, Pel-Ebstein, and Jausch-Herxheimer fevers are best forgotten. In today's hospital environment, these fevers can most likely be attributed to variations in oral, rectal, and axillary, or the unpredictable timing of, temperature-taking. Thus the technical and labor-related problems of clinical thermometry are perhaps most often responsible for typical or atypical patterns of this vital sign.

Chemical pyrogens of endogenous origin, including the cytokines—interleukin-1 (IL-1), interleukin-6 (IL-6), interleukin-2 (IL-2), tumor necrosis factor (TNF), interferon—and prostaglandin E_2 (PGE_2), are those best studied; by definition, they are capable of exciting the temperature controller directly. The best known exogenous pyrogen, endotoxin (the lipopolysaccharide complex in the cell wall of gram-negative bacteria), acts on the hypothalamus directly and causes endogenous pyrogen release from leukocytes, phagocytes, and other cells.

The increase in temperature causes an increase in all metabolic reactions (Q_{10} effect) (VO_2 changes about 11% per degree centigrade change in core temperature) and the attainment of a new homeostatic state. With phasic changes in pyrogen concentration as a result of biologic host factors or treatment with antibiotics or antipyretics, the original set-point returns and defervescence occurs as heat loss responses such as sweating are put into play. Approximately 100 ml of water must be evaporated to effect or prevent a 1°C fall or rise in temperature, respectively.

Pyrogenic responses are also mediated by the muramyl dipeptide component of the peptidoglycan layer of the cell wall in gram-positive organisms, which although also present in gram-negative bacteria is not as potent or abundant as their endotoxin; the biologic activity of the endotoxin lies in the lipid A moiety. Cell walls of fungi are also pyrogenic, but fever with viral infections appears to be exclusively a result of their activation of macrophages with subsequent release of inflammatory mediators acting as endogenous pyrogens.[10] Fever, however, is not a measure of pathogenicity, as the toxicity of endotoxin does not depend on the infectivity of the organism. Severe febrile reactions can be associated with pneumonias produced by bacteria of low pathogenicity. Patients with fatal septic syndromes and high fever may have otherwise trivial infections with negative blood cultures.

An awareness is now growing of the potential benefits of fever and fever therapy and the possible detrimental effects of antipyretics. It is argued that if fever was not beneficial it would not have survived through phylogeny, as it is a most metabolically expensive phenomenon, requiring a 20–30% increase in energy consumption for an increase in body temperature of 2°–3°C. Moreover, repeated reference is now made to infected lizards, which as poikilotherms move to a rock to "bask in the sun" in order to elevate their body temperatures, as their survival is

TABLE 7.2. Effects of fever on immunologic responses.

- Polymorphonuclear leukocyte function
  - Motility
    - Enhanced chemotaxis
      - Potentiates migration
      - Depression of emigration
  - Phagocytosis—increased killing rate
- Mononuclear phagocyte function
  - Proliferation
    - Increased responsiveness to cytokines
  - Phagocytosis
    - Increased killing zone, i.e, in warmer body regions
  - Cytokine production
    - Increased induction
- Antibody production
  - Enhances response of B cells, i.e., priming by T-helper cells
- Cell-mediated immunity
  - Increased generation T-helper and T-cytotoxic cells
  - Enhanced antigen recognition
  - Increased rate of IL-1, induced IL-2 release
  - Enhancement of IL-1/IL-2 cascade, i.e., higher rate and duration of secretion
- Cytokine activity
  - Augmentation with blocking of suppressor cell generation
  - Optimizes complement activation

correlated with "fever."[11] Thus reptiles and humans can regulate their body temperature by behavior as well as by the more classic physiologic thermoregulatory mechanisms. It has been found that fever also is associated with better prognosis in homeotherms such as humans during bacterial infection, whereas hypothermia has been associated with higher mortality.

Fever appears to affect leukocyte function in regard to the containment of bacterial infection (Table 7.2) by accelerating leukocyte responses; that is, it potentiates migration of leukocytes into areas of infection, and after the migration the leukocytes are more likely to remain at the site of inflammation and increase their killing effect (cytotoxicity). Temperature elevation enhances the processes involved in initial antigen recognition, that is, antigen presenting and functional interaction between antigen-presenting B cells (B-APC) and T-helper cells. The specific events that follow, such as the rate of IL-1-induced IL-2 release, has been also found to be temperature-dependent. These complex immunologic consequences of fever may then account for the observed decrease in the severity of acute inflammation such as rhinitis in human subjects treated with local hyperthermia (warm humidified air).[12]

Cardiovascular Effects of Fever

In response to an increase in the set-point of the central thermostat, an apparent decrease in environmental temperature is perceived and the body's primary thermogenic response, shivering (shaking chills), is initiated. Further protective mechanisms designed to protect the core temperature then dominate, most importantly central regulation of the cutaneous circulation. Whereas endogenous pyrogens have both a direct and a central action on the cardiovascular system, it is the sympathetic nervous system, with its high level of tonic activity, that is critical for homeostatic control and the characteristic cutaneous and systemic hemodynamic alterations that distinguish the rising, plateau, and defervescent phases of fever.

Acute Phase

Tonic sympathetic activity raising cutaneous vascular resistance normally limits skin perfusion to 5–10% of the cardiac output. In concert with the increase in heat production (shivering, Q_{10} effect), heat loss is diminished by further elevation of the cutaneous vascular resistance and the consequent curtailment of flow. The surface area functionally available for heat loss is thus diminished as a result of precapillary arteriolar and venoconstriction, diverting blood flow from superficial to more central vascular beds. This situation is similar to the circulatory adaptations with congestive heart failure, which in part are accountable for the associated low grade temperature elevations observed. Thus although the rigor serves as an immediate thermogenic mechanism, unlike the vascular alterations it is not essential for the elevation of temperature.[13] Furthermore, along with the withdrawal of vagal tone, the sympathetic discharge results in tachycardia and systemic vasoconstriction. However, the sympathetically mediated vasoconstrictor reflex to dependency is actively maintained. The net effect on flow is variable, serving to achieve the primary goal of maintaining the mean arterial pressure for organ perfusion.

Plateau Phase

As heat production attains its increased level, the thermoregulatory neurons allow the sympathetic tone to return to baseline levels, and cutaneous blood flow resumes its prefebrile levels. Heart rate may remain elevated as a result of a direct effect of elevated blood temperature on the sinoatrial node. Total peripheral vascular resistance (TPR) characteristically falls, and there is an increase in cardiac output in response to this decline in TPR and the residual elevation in sympathetic activity. The TPR falls as a result of the potent synergistic vasodilator actions of endogenous pyrogens, which are both direct and indirect through stimulation of the synthesis of prostanoid vasodilators. The action of IL-1 and TNF to diminish vascular smooth muscle responsiveness to catechols further explains the refractoriness to pressor agents. The hepatic blood flow in particular increases and is associated with an outpouring of cytokines produced by its Kupffer cells.

The peripheral cardiovascular action of the endogenous pyrogens in part explains the dissociation of fever and hemodynamic profiles. With lobar pneumonia, the pulse rate and core temperature are initially highly correlated, but the first sign of deterioration is a progressive rise in heart rate not accounted for by a rise in temperature, which may even be falling. Relative bradycardia, however, has long been thought to characterize enteric fevers. The decreased left ventricular afterload resulting from the reduced TPR is not as readily available to the right ventricle above and beyond the normal high complicance of the pulmonary vascular bed. Therefore it is in patients with preexisting right ventricular dysfunction and its associated pulmonary circulatory adaptation that sudden overt right ventricular failure might develop during fever.

Recovery

The link between sudomotor stimulation and cutaneous vasodilation is maximal during this phase, and the skin is converted to an arteriovenous fistula, with achievable flow rates as high as 50–70% of the cardiac output. The skin has a highly capacious vascular bed that can accommodate flows as high as 7–8 L/minute. The mean arterial pressure declines further, and thermal homeostasis takes precedence over the nonthermoregulatory reflexes necessary for maintenance of driving pressure. When blood flow is redistributed to the skin's compliant vascular bed, the venous capacity in other regions must be accordingly reduced if cardiac filling pressure is to be maintained; thus it appears that central thermoreceptors, through the sympathetic nervous system, trigger visceral vasoconstriction.[14] Ventricular performance returns to normal with decreased ventricular work and a return of both contractility and compliance to basal levels.

With pneumonia there is further complex interaction between thermoregulation and infection, as hypoxia elicits hypothermia. Teleologically, this adaptive response to decreased oxygen demand should promote survival and be beneficial for oxygen-sensitive organs such as the heart and brain. The heat loss observed in hypoxia is due to peripheral vasodilation. Furthermore, a normal thermogenic response to reduced temperature is depressed, as the set-point of the preoptic thermoregulatory neurons is altered. Arginine vasopressin has been suggested as the mediator responsible for this adaptation.[15] The apparent benefits of hypothermia in response to hypoxia are (1) a shift of the oxygen dissociation curve to the left, enhancing oxygen loading in the lung with increased oxygen affinity of the hemoglobin molecule; (2) decreased metabolic rate (Q_{10} effect); and (3) avoiding cardiac and pulmonary work that results from increasing flow and ventilation and the costly energy expenditures in response to hypoxic stimulation. Thus with pneumonia a complex integration of defense mechanisms to stress are operative, utilizing thermoregulatory control. A delicate balance is struck between immunologic imperatives, oxygen supply, and oxygen demand to minimize organ dysfunction and maximize survival.

Leukocyte Count

The classic reaction to bacterial pneumonia is mobilization of the marginated leukocytes as well as stimulation of the bone marrow. This response has been attributed to cytokine action, concurrent with alteration of thermoregulation, with a resultant leukocytosis greater than $15{,}000/mm^3$. Part of the definition of "atypical pneumonia" is failure of the leukocyte (WBC) count to exceed this value, which represents the upper limits of normal (95% confidence limit). The biorhythm for the WBC count is similar to that for body temperature, which can account for a variation in the WBC count of as much as 100% and in the differential count of 30%.

Physiologic leukocytosis under conditions of noninfectious stress is a well known phenomenon most readily reproduced in the laboratory by mental stress or exercise and in the emergency room by seizure activity.[16] The WBC count of spectators and "bench-warmers" of a football game remains normal despite their excitment, whereas that of the players increases almost 300% (Fig. 7.1). This increase occurs despite the fact that the ball is in play only 8 minutes of the 60-minute game, and it

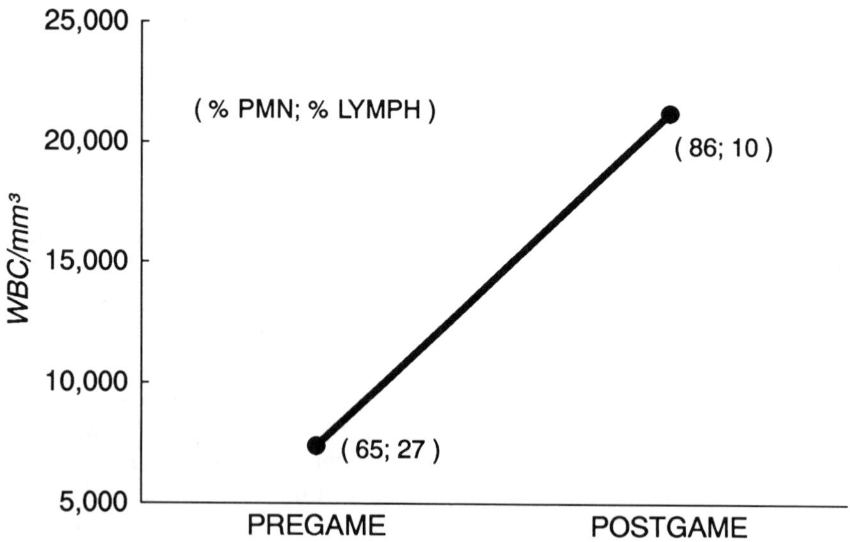

FIGURE 7.1. White blood cell (WBC) count increase in players following a football game. (Data from Edwards and Wood[16])

persists over the 2 hours of actual playing time. The duration and intensity of playing time correlates with the WBC count. The differential count shows an increase in the polymorphonuclear neutrophilic cells (PMNs) and a decrease in the percentage of lymphocytes, which also appears to be a function of the duration and intensity of the effort. The onset and recovery may range from minutes to hours and are characterized by the absence of band forms (no "shift to the left"). Thus there is no apparent output from the bone marrow, which serves to differentiate this "stress" or "demargination" response from that of an infectious stimulus. Nutritional factors, alcohol intake, and age have been associated with an impaired WBC response; and with pneumonia a "delayed" leukocytosis may be observed during recovery.

The leukocyte count resulting from viral infections in inoculated human volunteers who became ill tended to result in WBC counts greater than $10{,}000/mm^3$, associated with an initial increase in neutrophils followed by a rise in lymphocytes after an initial fall.[17] These responses appeared to be a function of the severity of the illness. Moreover, the results did not appear specific for a particular virus. It was also concluded that leukocytosis of $10{,}000–13{,}000/mm^3$ at the onset of illness occurs commonly enough with viral respiratory disease that the WBC count is not useful for differentiating bacterial from viral respiratory infections. It was suggested, however, that subsequent leukopenia favors a viral etiologic agent and leukocytosis a bacterial etiologic agent.[17] As previously noted for thermoregulation, leukocytosis is similarly a manifestation of the invasion or of activation of host macrophages that stimulates endogenous pyrogen release. In addition, cell death and subsequent tissue necrosis also result in pyrogen release and leukocyte mobilization.

An assessment of the WBC count and differential therefore does not have the commonly implied benefit of allowing differentiation between bacterial and nonbacterial disease. Using a WBC count threshold value of $15{,}000/mm^3$ for bacterial disease and less than $15{,}000/mm^3$ for nonbacterial disease, a study in children demonstrated 53% false positivity, 22% false negativity, and only 49% sensitivity.[18] The differential count fared even less well primarily because of an increased number of band forms with nonbacterial disease. Others have concluded that, statistically, an observed change in a patient's serial WBC differential is much more likely to be due to technical factors than to disease and can account for more than 75% of the total variance encountered.[19] It appears that frequent repeat differential counts are not only an unnecessary expense but an almost worthless indulgence.

Physical Examination—Auscultation

The production of sound at the surface of the chest wall generated within lung parenchyma and airways is a complex process. Efforts at exploring the scientific basis of auscultation have utilized recorders and computerized digital analyzers; although failing to displace the stethoscope, these methods have clearly indicated the poor correlation between noninvasiveness and specificity or sensitivity. A representative investigation into the agreement by observers on the presence or absence of physical signs has shown that interobserver repeatability of respiratory physical signs falls midway between chance and total agreement.[20] Similar studies of history taking have also shown considerable interobserver and intraobserver error for symptoms of cough, sputum production, and chest pain.

When the lung between the trachea and the point of auscultation is airless, the higher frequencies, including the formants of vowels, are transmitted, and speech becomes intelligible (the clarity of e.g., say the number ninety-nine). This process is known as *bronchophony*. A study of the frequency analysis of voice sound recorded from the chest wall of pneumonia patients and normal subjects has explained the e to a change over an area of consolidation that should allow the higher frequencies through.[21] It was found that even though higher frequencies were transmitted by consolidated lung (1000 Hz rather than 400 Hz) the higher frequencies of the sound e (2000–3500 Hz) did not pass, so the sound becomes an a; hence the apparent paradox of bronchophony was clarified.[21]

Breath sounds are produced in the turbulent zone of the respiratory tract from the mouth to the segmental bronchi. Normal lung parenchyma acts as an acoustic filter that attenuates and selectively filters breath sounds, normally allowing penetration of only low-frequency sounds, and their passage to the surface of the chest wall. As a result of consolidation, sounds produced in the large airways are much less altered, thus producing bronchial breathing, during which the higher frequencies are better preserved. The sounds heard on auscultation are probably generated at the level of the trachea. The low frequencies fall below the theshold of audibility early during expiration, but the high frequencies are audible throughout expiration as well as inspiration. Because the whisper lacks the low frequencies selectively transmitted through the normal chest, it is inaudible over air-containing lung. The high-pitched components of the noise of turbulence and the formants of vowels are, however, transmitted through airless lung, so whispered speech (*whispering pectoriloquy*) becomes intelligible.[22] It occurs under the same conditions as bronchial breathing and bronchophony and completes the triad of auscultatory signs of consolidation.

Crackles are produced by the sudden equalization of gas pressure and snapping open of air passages. It has been demonstrated that, at low lung volumes, dependent airways close.[23] Atelectasis is a direct consequence of such ventilation below closing capacity, and its occurrence is enhanced by prolonged shallow breathing such as occurs with pneumonia. The resulting decrease in compliance, or increased elastic recoil of the lung, leads to an increase in transpulmonary pressure. Crackles are then generated with the reopening of the distal atelectatic lung units as they are ventilated at end-inspiration. The more crackles, the greater the number of collapsed peripheral lung units.[23]

Pleural disease may also produce crackling, which at times is indistinguishable from that produced by parenchymal disease. A pleural crackle (*rub*) is produced by sudden jerky movements of the pleural surface momentarily delayed by friction.[24] The individual components of the crackling are produced by a sudden release of tangential tension in a superficial portion of the lung momentarily arrested in its sliding movements by a frictional force between the visceral and parietal pleura. These sounds may be expiratory as well as inspiratory, which serves to distinguish them from pulmonary crepitations. Fluid in the pleural space increases the acoustic barrier, and the breath sounds become fainter or inaudible over the chest, even in the presence of underlying consolidation. At the upper margin of a pleural effusion the thin layer of fluid still permits transmission of higher sound frequencies, giving the breath sounds a nasal quality termed *egophony*.[22] The bubbling sounds heard in the presence of copious secretions are presumably formed by bubbling of air through liquids, which repeatly form a thin film that breaks explosively. In patients with pneumonia, as with other conditions such as pulmonary edema, this bubbling occurs in the proximal airways, not at the alveolar level. The "inspiratory squawk" combines a crackle followed by a brief wheezing sound. Such sounds have been reported in patients with hypersensitivity pneumonitis. The sounds result from sudden opening of airways of differing sizes.

The value of auscultation, though limited, has been greatly enhanced by standardization of nomenclature corrupted by the passage of time, differences in translation, and qualitative descriptions.[25] Efforts to relate lung sounds to physiologic or pathophysiologic events rather than to anatomic changes has also enhanced their value.[22] Correct diagnostic testing is ensured by both a careful history and competent physical examination. Repeated studies have shown that pleural rub, decreased percussion note, and reduced breath sounds have physician agreement well in excess of chance, whereas signs such as whispering pectoriloquy and tactile vocal fremitus show agreement that is only a little better than chance.[26] Moreover, a comparison of diagnoses based on clincal findings with true diagnoses showed that 28% of diagnoses by physicians were incorrect.[26] It was further shown that the more often physicians differed from their peers regarding the presence or absence of signs, the more likely they were to make an incorrect diagnosis. Finally, although such variability appears unacceptable for diagnostic and therapeutic decisions, it has been pointed out that it is about the same as that found with clinical data collection in general, including interpretations of chest roentgenograms, and that it is with good reason that physicians rarely use single observations for clinical decision making.[27]

Pleuritic Chest Pain

Sharp, stabbing, localized pain related to inspiratory effort has been a classic sign of pneumonia commonly termed *pleurisy*. The visceral pleura does not have pain fibers, which has greatly clarified the mechanism of pleuritic chest pain and focused attention on the parietal pleura, which has abundant pain fibers. Several theories of the origin of pleuritic chest pain have been proposed.[28] The oldest and favorite of clinicians attributes the pain to friction produced by the opposition and movement of the two roughened, inflamed pleural surfaces. It has always been somewhat bothersome that pain is often present without, and independent of, the presence of a pleural friction rub. In fact, pain may be at its peak with a breathhold at the maximum inspiratory position only to be alleviated with an expiratory maneuver. Others have attributed the pain to contraction of hyperalgesic intercostal muscles. The pain has also been attributed to the traction of tissues immediately underlying the parietal pleura also served by the distribution of the intercostal nerves. Autopsy studies have failed to shown consistent evidence of pleuritis that would account for the pleurisy in fatal cases of lobar pneumonia.

Most observers have concluded that pain is initiated as the chest expands and exerts tension on the sensitive, edematous (if not inflamed) parietal pleura. With inspiration, the increasing tension brings the pain to its peak, and it subsides with expiration. Thus the tendency of the pain to be greatest in the lower thorax is attributed to the partitioning of the tidal breath and greater tension on the parietal pleura in this area. Such a mechanism is supported by the persistence of pain in the presence of an ipsilateral pleural effusion in patients with pneumonia or as reported after a therapeutic pneumothorax in patients with tuberculosis.

The lower chest, including the outer segment of the diaphragmatic pleura, is innervated by the lower six intercostal nerves, which also supply the abdominal wall. Pleuritic pain may therefore be referred to the abdomen. It is a surgeon's nightmare to have performed an exploratory laparotomy when the diagnosis is actually pneumonia. The central portion of the diaphragm is innervated by the phrenic nerve, which enters the spinal cord through the third, fourth, and fifth dorsal roots. Such pain may be referred homolaterally to the neck and tip of the shoulder (Capps' area).

It must be stressed that not all chest pain seemingly related to inspiration is pleuritic in origin. Pain in the chest wall that is musculoskeletal in origin must be differentiated. Classically, cough may result in an athlete's muscle strain or tear of an intercostal or "accessory" muscle of respiration because of the force involved—even a fracture of the bony or cartilagenous portion of a rib. Such coughing does not have to be violent; it may be only a minor, subtle episode in a mechanically predisposing position. The pain may be indistinguishable from one that is pleuritic in origin, timing, intensity, or quality. Its origin from chest wall structures is suggested by localized tenderness to direct palpation. Furthermore, on the basis of autopsy studies, roentgenograms show only about half the rib fractures that actually exist.

The mechanisms of pain production have been reviewed elsewhere.[29] The initiation of pain is the result of tissue injury with subsequent release of inflammatory mediators, including kinins, prostaglandins, and potassium, which stimulate pain receptors.[29] According to the specificity theory, the pain impulses are transmitted by fine myelinated and unmyelinated fibers contained in peripheral nerves. The intensity of reverberation in central circuits determine pain intensity; or as also proposed, the intensity of peripheral receptor excitation beyond some critical threshold level is determinant of pain intensity. Yet another thesis of "gate control" suggests a critical ratio between the inhibitory effects of fast-transmitting myelinated versus the enhancing effects of slow-transmitting unmyelinated fibers. Inflammatory mediators favor stimulation of the receptors of unmyelinated fibers. The neurotransmitters acting as synapses to enhance impulse conduction are unknown, but evidence has pointed to substance P. This neuropeptide is concentrated in pain-mediating neural cell bodies and terminals. This unadecapeptide has also been suggested as a chemical mediator of airway hyperreactivity associated with asthma. It may be responsible for pain, along with other, yet unspecified polypeptides, by influencing differentially the activity of myelinated and unmyelinated pain fibers.

In summary, because there are essentially no pain fibers in the lung parenchyma or visceral pleura the pain associated with pneumonia must be attributed to other structures. Its exacerbation by inspiration, coughing, limb movement, and postural changes tends to cause unilateral splinting and tachypnea with small tidal breaths influencing the movement of the chest wall. The altered partitioning of the tidal breath may contribute to the sensation of dyspnea, the appearance of atelectasis, and the auscultatory findings of crackles; it may also have a significant adverse effect on lung clearance mechanisms and gas exchange. Analgesics are indicated for these reasons and for symptomatic relief.

Radiologic Studies

The routine posteroanterior and lateral radiographs of the chest remain the initial studies for the radiologic diagnosis of pneumonia. Although a chest radiograph may be normal during early pneumonia, it is uncommon. Radiographic findings indicate definite or probable pneumonia in 2.6–28.0% of adults seen in various emergency rooms for acute respiratory illness. Several modern imaging modalities have been applied to the diagnosis and assessment of pneumonia. Among the radiologic armamentarium shown to have a real or potentially significant clinical role in chest diseases are computed tomography, nuclear medicine (nucleology), ultrasonography, magnetic resonance imaging, and digital radiography. In particular, strategems have been developed utilizing these techniques in the intensive care unit patient.

Chest Radiography

The pneumonias, by convention, have been divided into three types: lobar pneumonia, bronchopneumonia, and interstitial pneumonia. This division was based on postmortem findings and adapted to radiographic description. It is not surprising therefore that the descriptive utility frequently seems forced and artifactual, usually adding little specificity to the diagnosis. All pneumonias, regardless of etiology, present a spectrum of radiographic features resulting in a considerable overlap for specific bacterial infections and even making the differential diagnosis of viral from bacterial pneumonia inaccurate strictly on the basis of their radiographic apperance.[30] Despite this problem, continued efforts are made to relate specific pathogens to radiographic characteristics of focal and diffuse processes. With *Legionella* pneumonia, for example, a study of 14 fatal cases found no lobar predilection, whereas others have reported a predilection for the lower lobes.[30]

Organisms causing atypical pneumonia are by definition more likely to cause bilateral interstitial infiltrates without pleural effusions. However, pleural effusions are reported in 24–63% of cases of *Legionella*.[31] Radiographic features, similar to the "characteristic" clinical presentations for "atypical" pneumonia, are just as unreliable for distinguishing it from "typical" bacterial pneumonia, and this syndrome classification is falling into disuse. Upper lobe pneumonia has the same differential diagnosis as that for lower lobe pneumonia. Although pyogenic and *Mycoplasma* pneumonias occur more often in the lower lobes, their occurrence in the upper zone is still common enough that radiographic specificity is lost. Involvement of the upper lobes alone is uncommon with either staphylococcal or gram-negative infections. The most common diffuse pneumonias are those caused by viral agents; and in immunocompromised hosts with acquired immunodeficiency syndrome (AIDS), *Pneumocystis* is the first consideration. Confluence of patchy airspace infiltrates is seen with both *Pneumocystis* and influenzal pneumonia and, moreover, may be localized to a single lobe with segmental consolidation.

The relative sparing of the lung periphery seen in cardiac or noncardiac pictures of acute pulmonary edema is nonspecific. It has been suggested that the increased compliance of the lung "cortex" enhances lymphatic resorption, thus diminishing peripheral (relative to central) edema and giving rise to the "bat's wing" and "butterfly" patterns. This inability to differentiate cardiac from noncardiac pulmonary edema is especially apparent on supine portable films of patients with severe pulmonary edema.

Rounded pneumonia and possibly a related entity, round atelectasis, are frequently confused with tumor and are appreciated only after a response to bronchodilator therapy and antibiotics.[32] The causative agents are usually undefined, but an infectious process is thought to initiate a predominantly alveolar inflammation and exudation. The infiltrate spreads from a small peripheral alveolar locus centrifugally through the interalveolar channels (pores of Kohn and channels of Lambert), accounting for its initial nonsegmental distribution and spherical shape.

Once the diagnosis of pneumonia is established, chest roentgenograms are best used to follow the course of the pneumonia over the following days to weeks for either normal resolution or complications. There is poor correlation between the severity of the abnormalities seen radiographically and the prognosis. Resolution is highly variable but tends to be delayed with *Legionella pneumonia*.[31] Dehydration, often suggested to mask underlying pneumonia in the elderly, is associated with rapid progression of opacities with "early hydration." Both animal and clinical studies[33] have confirmed that the more appropriate term of this therapeutic if not diagnostic endeavor should be "early drowning."

Chest films are routinely obtained for the evaluation of fever in neutropenic patients, but their usefulness has been questioned and only recently clarified.[34] In such a population the chest film is abnormal in 22% of patients. However, 17% of patients had abnormalities in the absence of clinical findings of pneumonia, and the test resulted in changes in therapy in 61% of the episodes of persistent or recurrent fever, of which 40% resulted in clinical improvement. Morever, there was no evidence that neutropenic patients, as similarly suggested for dehydrated patients, were "unable to mount" an infiltrate with lung infection.[34]

Computed Tomography

Computed tomography (CT) scans have been suggested for management of patients with pneumonia when the conventional roentgenogram fails to clarify the presence, location, extent, or nature of the infection. The apparent clinical benefit of distinguishing airspace from interstitial disease radiologically is often lost on further pathologic analysis. There are no CT findings characteristic of a specific bacterial infection. It may be useful, though, in a patient whose chest film has not yet become abnormal. CT has been most frequently suggested for the early detection of *Pneumocystis* pneumonia in AIDS patients. Also it is used to facilitate percutaneous invasive procedures, including biopsies, aspirations, and tube thoracostomy placement for drainage.

The standard bedside portable chest film frequently fails to adequately define the retrocardiac, costophrenic, juxtadiaphragmatic, and paravertebral infiltrate and the extent of a fluid collection in the pleural space. It has been recognized that CT is a valuable tool for detecting the full extent of noncardiac pulmonary edama as well as the presence of nosocomial, drug, and radiation pneumonias. Complicated pneumonias with pleural involvement, abscess formation, and empyema with bronchopleural fistula are readily defined with CT scanning.

High-resolution CT, defined as thin-section CT optimized by using a high-spatial-resolution algorithm (1- to 2-mm collimation) in contrast to routine thick sections (10-mm collimation) emphasizes the secondary pulmonary lobule. It has been used for the evaluation of hypersensitivity pneumonitis; but unlike the characteristic change in lobular anatomy suggested for chronic interstitial disease, findings have been nonspecific for acute hypersensitivity pneumonitis.

Ultrasonography

The most frequent use of ultrasonography in patients with pneumonia is to identify the extent of pleural fluid collections and facilitate thoracentesis or tube drainage. Furthermore, the nature and aspiratability of the pleural collection may be determined. A hypoechoic collection is likely to be "complicated," distributed into fibrin-septated "loculated" subspaces; an anechoic collection is uncomplicated. The more complex the collection, the more likely (but not certain) it is that an empyema is present, whereas an anechoic collection may still be infected.

A significant number of echo-free pleural effusions, up to 20% in some reports, do not yield free fluid. Various explanations include high viscosity of an otherwise hypoechoic effusion that may be simple hemorrhage or pus. More frequently it represents a poorly reported entity first described in group A β-hemolytic streptococcal pneumonia termed *pleural edema*. This is potentially a totally reversibe anechoic phenomenon.

Nuclear Radiography

The use of scintigraphy to detect infectious and noninfectious inflammatory lung disease is expanding rapidly, made possible by the development of radiopharmaceuticals and methods as well as by the performance of controlled clinical trials.[35] Perfusion lung scans in patients with adult respiratory distress syndrome (ARDS) show nonsegmental focal perfusion deficits, mostly in the peripheral and dorsal portions of the lung, and a shift away from the dependent lung zones as a result of the gravity-dependent distribution of pulmonary edema. This finding is nonspecific for any form of pulmonary edema and reflects increased resistance in the microvasculature secondary to alveolar and perivascular edema with a gravitational gradient.

The use of gallium 67 citrate scans and indium 111 oxine-labeled granulocytes have become standard techniques for evaluating pulmonary infection in immunocompromised hosts, particularly those with AIDS or drug-induced immunosuppression, especially transplant recipients. More recently, technetium diethylenetriamine pentaacetic acid (^{99m}Tc-DTPA) aerosol clearance and thallium 201 chloride scans have been used to a limited extent. Gallium, a group III B metal, behaves like iron in vivo and binds to unsaturated serum transferrin in the serum; and localization of gallium in inflammatory processes may be due in part to the ability of the protein lactoferrin (with a stronger affinity for the radionuclide) to remove gallium from transferrin and its subsequent sequestration intracellularly. As a result of cell lysis, especially of granulocytes, phagocytosis of the protein complex occurs, particularly by lung macrophages. Also as a result of its binding at cellular surface receptors, retention in areas of inflammation occurs, a consequence of protein extravasation due to the associated increased permeability of lung vasculature.

There is nothing specific in the unptake pattern of gallium for any of the disease processes causing ARDS. However, the specificity of gallium uptake in AIDS patients for *Pneumocystis carinii* peumonia can be as high as 95% when intensity of lung uptake is considered. The evaluation of the heterogenicity of the gallium uptake also increases the positive predictive value to almost 90%.[35] Other patterns of gallium uptake also have utility, such as localized uptake, which most often is secondary to bacterial pneumonia and focal regional lymph node uptake, suggestive of mycobacterial infection.

Indium 111-labeled leukocyte scintigraphy, though not as sensitive as gallium 67 for the diagnosis of diffuse opportunistic pulmonary infections (e.g., *Pneumocystis*), has been shown to be superior for identifying focal pulmonary lesions. Neutophils circulate with an average lifetime of 6 hours, after which they marginate to various tissues, such as the lungs. The labeling procedures for indium is time-consuming and technically demanding; it requires harvesting the leukocytes (the patient must have an adequate leukocyte count, i.e., >4000 cells/μl) and subsequently labeling the cell suspension, centrifuging it, and delicately resuspending the indium 111-labeled leukocyte pellet for injection. Images are generally obtained within 24 hours of injection. Sequestration in the lung, as with gallium 67, may represent a nonspecific inflammatory response rather than infection. There are both specific and nonspecific sequestration mechanisms related to pulmonary vascular injury and enhanced pulmonary clearance of damaged cells by alveolar macrophages. Focal, in contract to diffuse, uptake, especially if of high intensity, identifies an infectious etiology in more than 50% of cases.

The disadvantage of gallium scanning is that after intravenous injection of the radiopharmaceutical at least 48 hours and sometimes even 96 hours are required for the blood pool to clear the chest; moreover, other nuclear radiographic procedures cannot be performed for 10–14 days. For this reason thallium scans have been introduced; not only are they readily available within 2 hours, but other nuclear scanning techniques may be initiated if required. Preliminary data suggest a high correlation with the gallium scans, with similar sensitivity and specificity.

Magnetic Resonance Imaging

The use of magnetic resonance imaging (MRI) for evaluating lung parenchyma has been limited by a poor signal-to-noise ratio and physiologic motion. The high T1-weighted signals seen with airspace consolidation resulting from alveolar hemorrhage was reported to allow differentiation of pulmonary infarction from pneumonia by MRI.[36] The aging hemorrhage, because of methemoglobin formation, produces a hyperintense T1-weighted signal. The utility of MRI profusion scores has also been reported to facilitate the early diagnosis of *Pneumocystis* pneumonia, whereas the T1 and T2 relaxation times were of no predictive value.[37] The potential for MRI to monitor disease activity reflecting progression or response to therapy makes it a technology whose expaned role in the assessment of pneumonia is to be anticipated.

Other Methods

Digital imaging, nuclear quantitation of amine receptors, and positron emission tomography scanning have not yet found significant clinical application in pneumonia patients. As technology, methodology, and clinical experience grow, this picture may be expected to change, with the radiologic asessment of pneumonia to be enhanced and the patient's presentation redefined.

Complications

Pleural Effusion

The normal pleural space is nonexistent, and the lung's visceral pleura is in contact with the chest wall's parietal pleura. The few milliliters of fluid normally present simultaneously provide lubrication and enhance the surface adherence properties while allowing mechanical coupling of the lung and chest wall. The mesothelial membranes are highly permeable, offering little resistance to fluid and electrolyte flux and resulting in a pleural fluid composition similar to that of interstitial fluid. The protein content of the liquid is, however, maintained lower than that of lymph and of the interstitial compartment. The parenchymal inflammatory process of pneumonia extending to the pleural surface alters pleural permeability, resulting in an elevated pleural fluid protein concentration. Moreover, the associated release of proteases and inflammatory mediators causes degeneration of the oncotic gradient across the pleural membranes.

The arterial blood supply of the parietal pleura is systemic, and primarily, if not entirely, for the visceral pleura via the bronchial arteries in humans (via the pulmonary arteries in the dog).[38] The venous return is predominantly to the left side of the heart from the visceral pleura and to the right artium from the parietal pleura. Drainage of normal or abnormal volumes of fluid, amounts of protein, or quantities of particulate or cellular material in the pleural space is now thought to be primarily via parietal pleural lymphatics.[39] The continuity of the parenchyma's interstitium with the visceral subpleural interstitium readily allows escape of fluid from this peripheral portion of the extravascular space of the lung into the pleural cavity.

The pleurolymphatic drainage of the parietal pleura is primarily to the right lymphatic duct. The parietal (in contrast to the visceral) submesothelial lymphatic system communicates directly with the pleural space via a variety of specialized anatomic pleurolymphatic structures in its surface, such as stomata and crevices. Moreover, costomedial and caudocephalic gradients of pleural liquid pressures are maintained and enhanced by diaphragmatic respiratory excursion and cardiac contraction. Thus the setting for bulk flow along a hydraulic pressure gradient exists, and the fluid dynamics are affected by postural gravity-dependent alterations as well. The importance of the rate and depth of respiration in facilitating removal of artificial hydrothorax has been demonstrated in anesthetized animals. Its clinical counterpart is readily apparent in the demonstrated diurnal variation seen in fluid removal via lymphatic absorption during the night.[40] This variation can be attributed to the relative hypoventilation during sleep, but because the rate of fluid formation persists unabated it may explain the phenomenon of paroxysmal nocturnal dyspnea in noncardiogenic and cardiogenic pleural effusions.

The appearance of a pleural effusion indicates the adverse effects of pneumonia and associated pleural inflammation, immunologic or infectious, on the forces governing the filtration and drainage of pleural fluid. The processes of Starling-dependent filtration and bulk transfer of liquid and protein from the lung interstitium become predominant over the sucking capability of lymphatic-dependent absorption. In this setting, the use of steroids therapeutically may affect the egress or ingress of inflammatory pleural effusions through pleural surfaces. With pneumonia, the high protein concentration of the pleural fluid reflects increased permeability, which may result from inflammatory injury to (1) the visceral pleural mesothelial cells or (2) the visceral pleural microcirculation. However, with increased-permeability pulmonary edema, or ARDS, the alveolar-epithelial barrier is disrupted and the resultant alveolar flooding decompresses the perivascular interstitial space, accounting for the infrequency of radiologically detectable or large pleural effusions. However, the frequency of pleural effusions with increased-permeability pulmonary edema has been reported to be nearly the same as that with hydrostatic pulmonary edema.[41]

The right and left pleural spaces do not communicate with each other, and their elimination by pleurectomy, pleurodesis, or phylogeny, as in the elephant, does not have a significant effect on respiratory function. Pleural effusion frequently causes a disproportionate degree of dyspnea in comparison to the magnitude of impairment of pulmonary function as reflected by decreases in lung volumes and arterial oxygenation.[42] The volume of pleural fluid present is partitioned between an increase in chest wall volume and a decrease in lung volume. Therefore although there is a significant relation between the size of the pleural effusion and the decrease in lung volume, the partitioning is apparent by the smaller increases in lung volumes relative to the volume of fluid removed with thoracentesis. This partitioning is determined by the relative compliances of the two structures: the lung and the chest wall (Fig. 7.2). With pneumonia the stiffer lung relative to the chest wall shows a smaller change in functional residual capacity.

The effects of pleural effusion on the lung and chest wall volumes are influenced by both the pleural liquid pressure at the level of the effusion

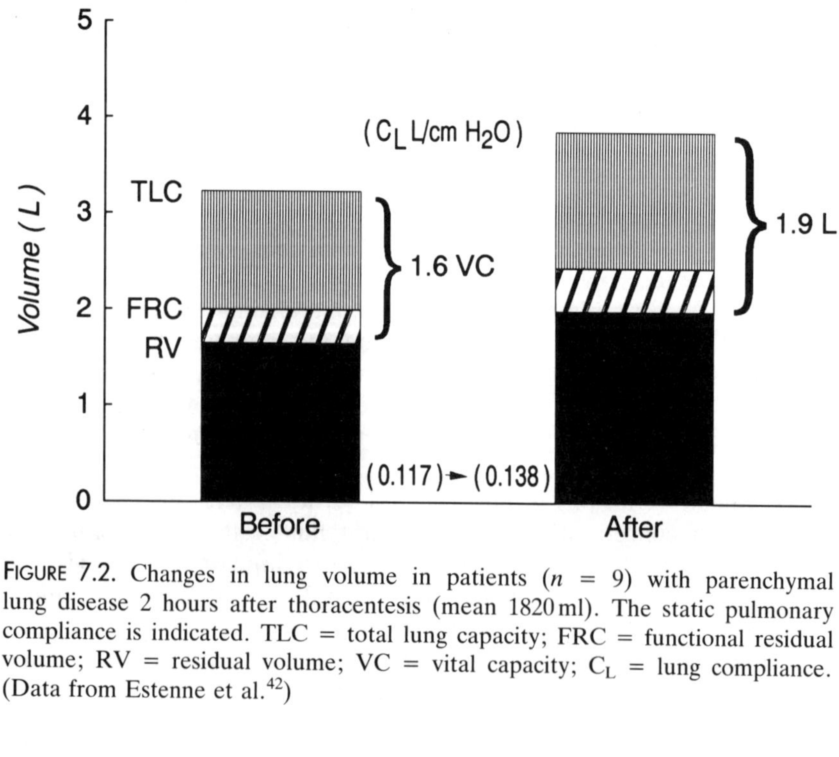

FIGURE 7.2. Changes in lung volume in patients (n = 9) with parenchymal lung disease 2 hours after thoracentesis (mean 1820 ml). The static pulmonary compliance is indicated. TLC = total lung capacity; FRC = functional residual volume; RV = residual volume; VC = vital capacity; C_L = lung compliance. (Data from Estenne et al.[42])

and the pleural surface pressure above the pleural effusion. Dyspnea appears to be related to the shortening of inspiratory muscles, which occurs when breathing at an increased chest wall volume. The shortened muscles operate on a disadvantageous portion of their length–tension curve, and neural-mechanical input–output mismatching occurs. This "length–tension inappropriateness" gives rise to the sensation of dyspnea and is alleviated with thoracentesis and lengthening of the inspiratory muscles at end-expiration and their placement on a more advantageous portion of their length–tension curve. The symptomatic alleviation of dyspnea is therefore found to be independent of and to correlate poorly with changes in either lung volumes or blood gases.

The pleural fluid PO_2 and PCO_2 are readily altered by changes in the FIO_2 and level of ventilation[43,44] (Fig. 7.3). This alteration illustrates the dynamic nature of the equilibrium between the pleura, lymphatics, underlying lung, and pleural fluid. Moreover, postural effects on cardiac and pulmonary function are magnified in the presence of a pleural effusion (Fig. 7.4). Thoracentesis is thus a potential effective therapeutic intervention for cardiac and pulmonary insufficiency.

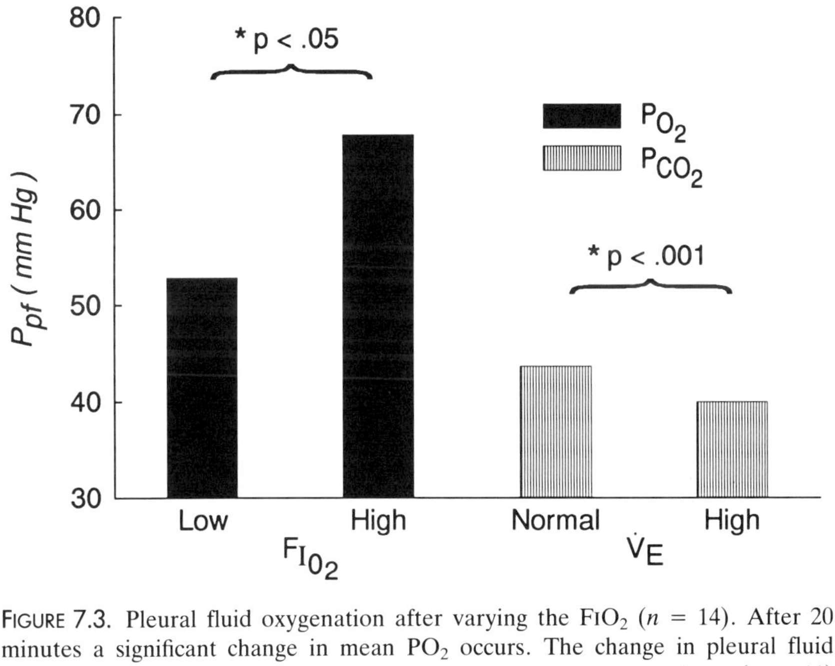

FIGURE 7.3. Pleural fluid oxygenation after varying the FIO_2 (n = 14). After 20 minutes a significant change in mean PO_2 occurs. The change in pleural fluid PCO_2 is also shown after 10 minutes of hyperventilation in patients (n = 11) being mechanically ventilated. The $PaCO_2$ was decreased from 36.7 mm Hg to 28.7 mm Hg. (Data from Zaman and Karetzky[43] and Brandstetter et al.[44])

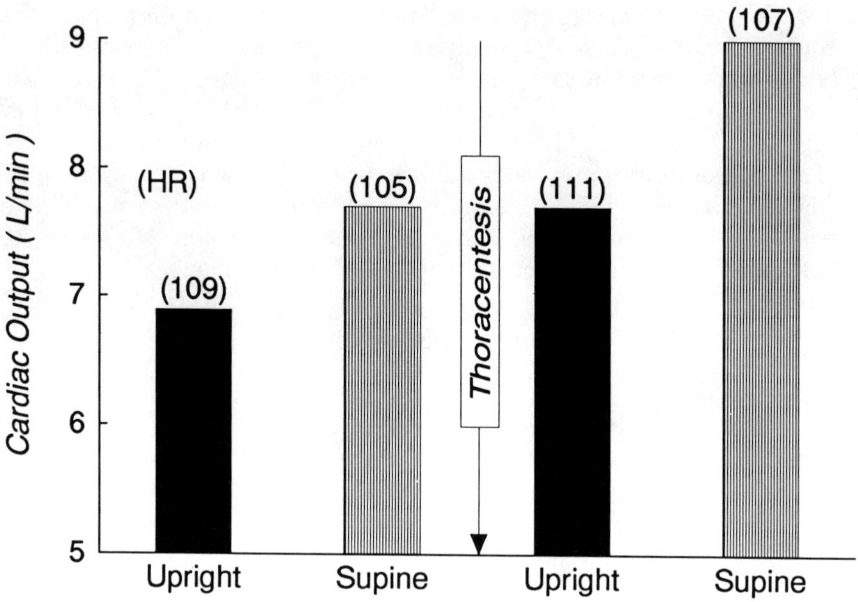

FIGURE 7.4. Hemodynamic consequences of thoracentesis in 12 patients in the upright and supine postures. The increase in cardiac output was due to an increase in stroke volume in response to decreases in both pulmonary and systemic vascular resistances.

Pneumothorax and Pneumomediastinum

Infection, as with other degenerative diseases of the lung, impairs the integrity of the walls of the distal bronchioloalveolar structures, including existing bullae, or pneumatoceles. It then allows escape (leakage) of air at less than the usual critical pressure gradient of the epithelial barrier, which in normal lungs is approximately 40 cm H_2O. The resulting interstitial air then dissects its way underneath or to the visceral pleural surface. It may remain there under various degrees of tension as a subpleural loculation (bleb, mediastinal emphysema); it may dissect further through extrathoracic tissue planes (subcutaneous emphysema); or it may "rupture" into the pleural cavity (pneumothorax).

The role of interstitial emphysema in pneumothorax formation has been defined in both the laboratory and clinical settings.[45] It is the transpulmonic pressure gradient between the alveoli and interstitial space due to inadequate venting and an elevated intraalveolar or lowered pulmonary intravascular pressure (or both), rather than the absolute intrathoracic pressure, that is responsible for interstitial air accumulation. Inflammation by damaging the epithelial barrier and impairing its integrity predisposes to infectious interstitial emphysema.[46]

The concurrent cough of pneumonia produces shearing forces that alter the topographic pressure profile along the pleural surface. The cough more importantly causes the critical pressure gradient across epithelium-lined intersitium to be exceeded, as intrathoracic pressures as high as 150 mm Hg may be produced. In addition, the extrapulmonary transmission of the airways' positive pressure may significantly impair venous return, serving to lower the pulmonary vascular hydrostatic and thus interstitial pressure. Hence apparent innocuous coughing represents a real determinant of the occurrence of pneumothorax. Consideration must also be given to the increase in surface tension resulting from the impaired synthesis and enhanced inactivation of surfactant that occurs in alveoli affected by pneumonia. Therefore a combination of increased hydrostatic and surface forces exerted on compromised parenchymal structures predisposes to the dissection of air, pneumothorax development, and the entity best termed infectious interstitial emphysema.

The pathophysiology of pneumothorax associated with the classic fluid-filled alveoli of lobar pneumonia is presumably related to the associated airway obstruction. This situation impairs pressure equilibration of entrapped alveolar gases, resulting in interstitial dissection of air and finally decompression into the pleural cavity. Pneumothorax occurs in patients with pneumonia and pulmonary alveolar proteinosis following bronchoalveolar lavage (BAL).[47] Approximately 40–60% of BAL fluid is not removed with suctioning, depending on the severity of the destructive parenchymal process. The retained fluid may promote local gas trapping as a consequence of the loss of the protective decompression mechanism of collateral ventilation acting via channels at both the alveolar and bronchiolar levels.[48] Collateral flow has similarly been observed to be impaired in the lung of a dog model when water is injected into a lobe.[49] Also, obstruction of the sublobar segments at low lung volumes in animal models results in a greater outward acting stress on the alveolar wall (alveolar pressure gradient) as a result of pulmonary interdependence.[50] The potential significance of these pathogenic mechanisms of pneumothorax are enhanced with middle lobe segmental involvement, as there is only a single interface with another segment.[47]

Attention has been given to the presentation of AIDS-related *Pneumocystis carinii* pneumonia with spontaneous pneumothorax. The occurrence of adventitious air was reported in association with *Pneumocystis* pneumonia in immunocompromised patients prior to the recognition of AIDS. This problem presented spontaneously as mediastinal emphysema, subcutaneous emphysema, or both unilateral and bilateral pneumothorax. Previously, attention to the role of infection in the pathogenesis of infectious interstitial emphysema was most clearly illustrated in patients with tuberculosis. *Mycobacterium tuberculosis* infection long has been considered to be a common cause of pneumothorax, particularly in its cavitary form; and in some reports it has been associated with as many as

60% of cases presenting as apparent spontaneous pneumothorax. Similarly, necrotizing pneumonias associated with aspiration have been shown to have a high incidence of pneumothorax and pneumomediastinum. These infections predispose to barotrauma if ventilatory support is required. Such injury occurs with both pressure and volume ventilators, and the incidence is further promoted with positive end-expiratory pressure (PEEP), though the peak inspiratory pressure is of prime importance.[51,52] The pressure range of assisted positive pressure or volume ventilators is usually a minimum of 20–25 cm H_2O. This level is often exceeded when patients expire out of phase with the instrument. Overexpansion of small airways and alveoli due to maldistribution of volume and pressure may result in occlusion of thin-walled microcirculatory elements in their walls. Thus mechanical ventilation, by increasing intraalveolar pressure, enhances the development of a local perivascular pressure gradient, which, especially with infection, does not have to exceed 40 cm H_2O to cause alveolar leakage and continuous escape of air from the alveoli to the interstitium and vascular sheaths.

Extrapulmonary air is not pathognomonic of any specific interstitial degenerative, inflammatory, or fibrotic process. However, the occurrence of pneumothorax in AIDS patients serves to demonstrate that a particularly invasive form of infection, with an especially destructive lesion of the distal lobule, alveoli, and terminal bronchioles, such as reported with *Pneumocystis* pneumonia, predisposes to pneumothorax. *P. carinii* pneumonia serves as a model for inflammatory interstitial emphysema originating in the bronchioloalveolar interstitial space as a result of disruption of the alveolar lining due to type I cell necrosis and denudation with breakdown of bronchioloalveolar septa. This situation would predispose to the more widely recognized entity of barotrauma, particularly pneumothorax complicating mechanical ventilation.

Lung Abscess

During the preantibiotic era, lung abscess was reported to be associated with a mortality of 60–100%, with the value of bronchoscopy difficult to assess. Mortality was reduced to 20% with surgical intervention; and for the nontuberculous abscess, thoracotomy for drainage, if not surgical resection, was considered obligatory.[53] Antibiotic therapy has reduced mortality to approximately 7%. The outstanding pathologic feature of lung abscess remains the rapidity with which necrosis goes on to liquefication and sloughing with sphacelus formation at its extreme. The necrotizing pneumonia that progresses to abscess formation cannot be distinguished initially by clinical features to be due to pyogenic or putrefactive organisms.

Aspiration of mouth organisms following states of unconsciousness, allowing for ongoing symbiosis of a polymicrobial flora in the lung, has long been recognized in the pathogenesis of lung abscess; and the rarity of such a putrid complication in edentulous people and children free of pyorrhea alveolaris has been repeatedly noted.[54] The unusual virulence demonstrated by the anaerobic organisms involved, which usually are of low pathogenicity, has been explained by synergy and the propitious conditions of the event. They include the liquid nature and volume of the aspirate and the concentration of organisms in the inoculum. Other factors are thought to include impaired upper airway protection (diminished gag reflex), lower mucociliary clearing, and impairment of basic immunologic defense mechanisms. Approximately one-third of lung abscesses are complicated by empyema, with or without bronchopleural fistula formation.

Patients present most frequently with pneumonitis of a dependent lung segment, indicating the importance of the laws of motion, specifically of gravitational forces (Newtonian pneumonia). Empiric definitions differentiate the necrotizing pneumonia, characterized by multiple cavitary lesions measuring less than 1 cm in diameter, from the larger usually solitary lung abscess. The bacterial flora is influenced by the patient's oropharyngeal colonization, which in turn is affected by location (i.e., community versus hospital) and underlying immune status. Radiologic evidence of abscess formation does not appear before 7 days (mean 15 days) from an identified aspiration event. The syndrome of aspiration pneumonia and its consequent stages of progression is considered to be initiated by a chemical pneumonitis followed in approximately one-third of patients by the development of a subsequent superimposed bacterial pneumonia, a phenomenon uninfluenced by antibiotic prophylaxis. An unknown percentage of such events, most of which were minimized by subsequent initiation of antibiotic therapy, develop into a complicated necrotizing suppurative pneumonia; alternatively, in a "select" group, the process degenerates into a lung abscess with the development in some of the final complication of the continuum, empyema.[55]

The bacteriology of the necrotizing pneumonia, lung abscess, and empyema of these patients is similar and has been described under the term anaerobic pleuropulmonary infection. The polymicrobial flora has been shown to be characterized by an overwhelming predominance of anaerobic and mixed anaerobic-aerobic isolates.[56] Advances in anaerobic technology has presumably clarified the true etiologic agents of the "nonspecific lung abscess." With antibiotic therapy, complete resolution is almost uniformly observed at the end of 3 months. The rate and success of resolution depends on the initial size of the cavity and the duration of symptoms. The importance of location has also been inferred with abscesses in the right upper lobe resolving more slowly than those in other locations but with no greater incidence of treatment failure.[57,58]

It has been observed, however, that, in contrast to the excellent prognosis for primary lung abscess, more than 75% of lung abscesses are fatal in patients with opportunistic suppurative infections.[59] With the increasing number of immunocompromised hosts, overall mortality due to lung abscess has been reported to be increasing since the 1960s to 28%,[60] with a resurgence of the classic pyogenic organisms such as group A β-hemolytic streptococci.[61]

Empyema

Infection may not be successfully confined to the parenchyma as simple pneumonia or even a lung abscess but can extend to and through the pleural surface as empyema (empyema thoracis). It may be by contiguous spread or by formation of a bronchopleural fistula. The relation of this pleuropulmonary complication to the anaerobic population of the normal oral flora was clearly established at the turn of the century. However, it was essentially forgotten as a result of the decreased incidence with effective antibiotic therapy of the primary pneumonia. The resurgence of interest and appreciation of the persistent pathogenic role of anaerobes in empyema resulted from the same technologic advances in laboratory methodology that clarified their role in lung abscess. Anaerobic bacteria are recovered in three of every four cases of empyema and are the exclusive isolate in one-third. As with aspiration pneumonia, the polymicrobial nature of the empyematous process is clearly reflected by combined anaerobic and aerobic cultures.[62] Thus despite the reduced incidence of this complication, the pathogenesis of empyema is little changed from the preantibiotic era, and anaerobic pleuropulmonary infections predominate.

Pleural effusions are common in pneumonia, but empyema is an unusual occurrence, its frequency dependent on definition. It is more than a semantic consideration, though, as treatment is affected and delay alters not only the duration of hospitalization and morbidity but the mortality. Clinical, radiographic, and laboratory criteria have been suggested to detect this complication, differentiate it from lung abscess, and detect the presence of a bronchopleural fistula. Many patients with anaerobic empyema have no other evidence of pneumonia on routine chest roentgenogram. CT scanning is reported to be sufficient to uniformly differentiate lung abscess from empyema. The most reliable CT features are wall characteristics (Table 7.3).[63] Xenon 133 gas lends itself well to the detection of bronchopleural fistulas. Detection of radioactive gas in the pleural space and its persistence on washout studies provides a simple and reliable test of communication. The initial characterization of the fluid and noninvasive serial monitoring may be achieved by MRI. Empyemas are more intense and show greater heterogenicity, reflecting the increasing cellular and chemical complexity of the fluid.[64]

The present definition of empyema includes cellular parameters (purulence), microbiologic findings (bacteriologic culture), and chemical charac-

TABLE 7.3. CT characteristics.

Measurement	Lung abscess	Empyema
Wall	Thick	Thin, smooth, uniform
Pleural separation	None	Split pleura
Chest wall angle	Acute	Obtuse
Shape	Round to oblong	Oblong to lenticular
Size	Small	Larger
Lung	Destroyed	Compressed
Luminal margin	Irregular	Smooth
Contrast	No effect	Enhancement
Posture	No effect	Gravitational change in shape
Bronchi/vessels	Abrupt termination	Compressed and distorted

teristics [pH, glucose, lactate dehydrogenase (LDH)] in relation to serum values. The term parapneumonic effusion has been coined to indicate the common occurrence of pleural effusion in association with pneumonia. Its further delineation as an empyema is dependent on criteria meant to suggest that a positive culture does not make an empyema, and an acellular fluid does not rule it out. The lower the pH and glucose, the higher the lactate, protein, and LDH levels and the WBC count; the more positive the Gram stain, the greater is the likelihood of the effusion being an empyema. The metabolic activities of the pathogenic organisms and the cellular components of the fluid play a relatively minor role in determining the pH of the fluid. In contrast, the metabolic activity of the pleural tissue and the ability of its metabolic products, carbon dioxide and lactic acid, to be transported out of and oxygen into the pleural compartment are found to be the primary determinants of the pleural fluid pH, PCO_2, and PO_2.[65,66]

The anatomic and immunologic barriers to infection of the pleural space are formidable. As with pneumonia presenting with an associated pneumothorax, if the destructive process is aggressive enough, the infected material may extend into the compartment beyond the containment barrier of visceral pleura. A breach in these defenses usually implies a necrotizing process. However, pleura may become infected directly also, via the visceral pleural capillaries, or the organism may be carried along a pressure gradient in the underlying contiguous interstitial space. The pleural lymphatic system provides not only for a dynamic fluid transport mechanism but an effective transport system for infective agents as well as for immunocompetent and phagocyte cells. Organisms are rapidly cleared unless the microbial onslaught is relentless and overwhelming or if the lymphatics of the parietal pleura are damaged by the inflammation process, interfering with their patency and ability to act as a delivery and drainage system.

A variety of immunologic mechanisms have been proposed in an effort to explain the persistence of microorganisms observed in empyema. It has been suggested that diminished local opsonization occurs because of the decreased complement-mediated opsonic activity, which may result from the release of granulocyte proteases, which inactivate C3 in purulent pleural fluids. Local consumption of complement has been shown to take place with empyema but not with benign parapneumonic effusions. With empyema, low values for hemolytic complement (CH50) along with large amounts of the C3d the Ba complement components have been reported and may prove to be of diagnostic significance.[67]

The likelihood of developing empyema is increased if treatment for pneumonia is delayed. Although postpneumonic empyema is uncommon, it accounts for 60% of the cases of empyema. As many as 40% of patients with bacterial pneumonia have an associated pleural effusion, but fewer than 1% of adults develop empyema. The incidence varies with the type of pneumonia, but its incidence is greatest in anaerobic infections. Aside from antibiotic therapy, management has not progressed much beyond facilitating spontaneous drainage through the chest wall (empyema necessitatis) seen commonly during the preantibiotic era. With all the treatment presently available, the mortality of patients with empyema is still high (variously reported at 9–50%). By excluding cases with underlying diseases, however, the mortality rate is between 2.9% and 5.8%.[67]

Adequate drainage is a prerequisite of successful treatment and may be achieved by repeat thoracentesis for "thin" effusions of small volumes. Small percutaneous catheters have been introduced, rather than large thoracostomy tubes or more extensive thoracostomies, and have been found to be as effective if not more so in selected cases. They may be inserted under ultrasound guidance allowing for multiple placements if necessary for different loculated compartments.[67]

Finally, instillation of streptokinase has been suggested for lysis of loculated effusions in order to avoid decortication. Its efficacy has been reported to be enhanced by instillation into the space around the emypema rather than intrapleurally directly into the loculation.[68]

Delayed Resolution; Chronic and Recurrent Pneumonia

Persistence of the radiologic manifestations of pneumonia for weeks rather than days with or without symptoms characterizes the entity of delayed resolution, or chronic pneumonia. It may be a complication of an infectious or a noninfectious etiology. Agents causing necrotizing acute processes such as gram-negative and anaerobic organisms do not predispose to delayed resolution other than their tendency to recur or persist with repeated aspiration. The underlying immunocompetence of the individual influences not only the specific type of pneumonia but its subsequent course as well.

During evaluation of the possible pathogenesis and etiology of this complication of the initial episode, the patient's environmental exposures are of prime consideration, including occupational, geographic, and social background (e.g. friends, family, and habitual predisposing factors, particularly use of drugs). Disease processes commonly associated with prolonged resolution are preexisting lung disease such as chronic obstructive pulmonary disease (COPD) and obstructing endobronchial carcinoma, alcoholism, diabetes, and AIDS. Whether aging should also come under the category of disease is a philosophical if not semantic question; it is important nonetheless when correlating the rate of resolution and the incidence of chronic, persistent pneumonia. No studies have been done regarding the incidence or frequency of the various predisposing factors to chronic infection.

The rate of resolution of pneumonia depends on the organisms' numbers and virulence and the hosts' local and systemic defense mechanisms. Defense includes immunologic and structural barriers in addition to the entire mucociliary transport system. The potential role and mechanism must be defined for each contributing factor to the persistent process whether it is of a continuous infectious nature or an inflammatory process that cannot or refuses to be turned off. Thus adding to the uncertainty of resolution is the nature of the process giving rise to a persistently abnormal chest film, usually in the absence of contining associated signs or symptoms of infection. Delayed radiographic clearing has been poorly differentiated in terms of whether the infection is chronic and persistent or recurrent.

With pneumococcal pneumonia, delayed resolution is common and is associated with initial bacteremia, upper, right, or multilobe involvement, advanced age, heart failure, prolonged leukocytosis, leukopenia, delayed treatment, alcoholism, and underlying COPD.[69] The presence of multiple factors, moreover, are additive in determining the likelihood of delayed resolution.[70] Advanced age has been the most consistent predictor, whereas the initial clinical picture is widely variable and does not predict speed of resolution, including the persistence of fever.[70] It must be emphasized, however, that delayed resolution is not synonymous with recovery; it means only that the chest film appears normal by 120 days rather than the usual 30 days.[70] Pneumonias uncommonly (approximately 4% of patients) have radiologic progression initially despite an otherwise appropriate clinical response.[71] *Legionella* pneumonia, in contrast to *Mycoplasma* pneumonia, is characterized not only by delayed resolution (up to 6–12 months) but by persistent functional abnormalities, especially in regard to diffusing capacity, fatigue, and dyspnea for up to 2 years after its onset.[72]

The persistence of radiographic abnormalities and symptoms for more than 1 month conveniently defines chronic pneumonia.[73] *Hemophilus influenzae* has been reported to be the most common cause of chronic pneumonia, and smoking is the most common predisposing factor.[73] It has been suggested that the course of *H. influenzae* pneumonia may be more likely to be prolonged because it has an increasing incidence of being the causative organism in the elderly with frequent associated illness and impaired host defense mechanisms.[74] Other associations are similar to those suggested for delayed resolution, and complete resolution occurs with appropriate long-term antibiotic therapy.

The terms relapsing or recurrent pneumonia are best utilized, then, using a 1-month asymptomatic interval, complete radiographic clearing of the acute infiltrate, or both for distinction.[75] *Mycoplasma* pneumonia, the prototype for atypical pneumonia, has in the past also been termed recurrent pneumonia. Weeks to years may separate recurrences, and the location and severity of the recurrence may vary with respect to the initial episode, inferring that immune protection developed to an inadequate degree following the initial infection. The role of antibiotic therapy for recurrence is not clear. The limited number of reports available suggest that recurrence is not rare, necessarily localized to the site of the initial pneumonia, and that there is no specificity for a particular etiologic agent.

The bacteriology of recurrent episodes is similar to that of initial episodes in terms of variability. Specifically, the causative agent of the initial episode does not correlate (other than pneumococcal infection remains predominant) with that isolated from the recurrent infection. Predisposing underlying illnesses are almost uniformly present; 93% of patients in one report had associated predisposing diseases, most commonly COPD and congestive heart failure.[75] Other considerations include inapparent aspiration of a foreign body, malignancy (especially endobronchial), alcoholism, and underlying immunodeficiency. Treatment remains similar to that for initial events, as does responsiveness and mortality.

In summary, it is important to differentiate delayed resolution from deterioration. Bronchogenic carcinoma is an uncommon cause of delayed resolution or recurrent pneumonia.[70,75] Continued observation is warranted with otherwise clinical improvement, whereas aggressive diagnostic measures are indicated with persistent or recurrent clinical signs and symptoms of pneumonia. Chronic, persistent inflammation may result in vascular proliferation and recurrent hemoptysis, causing severe anemia.[76] The fatality rate of recurrent pneumonia, despite the presence of associated illness, has been found to be similar to that of the initial infection.

Adult Respiratory Distress Syndrome

In the past the acute lung injury syndrome (ARDS) was characterized clinically by noncardiogenic (low pressure) pulmonary edema reflected by severe impairment of arterial oxygenation, a decrease in lung compliance, and diffuse infiltrates seen on roentgenography. More recently, it has been appreciated that the uniqueness of the impairment of pulmonary function is more apparent than real. The hypoxemia resulting from the lungs' failure to exchange oxygen, although a distinguishing feature initially suggesting that the lungs act as the target organ for inflammation, is in fact representative only of coexisting multiorgan dysfunction of varying degree. This defect in pulmonary gas exchange is associated with impaired peripheral oxygen extraction as well, which has been attributed to ill-defined factors of decreased delivery, increased diffusion path, decreased membrane penetration, and finally impaired cellular utilization of oxygen. The oxygen uptake may be increased and is found to be delivery-dependent when the driving pressure in the periphery is increased.

The syndrome is associated with a variety of organ and systemic insults, and the mortality varies greatly, affected by numerous confounders such as age and the primary underlying disease process. Death is only infrequently attributable to hypoxemic respiratory failure. ARDS occurs as a complication of both infectious and noninfectious pneumonia as well as nonpulmonary disease.[77] Mortality due to ARDS is greatest in patients with pneumonia (Fig. 7.5), which is a leading predisposing event for the development of ARDS. It may occur in patients with no apparent risk factor or preexisting disease. A variety of mediators of this neutrophil-induced lung injury have at different times held the forefront of the proposed variety of mechanisms resulting in an inflammatory cascade

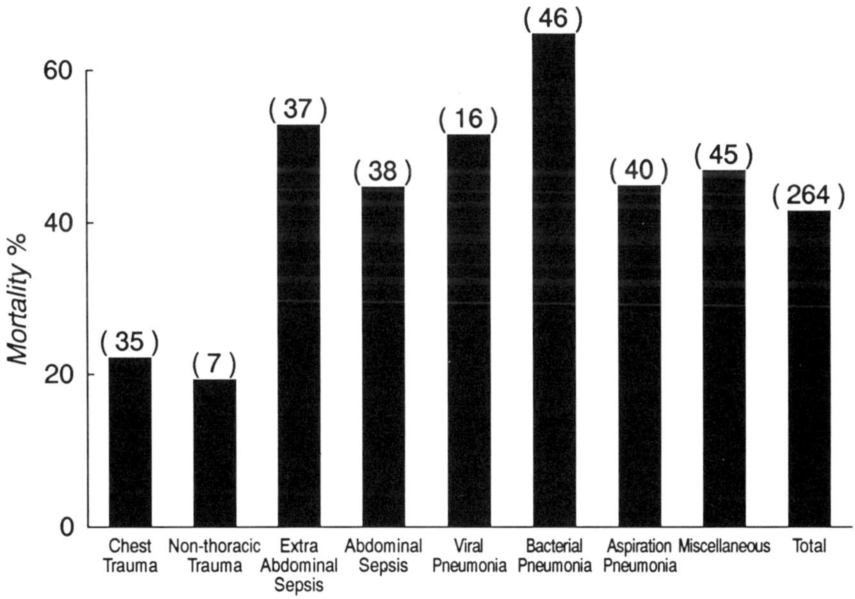

FIGURE 7.5. Mortality among 635 patients with ARDS. The numbers of patients are shown in parentheses. (Data from Zapol et al.[77])

causing the pathophysiologic findings of ARDS. The unifying hypothesis for the pathogenetic mechanisms responsible for their release and interaction continues to be enigmatic. The migration and aggregation of activated neutrophils and macrophages are thought to play interlocking roles in the destruction and damage of the alveolar epithelial and pulmonary capillary endothelial cells. Recruitment of PMN inflammatory cells appears to be due to directed chemotaxis. Neutrophils release preformed intracellular granules of cytotoxic proteases, generate cyclooxygenase and lipoxygenase metabolites of membrane-bound arachidonic acid, and together with other phagocytic cells have respiratory bursts, releasing cytotoxic reactive oxygen species.

It is becoming clear that although effective concentrations of oxygen at the tissue level allow the freedom of an aerobic life style, too much oxygen or inappropriate metabolism of oxygen can be toxic to cells. These reactive oxygen metabolites have accepted less than the usual four-electron reduction of oxygen to form water. The superoxide anion radical dismutates to produce hydrogen peroxide (H_2O_2). These metabolites in the presence of iron-containing compounds form the hydroxyl free radical; the most reactive free radical produced in biologic systems, it causes lipid peroxidation of polyunsaturated fatty acids of cell membranes, altering membrane fluidity and permeability. Hemoprotein peroxidases combine with H_2O_2 to form a halide or pseudohalide; these substances are potent oxidizing agents that are toxic to cells, bacteria, and viral particles through their actions of sulfhydryl oxidation, hemoprotein inactivation, protein and amino acid degradation, and inactivation of essential metabolic cofactors and DNA.

The naturally occurring antioxidant enzymes and scavengers are superoxide dismutase, catalase, and glutathione peroxidase. A second line of defense is composed of the nonenzymatic scavengers and quenchers, such as phenolic compounds (α-tocopherol), carotenoids (vitamin A), and sulfhydryl and thioether compounds. Activated neutrophils produce large amounts of reactive oxygen species to kill invading microbes. Unrestrained production of prooxidants and their release in the extracellular medium disturbs the delicate oxidant-antioxidant balance, resulting in an "oxidative attack" on the lung tissue. Initial studies in patients with ARDS indicate that plasma and red blood cell glutathione levels are decreased and that *N*-acetylcysteine administration, through its reduced sulfhydryl group, increases the levels of glutathione. There is no evidence, however, that its therapeutic administration decreases mortality or improves pulmonary function.

Previous emphasis has been on preformed proteases and newly generated leukotriene and prostanoid lipid mediators from the cell membrane via the arachidonic acid cascade. Among the various mediators currently being focused on are the numerous cytokines, such as tumor necrosis factor (TNF), which causes endothelial injury, and the interleukins, the best known of which is IL-1, which alters intrapulmonary hemodynamics. These inflammatory markers, the *cytokines*, are cell-derived peptide molecules that act as mediators of intra- and intercellular communications causing a target cell to alter its activities. The cytokines are immunomodulators that are bound by specific receptors on the membrane surface of the target cells, initiating internal receptor-coupled (signal transduction) second messages to generate a response. The cytokines are derived (secreted) from a variety of cell types, including endothelial cells, monocytes, and macrophages each with their own mediator profiles. The dynamics stimulating their synthesis and release are largely unknown but are related to the action and interaction of endotoxins, bacteria, eicosanoids, and the cytokines themselves on target cells. The arachidonate metabolites appear to be amplifiers or modulators and regulators that fine-tune the evolution and resolution of inflammatory sequences rather than causing them.

The temporal features of diffuse alveolar damage include an initial exudative phase of edema, infiltrating inflammatory cells, and hemorrhage as a result of loss of alveolar-capillary integrity. Destruction and death of the endothelial cells cause widening of the capillary gap junctions. Similarly, damage to the alveolar type I cells results in disappearance of the epithelial tight junctions, with their death and desquamation. In addition, gaps appear in the basement membrane, resulting in direct contact between the interstitium and the alveolar airspace. The diffusion barrier is dissipated with loss of the alveolar epithelial barrier. A subsequent proliferative phase of organization and repair follows, leading finally to a fibrotic phase attributable to the proliferation of fibroblasts and collagen deposition. The proliferative phase is characterized by capillary proliferation and remodeling through organization of intra-alveolar and interstitial exudate with proliferation of type II and cuboidal cells, suggesting an attempt at repair of the air–lung interface. The net intraacinar microvascular cross-sectional area is reduced, and both pulmonary vascular resistance and physiologic deadspace are increased.

The lungs are not synchronously or homogeneously affected; alveoli may be unaffected, nonfunctional, or recruitable. With ARDS the weight of overlying edematous lung on underlying regions induces collapse of healthy, dependent lung units. The beneficial mechanism of the action of PEEP probably consists in recruiting these deflated localized lung regions. Thus measurements of specific compliance in ARDS has been reported to be normal. Alleviation of compression atelectasis by PEEP provides for its primary therapeutic effect, which immediately enhances oxygenation by reducing the venous admixture ("shunt").[78] Lung mechanics reflect the decreased aerable volume, but the inhomogeneity of the process predisposes to barotrauma such as bronchiolectasis with mechanical ventilation. The chest CT scan shows areas of well aerated, normal-appearing lung interspersed with patches of edematous, infiltrated and destroyed parenchyma. Patients with ARDS demonstrate increases in both the restrictive and elastic work of breathing. Increased airway resistance results from airway flooding and the reduced lung volume. The increased viscoelastic properties are due to the decrease in aerated lung volume and the diffuse inflammatory process in the lung.

Abnormalities of pulmonary function occur following recovery from ARDS. The extent of impairment apart from minor flow and restrictive changes and decreased DLCO is rarely severe and does not correlate with the extent of histologic abnormalities found with open-lung biopsy performed during the acute stage. This lack of correlation has been attributed to the inhomogeneity of the histopathology as well as to the reversibility of the interstitial fibrotic process.[79] Similarly, no relation was found between the duration of mechanical ventilation or the amount of oxygen received and the capacity to normalize DLCO, though this subject remains controversial.

High levels of PEEP are harmful and must be balanced against the lack of evidence showing it to reduce mortality.[80] Although PEEP improves gas exchange in the exudative, and perhaps the proliferative, phase of ARDS, in late-stage ARDS patients, when the fibrosis phase is dominant, a beneficial response to PEEP is not observed. The risk of barotrauma (including pneumothorax, increased lung water, and epithelial damage) and perhaps bronchopulmonary dysplasia is now appreciated to be a matter of magnitude, no longer a question of occurrence. Pulmonary edema due to barotrauma results from increased permeability of the alveolar capillary barrier and is accompanied by alveolar cellular damage.[81] The damage results from distension of the alveolar-capillary unit (high tidal volume), not the associated pressure. The uneven distribution of the ARDS lesions lends itself to regional overdistension with mechanical ventilation. The normal lung is the most susceptible to such injury and would be indistinguishable from ARDS lesions.

Mortality is unpredictable, and prognosis varies with the nature of the initial insult, its severity, and any associated disease. The onset of the syndrome occurs within 24 hours of the precipitating event in 75% of patients, and intubation is required within 72 hours in 90% of patients. Ninety percent of the mortality occurs within 2 weeks, and less than 20% results from irreversible respiratory failure. Isolated respiratory failure as a cause of death is primarily seen in the elderly with superinfection- and sepsis-related multiple organ failure is the primary cause of death both early (<72 hours) and late (>72 hours). Acute lung injury scoring systems based on the severity of impairment of oxygenation, the magnitude of the roentgenographic abnormality, the loss of respiratory compliance, and the level of PEEP required to maintain adequate oxygenation have been developed to suggest a continuum of respiratory dysfunction and to aid prognostication. Other established predictors of survival are the severity of the initial metabolic acidosis, the ability of the bone marrow to release

PMNs in response to the initial inflammatory insult, and the renal reserve as reflected by the blood urea nitrogen level (BUN).

Pneumonia appears to be even more common as a complication of ARDS than as a precipitating event. It is primarily gram-negative in type but may be gram-positive or polymicrobial; the dominant pathogen is *Pseudomonas*. Most late deaths are associated with sepsis, and the primary site of origin of the sepsis is the lung. The diagnosis of pneumonia in ARDS patients is difficult to make on clinical grounds, with high incidences of both false positives and false negatives.[82] The usual clinical criteria for pneumonia in patients with ARDS are inaccurate. Fever and leukocytosis are present in ARDS patients with or without pneumonia. In a comparison of premortem clinical findings with postmortem examination of the lungs, the clinical diagnosis regarding the presence or absence of pneumonia was correct in only 70% of patients. An apparent response to antibiotic therapy as well as serial chest film findings had no predictive value.[82] Additionally, the adverse consequence of nosocomial pneumonia is illustrated by its presence in 70% of patients dying with ARDS; and in 80% of the patients with clinical sepsis, the sepsis is attributable to pneumonia.[82] These observations have prompted studies on the nature of the apparent impairment of the antibacterial defense mechanisms of the lung in ARDS, particularly the antibacterial efficiency of lung phagocytes.[83] Alterations have been found in neutrophil function with respect to the production of reactive oxygen products, microbicidal activity, and chemotaxis, which seems to increase susceptibility to pulmonary infection in the patient with ARDS.[83]

Much of the pathophysiology and management have concentrated on the pathophysiology of the oxygen supply–demand imbalance. This observation has not been universal, and controversy still exists whether it is indeed merely attributable to a methodologic error arising from mathematic coupling.[84] Reports of studies utilizing independent measures of oxygen consumption and cardiac output have failed to find delivery (supply)-dependent oxygen uptake even in the presence of increased concentrations of plasma lactate (Fig. 7.6). It is similarly subject to methodologic interpretation depending on whether the increased measured or decreased calculated cardiac output is used to determine the oxygen delivery. Aside from central factors of anemia and cardiac dysfunction, local mechanisms of impaired oxygen extraction and decreased recruitable capillary reserve have been suggested. The disordered peripheral vasoregulation characterized by a decrease in systemic vascular resistance is further complicated, as in the lung, by altered intraorgan distribution of blood flow, which may be further aggravated by PEEP. A theory of multisystem panendothelial injury has been proposed that alters permeability and real if not functional capillary density with interstitial edema and both endothelial and parenchymal cell injury impairing oxygen utilization and extraction. The current strategy of management has thus

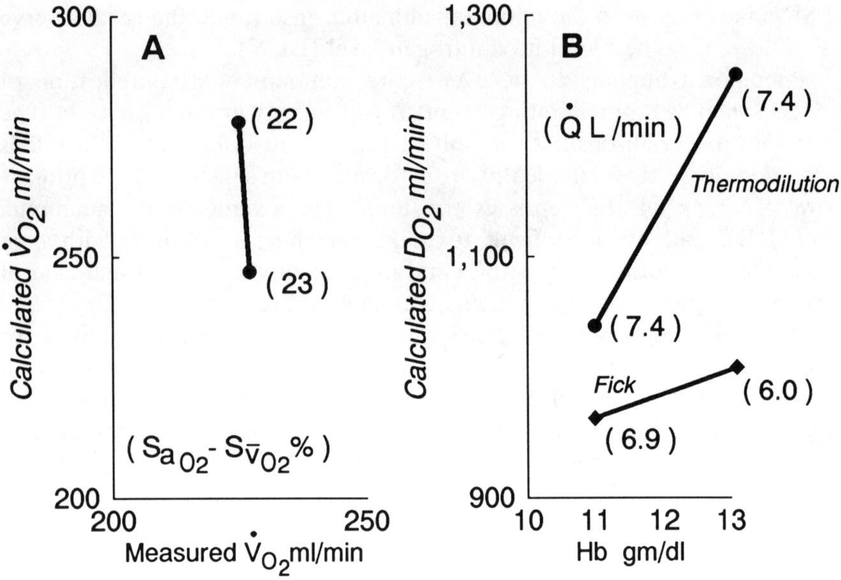

FIGURE 7.6. Lack of delivery-dependent oxygen uptake in patients with ARDS ($n = 17$). (A) Comparison of calculated versus measured oxygen uptake. (B) Oxygen delivery before and after transfusion of 600 ml of packed RBCs over a 1-hour period. The measured (thermodilution) cardiac output remains unchanged, whereas the calculated (Fick) cardiac output decreases. (Data from Ronco et al.[84])

both accepted and focused on the concept that oxygen uptake may not be equal to demand, and that tissues may be hypoxic in the presence of a normal supply.

References

1. Trenchard D, Gardner D, Guz A: Role of pulmonary vagal afferent nerve fibers in the development of rapid shallow breathing in lung inflammation. Clin Sci 1972;42:251–263.
2. Buller AJ: The muscle spindle and the control of movement. In Howell JBL, Campbell EJM (eds): Breathlessness. Philadelphia: Davis, 1966, pp. 11–17.
3. Tobin MJ: Dyspnea: pathophysiologic basis, clinical presentation, and management. Arch Intern Med 1990;150:1604–1613.
4. Killian KJ: Assessment of dyspnea. Eur Respir J 1988;1:195–197.
5. Burki NK: Dyspnea. Lung 1987;165:269–277.
6. Braga PC, Allegra L: Cough. New York: Raven Press, 1989, pp. 244.
7. Leith DE: Cough. In Brain JD, Proctor DF, Reid LM (eds): Lung Biology in Health and Disease. Respiratory Defense Mechanisms, Vol. 5. New York: Marcel Dekker, 1977, pp. 545–592.

8. Karlsson J-A, Sant Ambrogio G, Widdicombe J: Afferent neural pathways in cough and reflex bronchoconstriction. J Appl Physiol 1988;65:1007–1023.
9. Lindgren BR: New aspects on inflammatory reactions and cough following inhibition of angiotensin converting enzyme. Acta Physiol Scand Suppl 573 1988;133:1–60.
10. Murphy PA: Exogenous pyrogens. In Mackowiak PA (ed): Fever: Basic Mechanisms and Management. New York: Raven Press, 1991, pp. 49–58.
11. Kluger MJ, Ringler DH, Anver MR: Fever and survival. Science 1975;188: 166–168.
12. Robert NJ: The immunological consequences of fever. In Mackowiak PA (ed): Fever: Basic Mechanisms and Management. New York: Raven Press, 1991, pp. 125–142.
13. Greisman SE: Cardiovascular alterations during fever. In Mackowiak PA (ed): Fever: Basic Mechanisms and Management. New York: Raven Press, 1991, pp. 143–165.
14. Rowell LB: Human circulation: Regulation During Physical Stress. New York: Oxford University Press, 1986, pp. 416.
15. Wood SC: Interactions between hypoxia and hypothermia. Annu Rev Physiol 1991;53:71–85.
16. Edwards HT, Wood WB: A study of leukocytosis in exercise. Arbeitsphysiologie 1932;6:73–83.
17. Douglas RG Jr, Alford RH, Cate TR, Couch RC: The leukocyte response during viral respiratory illness in man. Ann Intern Med 1966;64:521–530.
18. Morens DM: WBC count and differential: value in predicting bacterial diseases in children. Am J Dis Child 1979;133:25–27.
19. Bull B, Korpman RA: Characterization of the WBC differential count. Blood Cells 1980;6:411–419.
20. Smyllie HC, Blendis LM, Armitage P: Observer disagreement in physical signs of the respiratory system. Lancet 1965;2:412–413.
21. Baughman RP, Loudon RG: Sound spectral analysis of voice transmitted sound. Am Rev Respir Dis 1986;134:167–169.
22. Forgacs P: Lung Sounds. London: Ballière Tindall, 1978, p. 72.
23. Ploysongsang Y, Schonfeld SA: Mechanism of production of crackles after atelectasis during low-volume breathing. Am Rev Respir Dis 1982;126:413–415.
24. Forgacs P: Crackles and wheezes. Lancet 1967;2:203–205.
25. Mikami R, Murao M, Cugell DW, et al: International symposium on lung sounds: synopsis of proceedings. Chest 1987;92:342–345.
26. Spiteri MA, Cook DG, Clarke SW: Reliability of eliciting physical signs in examination of the chest. Lancet 1988;1:873–875.
27. Loudon R, Murphy RLH Jr: Lung sounds. Am Rev Respir Dis 1984;130: 663–673.
28. Bray HA: An appraisal of the theories of pleuritic pain. Am Rev Tuberc 1954;69:634–635.
29. Cherniack NS: Chest pain. In Murray JF, Nadel JA (eds): Textbook of Respiratory Medicine. Philadelphia: Saunders, 1988, pp. 409–413.
30. Heckerling PS, Tape TG, Wigton RS, et al: Clinical prediction rule for pulmonary infiltrates. Ann Intern Med 1990;113:664–670.

31. Fairbank JT, Patel MM, Dietrich PA: Legionnaires disease. J Thorac Imaging 1991;6:6–13.
32. Hershey CO, Panaro V: Round pneumonia in adults. Arch Intern Med 1988;148:1155–1157.
33. Caldwell A, Glauser FL, Smith WR, et al: The effects of dehydration on the radiologic and pathologic appearance of experimental canine segmental pneumonia. Am Rev Respir Dis 1975;112:651–656.
34. Donowitz GR, Harman C, Pope T, Stewart M: The role of the chest roentgenogram in febrile neutropenic patients. Arch Intern Med 1991;151:701–704.
35. Kramer EL, Divgi CR: Pulmonary applications of nuclear medicine. Clin Chest Med 1991;12:55–75.
36. Kessler R, Fraisse P, Krause D, et al: Magnetic resonance imaging in the diagnosis of pulmonary infarction. Chest 1991;99:298–300.
37. McFadden RG, Carr TJ, Mackie IDF: Thoracic magnetic resonance imaging in the evaluation of HIV-1/AIDS pneumonitis. Chest 1992;101:371–374.
38. Pistolesi M, Miniati M, Giuntini C: Pleural liquid and solute exchange. Am Rev Respir Dis 1989;140:825–847.
39. Nakamura T, Tanaka Y, Fukabori T, et al: The role of lymphatics in removing pleural liquid in discrete hydrothorax. Eur Respir J 1988;1:826–831.
40. Stewart PB: The rate of formation and lymphatic removal of pleural fluid in pleural effusions. J Clin Invest 1963;42:258–262.
41. Wiener-Kronish JP, Matthay MA: Pleural effusions associated with hydrostatic and increased permeability pulmonary edema. Chest 1988;93:852–858.
42. Estenne M, Yernault J-C, DeTroyer A: Mechanism of relief of dyspnea after thoracentesis in patients with large pleural effusions. Am J Med 1983;74:813–819.
43. Zaman I, Karetzky, M: Effect of the inspired oxygen concentration on the oxygen tension of pleural fluid. Am Rev Respir Dis 1991;143(Suppl): A660.
44. Brandstetter R, Karetzy M, Viejo C, Zaman I: Effect of ventilation on the carbon dioxide tension of pleural fluid. Chest 1991;100:76S.
45. Macklin MT, Macklin CC: Malignant interstitial emphysema of the lungs and mediastinum as an important occult complication in many respiratory diseases and other conditions: an interpretation of the clinical literature in the light of laboratory experiment. Medicine (Baltimore) 1944;23:281–358.
46. Krueger JJ, Sayre VA, Karetzky M: Infectious interstitial emphysema in AIDS. N J Med 1987;84:489–491.
47. Krueger JJ, Sayre VA, Karetzky M: Bronchoalveolar lavage-induced pneumothorax. Chest 1988;94:440–441.
48. Menkes HA, Macklem PT: Collateral flow. In Geiger SR (ed): Handbook of Physiology. Sect. 3. The Respiratory System. Vol. III: Mechanics of Breathing, Part 2. Washington, DC: American Physiological Society, 1986, pp. 337–353.
49. Macklem PT: Airway obstruction and collateral ventilation. Physiol Rev 1971;51:368–436.
50. Menkes HA, Traystman R, Terry P: Collateral ventilation. Fed Proc 1979;38: 22–26.

51. Karetzky M: Asthma mortality associated with pneumothorax and intermittent positive-pressure breathing. Lancet 1975;1:828–829.
52. Latorre FJ, Tomasa A, Klamburg J, et al: Incidence of pneumothorax and pneumomediastinum in patients with aspiration pneumonia requiring ventilatory support. Chest 1977;72:141–144.
53. Whittemore W: The treatment of acute empyema and pulmonary abscess. N Engl J Med 1931;205:797–800.
54. Amberson JB: A clinical consideration of abscesses and cavities of the lung. Bull Johns Hopkins Hosp 1954;94:227–237.
55. Schweppe HI, Knowles JH, Kane L: Lung abscess: an analysis of the Massachusetts General Hospital cases from 1943 through 1956. N Engl J Med 1961;265:1039–1043.
56. Bartlett JG, Gorbach SL, Tally FP, Finegold SM: Bacteriology and treatment of primary lung abscess. Am Rev Respir Dis 1974;109:510–518.
57. Barnett TB, Herring CL: Lung abscess: initial and late results of medical therapy. Arch Intern Med 1971;127:217–227.
58. Weiss W: Cavity behavior in acute primary non-specific lung abscess. Am Rev Respir Dis 1973;198:1273–1275.
59. Schachter EN: Suppurative lung disease: old problems revisited. Clin Chest Med 1981;2:41–49.
60. Hagan JL, Hardy JD: Lung abscess revisited: a survey of 184 cases. Ann Surg 1983;197:755–762.
61. Frieden TR, Biebuyck J, Hierholzer WJ Jr: Lung abscess with group A β-hemolytic streptococcus: case report and review. Arch Intern Med 1991;151: 1655–1657.
62. Bartlett JG, Gorbach SL, Thadepalli H, Finegold SM: Bacteriology of empyema. Lancet 1974;1:338–340.
63. Stark DD, Federle MP, Goodman PC, et al: Differentiating lung abscess and empyema: radiography and computed tomography. AJR 1983;141:163–167.
64. Davis SD, Henschke CI, Yankelevitz DF, et al: MR imaging of pleural effusions. J Comput Assist Tomogr 1990;142:192–198.
65. Light RW, Luchsinger PC: Metabolic activity of pleural fluid. J Appl Physiol 1973;34:97–101.
66. Karetzky M, Kothari GA, Fourre JA, Khan AU: Effect of thoracentesis on arterial oxygen tension. Respiration 1978;36:96–103.
67. Vladutiu AO: Pleural Effusion. Mount Kisco, NY: Futura, 1986, p. 422.
68. Ogirala RG, Williams MH Jr: Streptokinase in a loculated pleural effusion: effectiveness determined by site of instillation. Chest 1988;94:884–886.
69. Van Metre TE Jr: Pneumococcal pneumonia treated with antibiotics: the prognostic significance of certain clinical findings. N Engl J Med 1954;251: 1048–1052.
70. Jay SJ, Johanson WJ Jr, Pierce AK: The radiographic resolution of Streptococcus pneumoniae pneumonia. N Engl J Med 1975;293:798–801.
71. Graham WGB, Bradley DA: Efficacy of chest physiotherapy and intermittent positive-pressure breathing in the resolution of pneumonia. N Engl J Med 1978;299:624–627.
72. Lattimer GL, Rhodes LV III, Salvent JS, et al: The Philadelphia epidemic of legionnaire's disease: clinical, pulmonary and serologic findings two years later. Ann Intern Med 1979;90;522–526.

73. Kirtland SH, Winterbauer RH: Slowly resolving, chronic and recurrent pneumonia. Clin Chest Med 1991;12:303–318.
74. Fein AM, Feinsilver S, Niederman MS: Slowly resolving pneumonia in the elderly. In Niederman MS (ed): Respiratory Infections in the Elderly. New York: Raven Press, 1991, pp. 293–324.
75. Winterbauer RH, Bedon GA, Ball WC Jr: Recurrent pneumonia: predisposing illness and clinical patterns in 158 patients. Ann Intern Med 1969;70: 689–700.
76. Nakazawa H, Tsuburaya T, Watanabe H, et al: Chronic bronchopneumonia with recurrent hemoptysis and resultant severe anemia. Respiration 1991;58: 332–334.
77. Zapol WM, Frikker MJ, Pontoppidan H, et al: The adult respiratory distress syndrome at Massachusetts General Hospital: etiology, progression and survival rates 1978–1988. In Zapol WM, Lemaire F (eds): Adult Respiratory Distress Syndrome. Lung Biology in Health and Disease, Vol. 50. New York: Marcel Dekker, 1991, pp. 367–380.
78. Gattinoni L, Pesenti A, Bombino M, et al: Relationships between lung computed tomographic density, gas exchange and PEEP in acute respiratory failure. Anesthesiology 1988;69:824–832.
79. Suchyta MR, Elliot CG, Colby T, et al: Open lung biopsy does not correlate with pulmonary function after the adult respiratory distress syndrome. Chest 1991;99:1232–1237.
80. Caroll GC, Tuman KJ, Braverman B, et al: Minimal positive end-expiratory pressure (PEEP) may be "best PEEP." Chest 1988;93:1020–1025.
81. Dreyfuss D, Soler P, Basset G, Saumon G: High inflation pressure pulmonary edema: respective effects of high airway pressure, high tidal volume, and positive end-expiratory pressure. Am Rev Respir Dis 1988;137:1159–1164.
82. Johanson WG Jr: Bacterial infection in adult respiratory distress syndrome. In Zapol WM, Lemaire F (eds): Adult Respiratory Distress Syndrome. Lung Biology in Health and Disease, Vol. 50. New York: Marcel Dekker, 1991, pp. 77–89.
83. Martin TR, Pistorese BP, Hudson LD, Maunder RJ: The function of lung and blood neutrophils in patients with the adult respiratory distress syndrome: implications for the pathogenesis of lung infections. Am Rev Respir Dis 1991;144:254–262.
84. Ronco JJ, Phang PT, Walley KR, et al: Oxygen consumption is independent of changes in oxygen delivery in severe adult respiratory distress syndrome. Am Rev Respir Dis 1991;143:1267–1273.

8 Pneumonia: Treatment and Prognosis

MONROE KARETZKY

Oxygen

The concentration of oxygen in the atmosphere has not changed since the turn of the century, and currently predictions are for it to remain constant for the foreseeable future. It does not, however, satisfy the needs of patients with pneumonia. The therapeutic potential of supplemental oxygen was immediately apparent to Priestly when he and his "volunteer" mice experienced the "high" of inspiring the "dephlogisticated air" he discovered 200 years ago. Following a dinner conversation shortly thereafter, Lavoisier subsequently elaborated on his colleague's findings. He demonstrated its uptake in the lungs and its respiratory function with the resultant carbon dioxide production. It was not until 1798, however, after a lapse of 25 years when Thomas Beddoes opened his Pneumatic Institute at Bristol, that the therapeutic potential of oxygen was pursued for a variety of ailments including lung disease. This spa (as well as the residential hotels established for hyperbaric oxygen therapy 150 years later), unfortunately did not prove to be a financially viable endeavor and could not be sustained on its scientific merit alone.

It was not until World War I, When oxygen was used to treat victims of gas poisoning, that it became an acceptable mode of therapy. Over the next 40 years high inspired concentrations of oxygen became firmly established as an essential component of therapeutic stratagems for management of patients with acute cardiopulmonary disease. The subsequent two decades witnessed the concept of high flow-controlled oxygen concentration therapy, which became a routine modification in treatment and, most recently, long-term domiciliary oxygen therapy for hypoxemic patients with chronic lung disease. Controlled studies showing improved survival have confirmed the anticipated benefits of continuous oxygen therapy in such patients. Their clinical response was characterized by increased exercise tolerance, reduction of pulmonary vascular resistance and pulmonary artery pressure, improved cardiac output, and improved neuropsychological function. Similar data regarding the use of oxygen for acute lung disease (pneumonia or otherwise), however, is not so readily available. Even the proclaimed benefit from its continuous administration in ambulatory patients with obstructive lung disease has been questioned and attributed not to enhanced oxygenation but to cessation of smoking.

Administration

It was the introduction of the technique of radial artery puncture that allowed assessment of arterial oxygenation in pneumonia.[1] Until this study of the cyanosis associated with pneumonia, only its relation to the saturation of venous blood had been analyzed, which of course made interpretation difficult. The arterial unsaturation (difference between oxygen content and total oxygen capacity) was found to be a valuable prognostic indicator, with fatal cases usually having an arterial saturation of less than 80% and nonfatal cases of greater than 80%.[1] Similarly, the observation was reported that in fatal cases of pneumonia the mean value of the venous unsaturation was 20% higher than in the nonfatal cases. The mechanism of cyanosis was correctly attributed to venous admixture or "incomplete oxygenation of the blood as it passes through the pulmonary capillaries or the passage of but part of the blood thru [*sic*] the lungs (as in congenital heart disease)."[1] Barach and Woodell, Stadie, and Meakins starting during the 1920s instituted the clinical use of oxygen,[2–4] and its value as a therapeutic agent, though initially debated, was subsequently firmly established.[5] It was administered by mask, in an oxygen chamber, and in a ventilated oxygen tent; and each mode was reported to provide a 40–50% inspired oxygen concentration. The arterial hypoxemia was relieved along with the associated cyanosis, dyspnea, tachycardia, restlessness, and delirium; and the life of the pneumonia patients was reported to be prolonged by this therapeutic intervention. The lower mortality rate was attributed to the additional time afforded for the patient to develop an immunity to the causative agent of the pneumonia by the avoidance of fatal hypoxemia.[6] Oxygen administration allowed limited compensation by the body's other organ systems for the lungs' diminution in redundancy resulting from pneumonia.

The development of high-pressure cylinders was stimulated by introduction of the ventilated oxygen tent, the double nasal catheter, and subsequently the double nasal cannula to treat moderately severe hypoxia necessitating a larger oxygen reservoir. The question of dosage considered critical to the administration of pharmacologic agents so as to provide the full therapeutic effect as well as to avoid toxicity is fully applicable but frequently ignored during the administration of oxygen. The observation that along with enhanced oxygenation there was an increase in the patients' carbon dioxide content[6] led to the suggestion that oxygen enrichment with alleviation of the hypoxic drive may depress ventilation.[7] This observation resulted in evolution of the concept of "controlled' oxygen therapy and led to the widespread practice of inappropriate administration of limited-flow high concentration (nasal cannula) or high-flow fixed inspired concentrations (Venturi masks) that frequently fail to achieve adequate levels of arterial oxygenation.[8]

It became readily apparent that physiologic concepts rather than controlled clinical data would have to serve as therapeutic guidelines, as withdrawal or withholding of oxygen therapy was immediately appreciated as ethically impossible. The benefits of oxygen therapy in the absence of cyanosis, confusion, and cardiovascular collapse are difficult to rationalize physiologically or to document clinically[9] (Table 8.1). Efficacy also depends on the adequacy of the other determinants of oxygen delivery—flow (cardiac output) and distribution—as well as oxygen binding capacity (hemoglobin concentration), the affinity of hemoglobin for oxygen, and finally the enigmatic actual oxygen uptake versus the need concept of pathologic supply dependence.

Availability

An aspect of oxygen transport unique to states of severe hypoxemia associated with dyspnea and alveolar hyperventilation such as pneumonia is the variable left shift in the oxygen dissociation curve caused by respiratory alkalosis. It was found to be an essential feature of effective oxygen transport in the Peruvian Andes and on the summit of Mt. Everest.[10] The advantage of an increase in oxygen affinity is thought to be analogous to the altered position of the oxygen dissociation curve of the blood in the placental circulation where fetal hemoglobin has a higher affinity for oxygen than does maternal hemoglobin, protecting the fetal "arterial" saturation. This adaptation during pneumonia favors oxygen

TABLE 8.1. Effect of oxygen therapy on oxygenation.[a]

Measurement	$PvO_2 > 32$ mm Hg ($n = 12$)			$PvO_2 < 32$ mm Hg ($n = 10$)			
	Room air	O_2	p1	Room air	O_2	p2	p3
PaO_2 (mm Hg)	71.9	124.4	*	65.1	138.8	*	NS
SaO_2 (%)	92.2	95.4	*	87.2	96.9	*	NS
PvO_2 (mm Hg)	35.8	38.2	NS	28.9	34.2	*	*
SvO_2 (mm Hg)	64.1	68.1	NS	54.8	61.9	*	*
Q (L/min)	7.90	7.50	NS	6.30	5.70	NS	NS
$(a-v)O_2$ (ml/dl)	3.82	3.52	NS	4.18	4.40	NS	NS

p1, p2 = oxygen versus room air value within each PvO_2 group; p3 = room air values between groups; NS = $p > 0.05$.

[a] The effects of an enriched inspired oxygen concentration on mixed venous oxygenation: oxygen and hemodynamic profiles in 22 critically ill patients according to the severity of tissue hypoxia.[9] Apparent benefit appears to be due to increased CaO_2 with unpredictable changes in mixed venous saturation.

* $p < 0.05$.

loading in the lungs rather than unloading in the tissues as an otherwise predicted increase in P_{50} would do. This situation stands in contrast to the effect of the reduced oxygen affinity observed under conditions of decreased carrying capacity when arterial oxygenation is adequate, such as with anemia, which serves to improve oxygen delivery to tissues. With other lung diseases as well, because of increased venous admixture from V/Q abnormalities, increased shunting and diffusion limitation of oxygen uptake in the lung, increased oxygen affinity seems appropriate to enhance uptake. Presumably, this advantage is not offset by the resulting impaired tissue unloading caused by excessively low venous PO_2, which reflects the driving pressure to cell mitochondria. Similarly, the benefits of the 2,3-diphosphoglycerate (2,3-DPG) effect for tissue oxygenation in the presence of normal lung function is not applicable in patients with pneumonia.

In addition, the "optimal hematocrit" for oxygen transport in the presence of disease must balance viscosity against oxygen-carrying capacity. In general, increased hematocrit resulting from dehydration increases the vascular resistance to flow, requiring increased blood pressure and left atrial filling pressure until a new homeostatic state is reached. Furthermore, "blood doping" with hypertransfusion is rheologically disadvantageous, leading to a decrease in cardiac output. Humans are unlike the Weddell seal, a mammal with the ability to breath-hold for an hour with a hemoglobin concentration of 27 g/dl. This phenomenon is made possible by maximal cerebral and coronary vasodilation of a magnitude capable of neutralizing the adverse affects of increased viscosity.

Tissue oxygenation utilizing classic parameters, still, even with disease, is a concept that appears simple enough. Difficulty with its application, however, arises immediately with the appreciation that heterogeneity of distribution to organs and to regions within a tissue exists normally and varies in addition as a function of physiologic stress, both normal and pathologic[11] (Table 8.2). It is further exaggerated in the pneumonic lung

TABLE 8.2. Proportion of basal blood flow and $\dot{V}O_2$ to organs in man.[a]

Organ	Blood flow (%)	$\dot{V}O_2$ (%)	COD
Mesenteric viscera	27	23	1.2
Kidney	25	9	2.8
Muscle	18	21	0.9
Brain	15	28	0.5
Heart	4	11	0.4
Other	11	8	1.4

[a] Distribution of blood flow as the percent of basal cardiac output (5.5 L/minute) and oxygen consumption as percent of basal metabolic rate (240 ml/O_2/minute). The ratio of oxygen delivery as reflected by blood flow to oxygen utilization is indicated by the utilization fraction, the coefficient of oxygen delivery (COD).[11]

owing to the reported increase in its metabolic rate caused by the inflammatory response.[12] The vast infiltration of metabolically active cells, particularly polymorphonuclear leukocytes (PMNs), significantly increases the organ's apparent oxygen consumption, found to be as much as 13–15% of whole-body VO_2 in the dog.[12] Moreover, this additional oxygen extraction increases the resulting arterial hypoxemia as well owing to the admixture of pulmonary or bronchial venous blood that is even more desaturated than pulmonary arterial blood.

Delivery

Metabolic inhomogeneity within organs exists normally and may be pathologically exaggerated with hypoxia when loci of critical oxygen pressures arise. In these tissues VO_2 depends on regional PO_2. Tissues such as the cerebral cortex contain regions that in the basal physiologic state operate near their critical PO_2 (approximately 20 mm Hg); the kidneys' medullary thick limb of the loop of Henle has a high metabolic rate of oxygen consumption and may be limited by oxygen availability. These compromised tissue beds are readily apparent by clinical and laboratory manifestations of cerebral (confusion) or renal ("prerenal") dysfunction. Thus it is recognition of the nature as well as the existence of tissue hypoxia that dictates appropriate therapy to increase oxygen delivery. Such therapy might include increasing the arterial oxygenation by increasing FIO_2; increasing the blood's oxygen-carrying capacity with transfusion; or increasing flow (cardiac output) directly with ionotropes or indirectly by influencing its distribution with selective vasoactive agents.

It can be shown mathematically that with severe arterial hypoxemia it is not possible physiologically by simply increasing the cardiac output to raise the oxygen delivery or coefficient of oxygen delivery to a level that prevents a fall in mixed venous oxygen saturation below normal.[11] Similarly, analogous with the critical shortening of pulmonary transit time in the lung, diffusion limitation may also exist at the tissue level, precluding the attainment of gas equilibration. Heterogeneity of capillary lengths (and therefore oxygen release time) impairs unloading; and the effluent blood from these capillaries constitutes a convective shunt (arterial admixture) and contributes to an "elevated" PvO_2. Such "impaired extraction" limits the value of mixed venous oxygen monitoring as a sensitive indicator of the adequacy of tissue oxygenation. Thus oxygen delivery is not synonymous with "oxygen availability" and tissue oxygenation.

Distribution

A further adaptation to hypoxic stress is relaxation of precapillary sphincters and recruitment of capillaries into the perfused network to shorten the oxygen diffusion path. The recruitment of systemic capillaries brings transit times and rate of oxygen release into balance, similar to the autoregulatory phenomena that are effective in the lung with pneumonia to enhance pulmonary gas exchange in uninvolved areas. The movement of oxygen from capillary to cell is the final step in the oxygen delivery system. Although mitochondria require oxygen tensions of less than 3 mm Hg, a "critical" PO_2 is presumed to exist below which mitochondrial respiration is compromised. It would be affected not only by failure of the delivery system but by an up-regulation of the cells' "oxygen sink" as well (i.e., metabolic rate or tissue oxygen consumption).

When oxygen supply is limited relative to demand, flow is restricted to tissues with low oxygen extraction, such as kidney and mesenteric organs in favor of tissues with high extraction, such as heart and brain. Thus renal and mesenteric blood flow are diminished during exercise and arterial hypoxemia. Flow limitation to these "core" organs, because of impaired coronary or cerebral vessel patency, would defeat these homeostatic mechanisms. Hypoxia alone, in contrast to asphyxia, has a weak effect on the magnitude of splanchnic vasoconstriction and alteration in arterial pressure as a result of systemic vasoconstriction. It may be attributable to local unopposed "prejunctional" effects of adenosine and potassium. Accordingly, just as exercise with hypoxemia induces sympathetic adrenergic stimulation and the release of norepinephrine, the role of the associated release of inflammatory mediators, such as the prostenoids and cytokines in pneumonia patients appears to be critical to the redistribution of blood flow and oxygen availability to different tissue beds.

One report demonstrated an oxygen delivery-independent effect of blood flow on a canine model of diaphragm fatigue.[13] It was suggested that oxygen availability to contracting myocytes is more than the sum of the whole (i.e., a function of total muscle delivery). Such compensatory enhancement of membrane transport (permeability) and local microvascular control with alterations in venous PO_2 serve to maintain tissue oxygenation. In skeletal muscle such regional control is thought to depend on perfusion pressure rather than blood flow (i.e., a more homogeneous flow pattern may increase the proportion of flow directed through nutrient vessels) and the recruitment of new capillary channels, shortening the oxygen diffusion path. Furthermore, intraluminal pressure is a critical determinant, especially in pathologic states associated with increased interstitial pressure for sustaining a transmural pressure adequate to maintain vascular patency.

It is thus integration of a complex series of homeostatic reflex mechanisms and stress factors that is responsible for regional vasoconstriction and the overall conservation of oxygen for focused delivery to the organs most susceptible to hypoxia: brain and heart. Furthermore, intraorgan distribution appears to be a function of perfusion pressure interaction, with metabolic and endothelial factors controlling the capillary surface area available for oxygen diffusion. Teleologically, the high-flow–low extraction areas of the circulation constitute an oxygen reserve system that may be called on at times of stress. If prolonged, signs of organ ischemia (e.g., renal, mesenteric, and muscle dysfunction) become apparent and are interpreted as stress bleeding, prerenal failure, non-infectious (ischemic) hepatitis, pancreatitis, and diaphragmatic fatigue.

Mechanical Ventilation

Modes of Ventilatory Support

Indications

The evolution of technologic advances in mechanical ventilation has not been accompanied by the necessary scientific support to establish their value. Patients with pneumonia, community-acquired or otherwise, who have respiratory failure with severe refractory hypoxemia are widely believed, on the basis of uncontrolled trials and anecdotal reports, to have increased survival with assisted ventilation. Clinical studies showing still greater advantages of newer ventilatory modes are similarly nonexistent. The most apparent examples of these unsubstantiated benefits are the use of positive end-expiratory pressure (PEEP) in patients with acute lung injury syndrome (adult respiratory distress syndrome, or ARDS) and intermittent mandatory ventilation (IMV) and pressure support ventilation for weaning a patient from mechanical assistance. Proposed advantages of IMV over assisted ventilation include eliminating respiratory alkalosis, enhancing hemodynamics, and reducing weaning time, all of which are without substantial support. There is similarly no evidence for the value of PEEP in reducing the incidence of pulmonary oxygen toxicity and increasing survival of ARDS patients. The administration of PEEP has also not been found to be of value, as reflected by increased survival in one report of its use in bacterial pneumonia.[14] Studies have also failed to show the benefit initially reported for the prophylactic use of PEEP to avoid the development of ARDS in predisposing clinical states or to avoid atelectasis or pneumonia in postoperative patients.

Recruitment, Derecruitment, Hyperrecruitment

Therapeutic concepts of mechanical support are potentially in conflict in pneumonia patients, complicating the strategies of management if the acute inflammatory process is superimposed on underlying lung disease. The goal of increasing functional residual capacity (FRC) in ARDS patients runs counter to the ventilation goals for obstructive lung disease, as such volume recruitment contradicts the therapeutic concept of avoiding further or diminishing existing gas trapping and dynamic hyperinflation. Dynamic hyperinflation occurs when insufficient expiratory time is allocated between tidal breathing cycles to reestablish the relaxed equilibrium position between the forces of chest wall expansion and lung recoil. In the nonpassive state increased work is required to halt flow and apply an increased negative inspiratory force with the inspiratory muscles, which because of hyperinflation are at a mechanical disadvantage in generating the pressure necessary to accomplish this work. Thus in the presence of airways obstruction, the peak inspiratory flow rate is maximized to prolong the expiratory time (T_E), whereas with the restrictive disease of pneumonia therapeutic reversal of the inspiratory and expiratory times (T_I/T_E) has been attempted to enhance gas exchange. The actual pattern of inspiratory gas flow is of little consequence for determining uniformity of gas distribution. Inspiratory time is the important factor, especially in the presence of a population of lung units exhibiting long time constants when prolongation of T_E is of importance in order to limit gas trapping.

The use of dual ventilators with a double-lumen endotracheal tube for differential (independent) lung ventilation remains a concept of continuing interest. Here again, although the personal clinical observations showing benefit are well reported, the overall advantages in terms of survival and decreased morbidity have not been substantiated. In the presence of asymmetric lung disease, as with unilateral pneumonia, the logic of treating each lung differently is apparent. Overdistension (hyperrecruitment) of the alveoli of the unaffected lung constricts the vascular elements in their septal walls, increasing vascular resistance, with the consequence of enhancing flow to the involved lung and increasing venous admixture. This gross difference of involvement with unilateral pneumonia is always obvious in lung units at the microscopic level in bilateral bronchopneumonia, and full recruitment with PEEP may be readily achieved, especially during the proliferative stage of ARDS and beyond, with minimal pressure requirement for aerodynamic strutting. Further increases in lung volume, then, tend only to reduce effective compliance, as with unselective inflation the less affected (more compliant) lung units and the chest wall approach their elastic limits. Determination of the best "recruitment" pressure is controversial in part because of the implied suggestion that it has a built-in factor presumed to reflect the number of alveoli being therapeutically recruited. The reality, rather than just the potential, for morbidity to result from barotrauma is becoming more appreciated.

Tracheal Intubation

The use of mechanical ventilation generally requires an endotracheal tube. Intubation, while reducing the normal 72-ml upper airway volume with a 15-ml endotracheal tube, also interjects a tube of 7.5–9.0 mm internal diameter as a fixed inspiratory and expiratory resistor.[15] Tube resistance at low rates of laminar steady flow is inversely related to the fourth power of the radius and directly to its length. For high flow rates with increased ventilation, not only does the increased flow directly increase the pressure gradient required but when the Reynolds number is exceeded, which is the usual situation, turbulent flow results, further increasing the effective resistance. Bending of the tube and pooled secretions also serve to increase work. The potential advantages of a shorter orotracheal tube over a narrower nasotracheal tube is therefore apparent. However, with all the various determinants involved, there is little if any difference between an endotracheal tube and a tracheostomy tube despite the differences in length and radius. Intubation also serves only to retard the rate of return to FRC; it does not diminish the actual FRC, indicating that the widely held concept of "natural" PEEP is incorrect.[15] It should be expected, as observed not infrequently in the clinical setting, that extubation may allow successful weaning from machine support in certain intubated patients who otherwise would not have been predicted to be able to tolerate the breathing circuit independently.

Hemodynamics

Pulmonary Circulation

The hemodynamic consequences of spontaneous ventilation on "the pump within a pump" may frequently be enhancing, such as with spontaneous hyperventilation; but with mechanical ventilation they are primarily determined by alterations in lung volume and intrathoracic pressure. The pulmonary circulation consists of alveolar and interstitial vascular beds, each influencing the total pulmonary vascular resistance "independently"; but the effect of the alveolar vessels is predominant over the extraalveolar vessels. Lung inflation has a complex effect on pulmonary vascular resistance, as the small vascular elements in the alveolar septa are primarily influenced by alveolar pressure, and alveolar overdistension leads to their occlusion. At low lung volumes alveolar instability is promoted and collapse occurs, which is only in part attributable to the loss of interstitial traction forces. Alveolar vessels then become narrower as a result of alveolar wall collapse or an active process of hypoxic vasoconstriction. In the presence of an acute lung injury syndrome, however, dependence on maintenance of the integrity of such an interactive homeostatic autoregulatory control mechanism seems unlikely.

The extraalveolar vessels are larger, and their patency is a function of interstitial forces, a primary determinant of which is intrathoracic pressure (lung-vascular interdependence). The degree of radial interstitial traction on these vessels is also influenced by the actual lung volume, with the promotion of luminal narrowing and collapse at low lung volumes.

Thus deflating the lung has a complex effect on the pulmonary vascular resistance, which is minimal at normal FRC.

The bronchial vasculature is similarly highly sensitive to the effect of both lung inflation and airway pressure. Increases in bronchial vascular resistance are related to its primary drainage into the pulmonary capillaries and other vessels that connect the peribronchial arterial and submucosal vessels.[16] PEEP has been shown to eliminate virtually all bronchial blood flow, suggesting that patients with ARDS who have occlusive lesions of their pulmonary capillaries are at risk for additional tissue damage and lung infarction with the administration of PEEP.

Ventricular Function

An additional mechanical effect of lung volume is direct compression of the heart between the expanding lungs. The heart is in effect trapped in the cardiac fossa subject to the consequences of overdistension and mechanical heart–lung interaction. This situation may result in significant impairment of ventricular relaxation and filling (preload), especially in states of decreased ventricular "reserve." In patients being mechanically ventilated, the cardiac output, which primarily depends on venous return, may also be decreased as a result of the adverse effect on venous return of increased intrathoracic pressure. The venous return is further impaired with increases in lung volume, which raises pulmonary vascular resistance and the back-pressure to venous blood flow. Fluid resuscitation, preferably transfusion, is the usual means for enhancing venous return, and therefore the hemodynamic status must be carefully monitored with weaning for signs of acute circulatory overload.

The decrease in right ventricular transmural pressure resulting from the increases in intrathoracic pressure associated with positive-pressure lung inflation is unpredictable. It is attributable to the variable effect on juxtapericardial pressure that has been observed and the nonuniformity of its regional distribution over the surface of the heart—which in turn is related to the variety of factors responsible for transmission of the pressure. These factors include lung compliance and mediastinal compression[17] and a tethering effect of diaphragmatic descent on the pericardium,[18] as there are areas of pleural surface contiguous with the pericardium. Moreover, because of the sharing of a common interventricular wall and elastic pericardial compartment (sac) there is interdependence with the left ventricle. In addition, the right ventricular outflow is mechanically coupled to left ventricular inflow via the pulmonary circulation.[17]

Distension of the right ventricle therefore impairs left ventricular compliance and filling. Continuous positive-pressure breathing by increasing the left ventricular surface pressure, however, decreases the left ventricular afterload and may improve left ventricular performance. If this unloading effect is acutely eliminated by weaning, the patient with borderline "reserve" may experience acute left heart failure as a result of the reinstitution of negative intrathoracic pressure. Further stress on a limited oxygen delivery system is caused by the redistribution of blood flow to a now working, if not overstressed, diaphragm in the presence of an increase in the work of breathing. Another mechanism of lung–heart interdependence exaggerated by ventilator management in the presence of pneumonia is attributable to the inhomogeneous distribution of pulmonary compliance, allowing the overdistended, more compliant lung units to compress juxtaposed alveolar vascular elements. This condition is associated with a decrease in pulmonary blood volume and the usual transfer of blood volume from the right to the left side of the circulation during inspiration being enhanced by positive pressure, with a resultant increase in left ventricular preload and cardiac output.[18]

Peripheral Circulation

Because most deaths associated with respiratory failure are nonpulmonary in nature, the effects of increases in intrathoracic pressure on cerebral, hepatic, renal, and splanchnic perfusion are of great significance[19] (Table 8.3). Increased airway pressure has been implicated as a significant factor responsible for the high incidence of hepatic dysfunction observed in patients treated with positive-pressure ventilation. In one report, 77% of patients had a serum bilirubin higher than 2.5 mg/dl.[20] Descent of the diaphragm increases intraabdominal pressure, in turn increasing portal vein pressure and decreasing portal venous flow. The observed increase in splanchnic resistance and decrease in splanchnic blood flow is directly proportional to the tidal volume with an associated decrease in oxygen delivery to the mesenteric organs. Thus adequate oxygenation depends on the varying abilities of the abdominal viscera to increase oxygen

TABLE 8.3. Effect of PEEP (10 cm H_2O) on distribution of blood flow in dogs.

Measurement or site	Blood flow (% of control)
Cardiac output	53
Mean artrial pressure	80
Heart rate	93
Kidney	55
Brain	106
Adrenal	62
Gastric	40
Liver	57
Pancreas	28
Bronchial	28
Coronary	60

Source: Modified from data of Cassidy and Schwiep.[19]

extraction. Continuous PEEP has, as would be expected, a much greater adverse effect on flow than an intermittent positive-pressure (IPPB) ventilatory mode.

Positive end-expiratory pressure is also associated with decreased urine output and salt and water retention as a result of the release of antidiuretic hormone (ADH) and alterations in the pattern of intrarenal perfusion. This reaction is characterized by weight gain, positive water balance, hyponatremia, and decreased hemoglobin concentration. The distribution of renal blood flow, rather than total renal blood flow, is primarily affected, with preservation of flow to the inner cortex and medullary zones (juxtamedullary nephrons) at the expense of flow to the outer cortex (cortical nephrons). This redistribution of blood flow exaggerates the normal nonhomogeneous distribution of intrarenal blood flow superimposed on nephron heterogeneity to result in renal dysfunction. The antidiuresis and antinatriuresis caused by PEEP may also be the result of a decrease in glomerular filtration rate, which is reversed with fluid administration, and a baroreflex-dependent mechanism that has been demonstrated in animals by its reversal with renal denervation.[19]

The decrease in splanchnic blood flow presumably predisposes to gastrointestinal bleeding from such well recognized entities as "stress" gastric ulcers and ischemic colitis. Another event that is a routine accompaniment of mechanical ventilation, even in the presence of a competent endotracheal tube cuff, is *meteorism*, commonly termed *aerophagia*. If excessive, the intraluminal pressure distends bowel loops to an extent that may be extensive enough to occlude the vascular elements in the bowel wall and cause ischemia in the bowel segments. It is also of interest to speculate on the hemodynamic effects of enteric feeding, as food intake normally increases mesenteric blood flow. Thus during weaning the postprandial increase in blood flow to the gastrointestinal tract may be of significance if it compromises diaphragmatic blood flow.

The increase in intrathoracic pressure acts to impede cerebral venous return, promoting an increase in intracerebral pressure. This tendency for impaired cardiac output and increased intracranial pressure results in a decrease in cerebral perfusion pressure. Thus increased tissue pressure, impeding inflow of a reduced cardiac output with blood having a decreased oxygen tension, sets the stage for cerebral dysfunction and a toxic metabolic encephalopathy due to cerebral hypoxia.

Ventilatory Monitoring

Arterial blood gas determinations remain the standard for respirator management. As with any parameter, it is the absolute value as well as the relative value that is of importance. The PaO_2 is compared to a norm or preceding result using the same or an interpolated PaO_2 for a varying

TABLE 8.4. Derived oxygen exchange indices.

Abbreviation	Index
Q_{Va}/Q_T	Venous admixture (any FIO_2)
Q_s/Q_T	Shunt flow ($FIO_2 = 1.0$)
$(A\text{-}a)D_O$	Alveolar-arterial oxygen gradient
PaO_2/PAO_2	Arterial/alveolar oxygen ratio
PaO_2/FIO_2	Arterial/inspired oxygen ratio
$(A\text{-}a)DO_2/PaO_2$	Respiratory index

FIO_2 from a nomogram. Other derived parameters of oxygen exchange have been suggested as well (Table 8.4), but PaO_2 remains the standard guide for tissue oxygenation and a reflection of the adequacy of pulmonary gas exchange. Tissue oxygenation is more closely reflected by $P\dot{V}O_2$ and $\dot{V}O_2$ as well as oxygen delivery. The sensitivities of these parameters are frequently seriously compromised and have been shown to be inadequate because of variabilities in the distribution of blood flow and the failure of the actual $\dot{V}O_2$ to be the required $\dot{V}O_2$ to meet the energy demands of all of the transport and metabolic processes of the body's organs. Similarly, arterial oxygenation cannot be equated with oxygen transport, as blood flow is frequently impaired by techniques used to enhance the PaO_2 (i.e., PEEP). When considering the adequacy of oxygen transport, the total hemoglobin concentration must also be closely monitored. Noninvasive and continuous methods to monitor arterial oxygenation (including pulse oximetry and transcutaneous blood gas measurements) have variable accuracy, undetermined clinical usefulness, and unproved savings for cost containment. The accuracy of such measurements of tissue oxygenation in critically ill patients is related to oxygen delivery[21] (Fig. 8.1).

The "amount of ventilator" required to achieve the level of oxygenation and ventilation ($PaCO_2$) desired has prognostic significance, especially if used in a monitored fashion. For a given tidal volume and inspiratory flow rate, the peak inspiratory pressure serves as a measure of the "effective dynamic compliance." With an "inspiratory hold" maneuver, the "plateau," or distending, pressure of the system at end-inflation reflects the static elastic recoil force. The greater the airway resistance, the lower is the dynamic compliance in comparison to the compliance measured at plateau pressure. Finally, the level of auto-PEEP may be determined at end-expiration, and the severity of dynamic hyperinflation and "gas trapping" may be monitored.

Weaning

The concept of partial ventilatory support for weaning from mechanical ventilation evolved from the desire to diminish the work of breathing

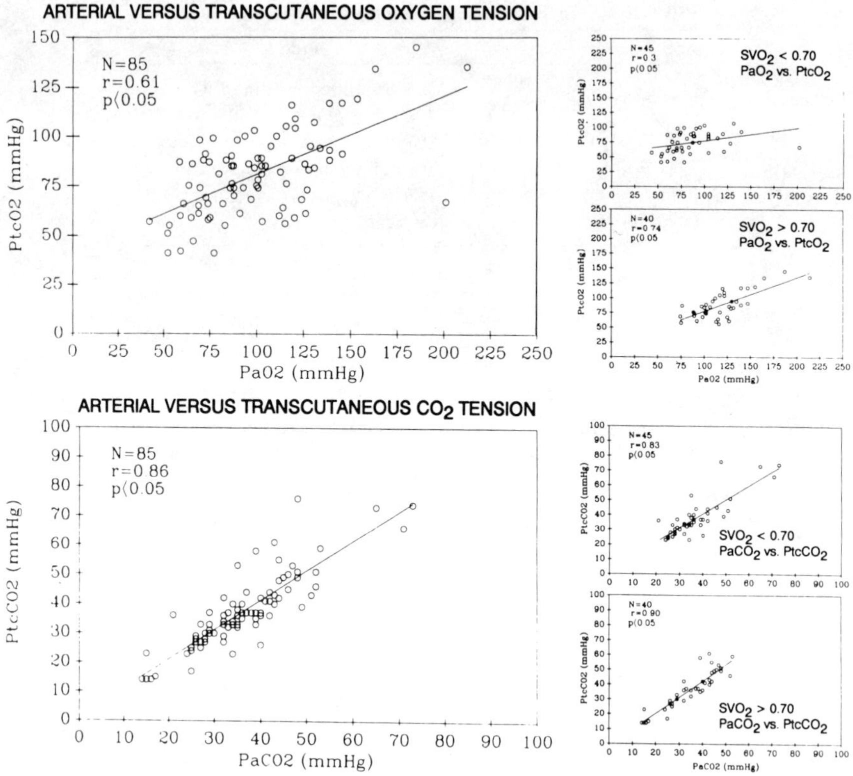

FIGURE 8.1. Transcutaneous (tc) oxygen and carbon dioxide measurements ($n = 85$) in 26 critically ill patients shown with simultaneous arterial blood gas values (39 on ventilator). Cardiac output and mixed venous blood gases were also determined, allowing calculation of oxygen delivery (OD) and measurement of SO_2. In group with $SO_2 < 70\%$ OD = 865 ml/minute and with $SO_2 > 70\%$ OD = 1035 ml/minute. (Data from Zaman et al.[21])

through the utilization of interactive modes. Such patient–ventilator interaction has the goal of amplifying patient effort to normalize its relation to ventilatory reward. In keeping with this thesis, yet another "weaning mode" has been described; termed proportional assist ventilation, the pressure delivered to the airway increases in proportion to inspiratory effort. Other noninvasive support techniques, such as nasal continuous and patient-triggered nasal intermittent positive-pressure ventilation, have been anecdotally reported to be successful.

Technical advances have not been shown to enhance weaning efforts and decrease the time required for assisted ventilation. Parameters usually monitored on "T-bar trials" include the tidal volume (V_T), respiratory frequency (f), minute ventilation (V_E), vital capacity (VC), maximum voluntary ventilation (MVV), and maximum inspiratory (P_Imax) and expiratory (P_Emax) forces.

Following tracheal intubation, especially if prolonged (>72 hours), complications can ensue with extubation, such as the sudden development of laryngeal (glottic) edema. The edema may be in the supraglottal or subglottal tissue or in the glottis itself. The pathogenesis of this entity is unclear, but several possibilities have been suggested including acute ulceration, acute laryngitis, sudden heart failure, epiglottitis, and even allergy to rubber.[20]

Laryngeal edema is usually readily apparent within minutes after extubation as the patient develops respiratory distress accompanied by inspiratory stridor. Uncontrolled observations have suggested benefit from corticosteroids and racemic epinephrine acutely as well as the administration of a helium-oxygen mixture. A simple comparison of "weaning parameters" before and after deflation of the cuff of the endotracheal tube may be a reliable method for predicting success or failure when weaning[22] (Table 8.5). The greater the entrainment of room air around the cuff, the lower is the PaO_2 and the more unlikely the presence of laryngeal edema.

The smaller the spontaneous V_T (<300 ml) and the greater the f (>25 breaths/minute) the poorer the outlook for successful weaning. Despite

TABLE 8.5. Weaning parameters on T-bar before and after cuff deflation.

Parametir	Entire group		Success		Extubation outcome: fail/not tried	
	Inf	Def	Inf	Def	Inf	Def
No.	55	55	32	32	23	23
pH	7.43	7.41	7.43	7.42	7.42	7.41
$PaCO_2$ (mm Hg)	42	43	40	40	46	47
PaO_2 (mm Hg)	121	101*	140	113*	95	84
HR (beaths/min)	103	105	103	103	104	107
f (breaths/min)	26	28*	24	25	29	31*
BP—syst. (mm Hg)	137	134	139	134	134	134
BP—diast. (mm Hg)	68	68	72	72	63	63
$\Delta PaCO_2$ (mm Hg)	0.8		0.8		0.8	
ΔPaO_2 (mm Hg)	20		26		11	
VC (L)	1.63		1.57		1.78	
V_T (ml)	433		513		334	
V_E (L/min)	10.1		10.7		9.4	
P_Imax (cm H_2O)	31.5		31.7		31.1	

Source: Data from Zaman et al.[22]

The successfully extubated group had a statistially significant fall in PaO_2 with cuff deflation ($p = 0.001$). The failed/not attempted extubation group did not have a statistically significant decrease in PaO_2 following cuff deflation ($p > 0.05$).

Inf = inflated; Def = deflated; V_T = tidal volume; VC = vital capacity; P_Imax = maximal inspiratory force.

* $p < 0.05$ in comparison to Inf value.

its ease of measurement (i.e., counting) the breathing frequency has been shown to be a notoriously inaccurate determination, as has the clinical estimation of tidal volume.[23] In general, the respiratory rate is elevated in proportion to the severity of the underlying lung disease, presumably to minimize inspiratory muscle effort. It has been equated with the magnitude of ventilatory muscle load, and the roles of mechanical and irritant receptors have been ignored. It has not been shown that the work or energy cost of breathing is higher in patients who are "weaning" failures. Current theses about weaning depend on the "jogger's mentality" of deconditioned respiratory muscles in the presence of increased respiratory loads. Ventilatory modes are used that theoretically reload the muscles of the respiratory pump in a tolerable, efficient, and synchronous manner.

Compartmental movement as determined by physical examination or technical recordings have also been used to predict weaning failures. Asynchronous motion (respiratory alternans), defining a time lag between the thoracoabdominal compartments and paradoxical motion (abdominal paradox), when the two compartments are completely out of phase and moving in opposite directions, have been suggested to reflect inspiratory muscle fatigue. These parameters are not universally accepted, however. Others have not found them to be reliable or sensitive signs of impending weaning failure, perhaps indicating that they are mere reflections of an increased respiratory work load rather than progressive fatigue.

Most patients who fail a weaning trial do not do so for their lack of effort. They generally display an elevated respiratory drive, as reflected by an increased mean inspiratory flow, tidal volume/inspiratory time (V_T/T_I), or $P_{0.1}$.[24] In general, weaning failure is not due to carbon dioxide retention, reflecting impaired drive, or failure of the diaphragm as a pressure generator. Rarely, carbon dioxide retention presents not from excessive carbon dioxide production resulting from the work of breathing but from therapeutic misadventures, classically with excessive parenteral rather than enteral nutrition, especially with a formula that has a high carbohydrate composition.

It is not difficult to understand the uniform failure of the variety of physiologic indices suggested to predict the success of weaning efforts. The studies use patients not only with varying severity of disease but different underlying causes of respiratory failure, varying durations of mechanical support and preceding weaning attempts, and the general absence of standardized objective criteria of weaning failure. The indices should be used as indicators of how closely to monitor the patient's independent ventilatory efforts not whether to initiate or even terminate them unless they fall within predefined "failure" limits. Whether these indicators should be the same as those used for initiating mechanical ventilatory support is not any clearer than which indicators should be used for initiating support short of complete cardiorespiratory collapse.

The best regimen for controlling a ventilator and then its discontinuation is never starting it in the first place.

Nutritional and Metabolic Support

Nutritional repletion has achieved the exalted status of qualifying as a legitimate "stratagem" in the therapeutic management of respiratory disease. The role of the calorie in the armamentarium of the pulmonary clinician has assumed a significance equivalent to that of spinach for the cartoonist's Popeye cult. The quantitative and qualitative appropriateness of the caloric intake has been enthusiastically, if not discriminately, endorsed as a means of both avoiding and treating respiratory insufficiency. This thesis has been suggested for patients with and without preexisting lung disease. It has been applied to the management of patients being weaned from mechanical ventilators and, more importantly, as a prophylactic measure to avoid the need for such devices by inadvertently precipitating ventilatory failure through "nutritional oversight."

Nutritional therapy for ambulatory, in contrast to hospitalized, patients has as its dual goals enhancement of ventilatory reserve and alleviation of dyspnea. Moreover, infection causes superimposed alterations in host metabolism and anorexia with decreased nutrient intake in the face of an increased metabolic demand due to fever. The need for gluconeogenesis because of carbohydrate depletion and inefficient fat utilization results in proteolysis manifested as myalgia and muscle weakness. This section attempts to correlate and place in perspective proposed effects of observed metabolic phenomena on parameters of respiration and immune function with reported clinical realities.

Respiratory Function

Muscle Strength

The potential benefits of nutritional support in enhancing pulmonary function by increasing the mass, strength, and endurance of the inspiratory muscles have been inferred from the clinical correlates of autopsy studies.[25] The size of the most important muscle of inspiration, the diaphragm, expressed in terms of thickness (centimeters), mass (grams), or area (square centimeters), has been found to be proportional to body weight in normal subjects and in patients who have no evidence of lung disease (Fig. 8.2).

In patients with emphysema, the diaphragmatic weight and total body weight decrease in proportion to the severity of the apparent airway obstruction; but the relative loss of diaphragmatic mass exceeds that of the rest of the body[26] (Fig. 8.3). The implied deterioration of muscle

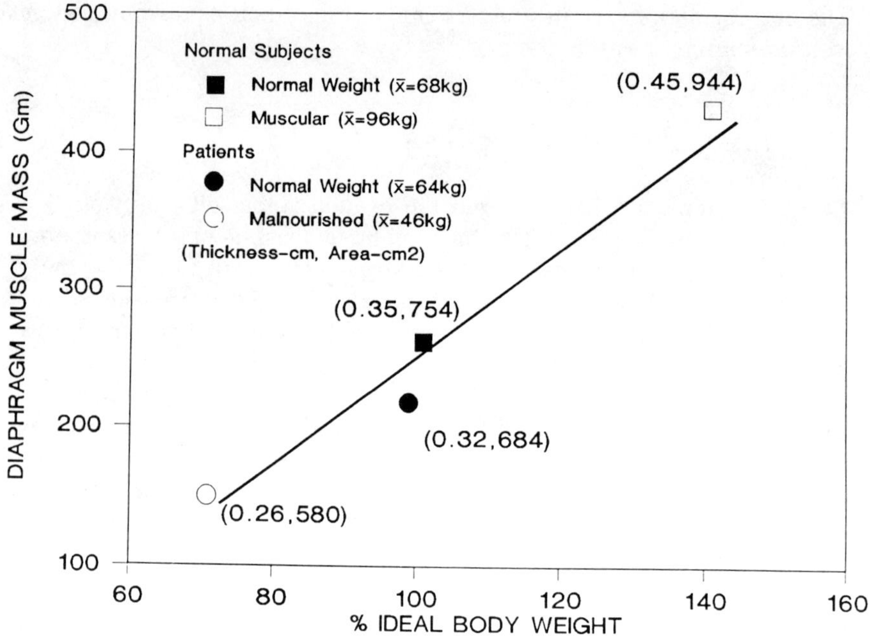

FIGURE 8.2. Mean values of diaphragmatic weight, thickness, and surface area of 33 normal subjects and 37 patients with various nonpulmonary diseases studied at autopsy. They are grouped according to estimates of the state of nutrition as determined from body weight. (Data from Rochester.[25])

performance in relation to nutritional status is also demonstrable in patients without lung disease by objective tests of pulmonary function.[27] The vital capacity (VC), maximum voluntary ventilation (MVV), and maximum inspiratory ($P_I$max) or expiratory ($P_E$max) pressures, inferring muscle strength, endurance, and force-generating capacity, respectively, of the respiratory muscles are reduced in association with weight loss (Fig. 8.4) Just as the loss of diaphragmatic muscle mass has been observed in autopsy studies to be relatively greater than the reduction in total body weight in patients with or without lung disease,[25,26] the impairment of inspiratory muscle strength has been found to be out of proportion to and to exceed that which would be predicted from loss of muscle mass alone, suggesting a superimposed nutritional myopathy.[27]

Ventilatory Control

The ventilatory response to an appropriate stimulus, in the absence of pulmonary or neuromuscular disease, is used as a measure of the chemosensitivity of the respiratory control mechanism. It may, however, be influenced by alterations in muscle strength. Both resting ventilation

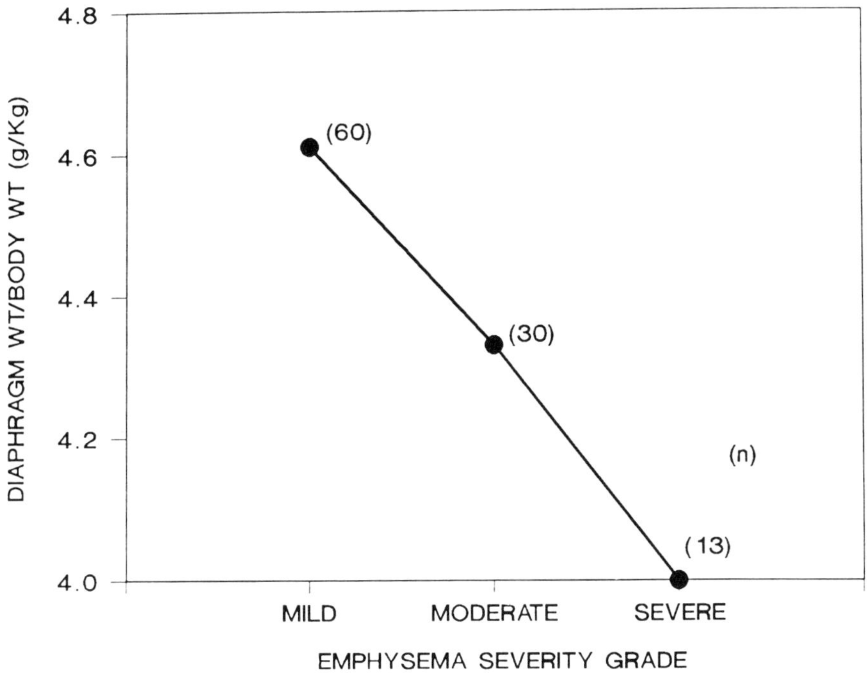

FIGURE 8.3. Mean values of the diaphragmatic/total body weight ratio found at autopsy in 103 male patients grouped according to severity of emphysema as determined by septal destruction and measured flow rates. The number (n) of patients in each group is shown in parentheses. (Data from Thurlbeck[26])

and the hypoxic ventilatory response decrease with caloric deprivation in direct relation to the magnitude of the associated fall in metabolic rate[28,29] (Fig. 8.5). In contrast, the effect of starvation on the ventilatory response to carbon dioxide is variable. This variability in part appears to be related to diet composition (Fig. 8.5).

The relation between the regulation of ventilation and metabolic activity has been previously studied, but only recently have primary alterations in metabolism as a consequence of nutrition been related to the central respiratory controller's "black box." The hypoxic response is readily restored by refeeding. However, calories supplied by amino acids alone, though they may be adequate to sustain nitrogen balance and enhance the ventilatory response to carbon dioxide, do not suffice to normalize chemosensitivity (Fig. 8.5). Normal ventilatory control can be fully restored only if total metabolism ($\dot{V}O_2$) is also returned to normal levels with calorie supplementation from additional sources such as fatty acids.[29]

This linkage of chemosensitivity to metabolism is also apparent with maneuvers inducing hypermetabolic states, as is seen with the thermogenic

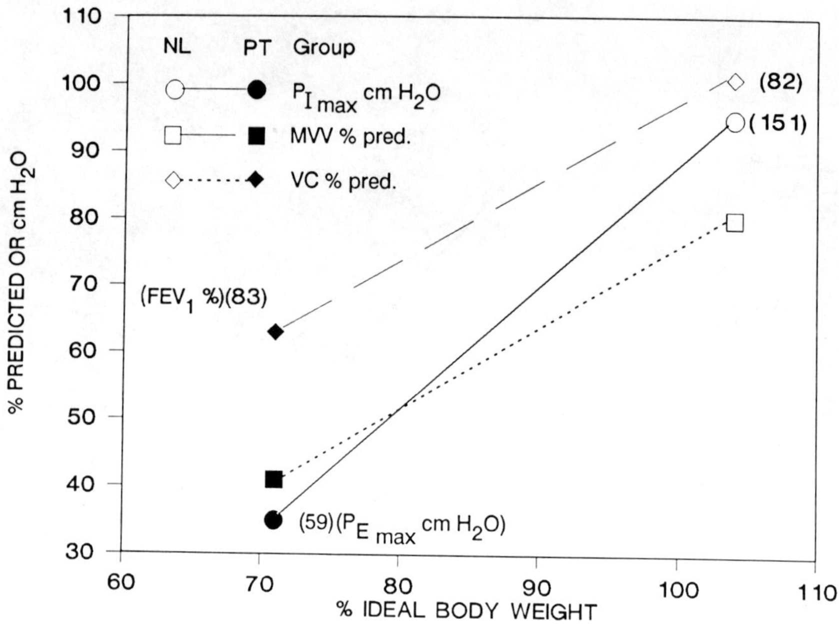

FIGURE 8.4. Mean values of tests of pulmonary function reflecting muscle strength in 16 normal subjects (NL) and 16 poorly nourished patients (PT) without cardiopulmonary disease. PImax (PEmax) = maximum inspiratory (expiratory) force; MVV = maximum voluntary ventilation; VC = vital capacity; $FEV_1\%$ = FEV_1/VC. (Data from Arora and Rochester.[27])

responses to exercise and overfeeding. The resting ventilation and hypoxic ventilatory response are enhanced in proportion to the immediate increases in metabolism induced by either carbohydrate (CHO) or protein administration.[30] However, for isocaloric intake, protein but not CHO enhances carbon dioxide chemosensitivity (Fig. 8.6).

The stimulatory effect of protein on neuromuscular drive, unlike that for CHO or lipid, does not totally depend on a rise in metabolic rate. This dynamic property of protein manifests by enhancing the sensitivity to carbon dioxide, as reflected by a shift of the intercept of the carbon dioxide response curve to the left (decreased threshold or carbon dioxide set-point), and the responsiveness (gain or slope) of the chemoreceptors to carbon dioxide. This effect is further characterized by greater flow rates (V_T/T_I) for a given PCO_2 (slope). The inspiratory timing mechanism (duty cycle), or duration of inspiration, expressed as a percentage of the total respiratory cycle (T_I/T_{TOT}), however, remains unchanged. CHO also tends to decrease the carbon dioxide threshold but less so than a calorically equivalent amino acid meal and without an associated change in flow rates. Thus the ventilatory stimulus of parenteral nutrition is

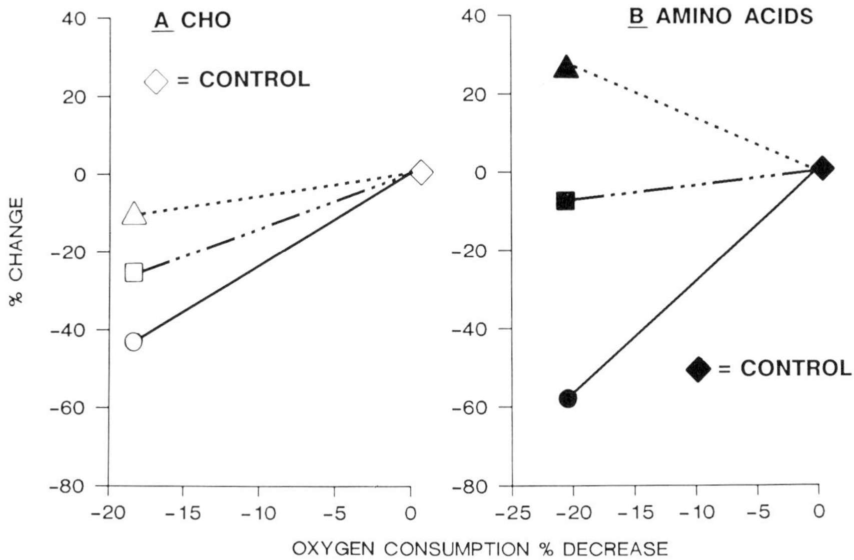

FIGURE 8.5. Mean changes in resting ventilation (□), carbon dioxide (△), and hypoxic (○) ventilatory responses in normal subjects after 10 days of semi-starvation on a daily diet of (A) 500 kcal glucose given daily (n = 7, open figures)[28] and (B) 550 kcal amino acids given parenterally (n = 6, solid figures)[29] in relation to the associated decrease in metabolic rate ($\dot{V}O_2$). (Data from Doekel et al.[28] and Baier and Somani.[29])

primarily due to the neurodynamic action of protein magnifying the ventilatory response to the carbon dioxide and thermogenic loads resulting from the oxidation of CHO.

The ventilatory response to caloric intake represents the efferent limb of a stimulus influenced by a number of factors, including nutrient composition, quantity, rate, and even route of administration. The afferent axis further depends on the subject's preexisting metabolic and nutritional status. The net magnitude of the resulting response is a complex function of the metabolic deposition of the caloric substrate and its intrinsic thermogenic contribution to the metabolic rate. If a given metabolic load is associated with a rise in $\dot{V}O_2$ and $\dot{V}CO_2$, the resulting ventilatory stimulus would be greater than if an increase in only $\dot{V}CO_2$ occurred. The pattern of the observed ventilatory response tends to be frequency-dependent in acutely ill patients but volume (V_T)-dependent in normal subjects and patients with normal lungs and stable metabolic profiles.[30] It may be postulated that the "impaired" neuromuscular drive and metabolic "dumping" associated with starvation serve a teleologic role when pulmonary function is impaired, and the potential adverse consequences of nutritional therapy are heralded clinically by dyspnea initially and, at its extreme, by the dreaded "weaning" failure.

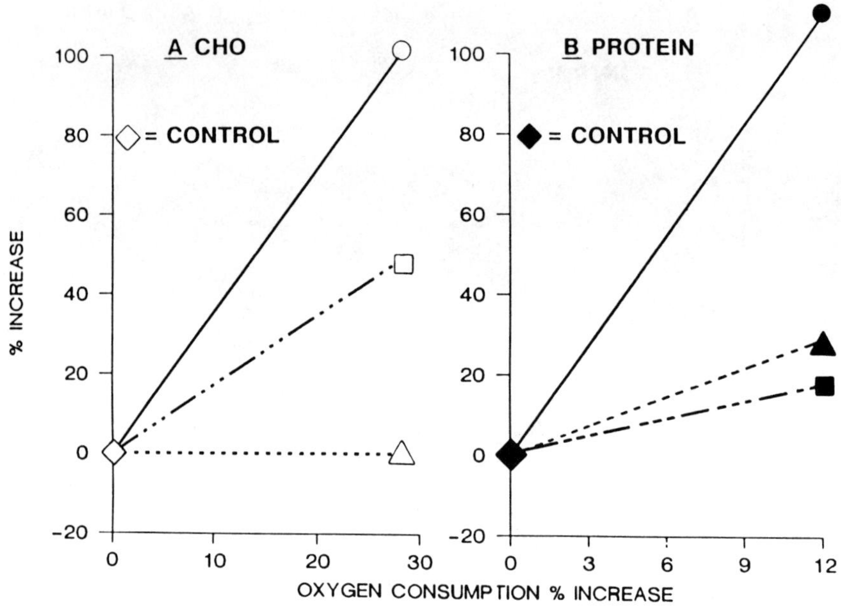

FIGURE 8.6. Mean changes in resting ventilation (□), carbon dioxide (△), and hypoxic (○) ventilatory responses in 6 normal subjects 3 hours after a 1000-kcal enteric bolus of (A) glucose (open figures) and (B) egg albumin (solid figures) in relation to the associated increase in metabolic rate ($\dot{V}O_2$). (Data from Zwillich et al.[30])

Acute Ventilatory Failure

Caloric repletion enhances ventilation in patients with respiratory insufficiency not only by increasing central neuromuscular drive but, if it results in a gain in body mass, by an increase in inspiratory force as well. Thus it has been proposed that the nutritional state of patients with respiratory failure should be optimized to maximize the bellows function of the respiratory apparatus. Others have clarified the important roles of the Mg^{2+} and PO_4^{2-} ions in muscle metabolism. Muscle weakness and respiratory failure may be precipitated by depletion of these ions, as they are essential for synthesis of the high-energy phosphate compounds adenosine triphosphate and creatine phosphate, which serve as sources for the immediate energy requirements of muscle contraction. The stores of both these compounds are depleted from respiratory and nonrespiratory skeletal muscle during episodes of respiratory failure.

The composition of the caloric regimen utilized is also of added significance in ventilatory failure because of the potential carbon dioxide load resulting from CHO metabolism. The burden is greater with CHO

TABLE 8.6. Metabolic pathways and resultant respiratory quotients.

Process	Reaction	RQ
Oxidation	CHO + 10 O_2 = 10 CO_2 + H_2O	1.0
Oxidation	Fat + 10 O_2 = 7 CO_2 + H_2O	0.7
Lipogenesis	CHO + 10 O_2 = 80 CO_2 + Fat	8.0+

relative to fat with complete oxidative metabolism [respiratory quotient (RQ) 1.0 versus 0.7]. The adverse consequences of administering excessive calories in the form of CHO are potentially even greater owing to the potential for "futile cycling" and because a progressively massive carbon dioxide load results, as lipogenesis (with an RQ far in excess of 1.0), rather than oxidation, becomes the predominant metabolic pathway (Table 8.6).

In patients whose ventilation is absolutely or relatively fixed owing to either dependence on mechanical ventilation or intrinsic pulmonary disease, this additional metabolic burden may result in overt respiratory failure or an inability to be successfully "weaned" from a ventilator. The stratagem of maximizing the fat content of nutritional supplementation must, however, also allow for an increase, albeit not as great, in ventilation, as for CHO loads[31] (Fig. 8.7).

In summary, a good deal of information has accumulated pertaining to the effects of nutritional interpositions on ventilation and respiration. Unfortunately, much of the evidence is contradictory and does not clearly indicate the role of nutrition in pulmonary dysfunction. With this approach to treatment, as with others, it is important to appreciate not only the well recognized side effects but the disputed benefits and then attempt to estimate the risk/benefit ratio.

Immunity

Cell and Humoral Mechanisms

Malnutrition is clinically associated with altered immune function (secondary immunodeficiency), increased respiratory tract infections, and increased mortality, yet the scientific relation between the cellular defense mechanisms and nutrition is complex and remains unclear. There is a well recognized linkage between infection and malnutrition, with bronchopneumonia commonly found at autopsy in children dying with severe malnutrition; its frequency correlates with the severity of malnutrition.

Changes in B cell number and function are inconsistent. Humoral immunity is less sensitive than cellular immunity to effects of protein

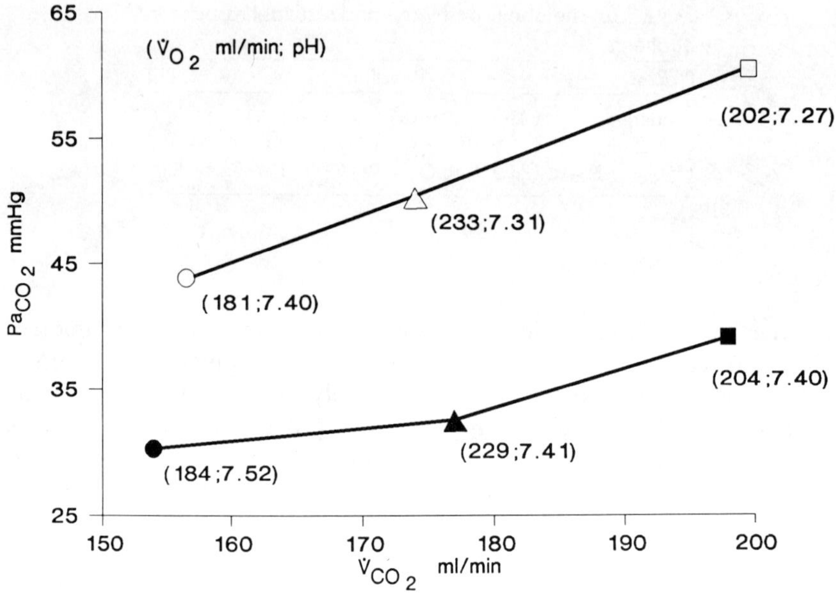

FIGURE 8.7. Mean control values (○) of arterial PCO_2 in 514 patients with COPD on mechanical ventilatory support measured at a fixed V_E of 6 L/minute (open figures) and 10 L/minute (solid figures) and 48 hours after a 1500 ml 50% glucose (2550 kcal/day) (□) or 1500 ml 20% fat emulsion (3000 kcal/day) (△). (Data from Herve et al.[31])

deficiency. Studies tend to indicate that nutritional deprivation decreases the humoral immune response to both viral and bacterial vaccines; the response is variable, however, and refeeding can correct the abnormality. B cell regions in lymphoid tissue are histologically preserved, and normal numbers of circulating B cells are present in the peripheral blood of patients with protein-calorie malnutrition.

Primary and secondary lymphoid tissue is altered with malnutrition. The thymus becomes atrophic, tonsillar size is grossly decreased, and the weight of the spleen can be reduced to one-third normal. Histologic examination of lymph nodes shows diminished cellularity of both germinal centers and the T-cell-dependent paracortical areas, but the latter are more severely affected. Peripheral blood lymphocytopenia with reduction of T4-helper and T8-suppressor lymphocytes and natural killer cells are reported, but there are also reports that lymphocyte populations may be normal, especially circulating suppressor T lymphocytes. Cell-mediated immunity and other T-cell functions have been reported to be impaired. The most consistent finding is impairment of cutaneous delayed hypersensitivity reactions. These abnormalities of cell-mediated immune function are reversible with nutritional repletion. Although early steps in PMN activation may be impaired, phagocytic activity and bactericidal capacity remain intact.

Repletion

It is difficult to attribute the state of nutrition to infection or reversal of the nutritional state to a return of immune function. It appears that nutritional support, enteric or parenteral, allows protein sparing and decreased infection and mortality in malnourished patients. It has been shown that during infections in protein-deficient patients antibody synthesis is maintained despite the reduction in synthesis of other serum proteins such as albumin. It appears that the quality as well as the quantity of the amino acid content of the protein is also important. Specific amino acid deficiencies (e.g., isoleucine, valine, and other essential amino acids) impair lymphopoiesis and cellular immunologic competence.

Enteric feedings are thought by many to be superior to total parenteral nutrition (TPN) for maintaining gut integrity and preventing septic complications presumably by the mechanism of translocation. Regardless of the route of repletion, few data are available to validate the intuitive benefit of nutritional therapy. This point is particularly pertinent to infections in general and lung infection in particular, which have not been used as clinical endpoints in the human studies that are available. Immunocompetence, though it reveals aberrant parameters in anorexia nervosa, is seldom reported to be impaired to a degree of such severity as to be associated with an impressive increase in infectious disease.

Similarly, perioperative nutritional supplementation (TPN) appears to benefit only those severely malnourished, whereas those identified as having only mild malnutrition (after stratification) have an increased incidence of infection.[32] The increase in bacterial complications are not catheter-related but are wound infections and pneumonia. Although TPN has not previously been shown to be causally related to an increased rate of other than catheter-related infection, concern has been expressed that, rather than supporting host defense mechanisms, TPN might have the opposite effect and in critically ill patients may cause further impairment of the host's defense. Lipids in particular have been suggested to have a possible detrimental effect on the immune system. This suggestion has not been substantiated to date, and questions remain particularly regarding overload of the reticular endothelium system and how the various fatty acids in fat emulsions may adversely modulate immunity. The difficulty of assessing outcomes is the synergistic interaction between nutrition and the immune response to infectious disease. This interaction is bidirectional: Nutritional status influences host immunologic responsiveness, and infectious disease has a detrimental influence on nutritional status.

Physical Therapy

Antibiotic regimens are frequently supplemented with adjuvant modes of therapy that are meant to augment the lung's defense mechanisms, enhance gas exchange, and ameliorate symptoms. Their efficacy has been challenged; and as soon as one therapeutic modality has been irrevocably put into disrepute it is replaced by another unproved supportive measure that rapidly becomes a standard of care through usage and intuitivism.

Chest Physiotherapy

Supportive measures in addition to expectorants and mucolytics to improve pulmonary toilet have classically included chest percussion and postural manipulation to enhance gravity drainage. Chest physiotherapy consisting of postural drainage was introduced as a therapeutic intervention at the turn of the century. After World War I, chest percussion and vibration were used concomitantly and subsequently with intermittent positive-pressure breathing (IPPB), which had been developed prior to World War II but was not widely utilized until the 1950s. These modes of therapy, though vigorously advocated, have not been shown to have a beneficial effect on pneumonia patients with respect to mortality, radiologic clearing, duration of fever, or hospitalization.[33]

Even more discouraging are the results of a study in patients with pneumonia that revealed regular chest physiotherapy to be associated with prolonged duration of fever and increased hospital stay when compared to verbal advice on the need for expectoration and deep breathing.[34] Airway obstruction as determined by the forced experatory volume in 1 second (FEV_1) also showed no benefit from therapy. As might be expected, responses from patients who received physiotherapy, when contacted 5 months after discharge, were all "positive" or "very positive" in regard to the value of the physiotherapy for the healing process.[34] The prolonged fever in the treatment group was attributed to the spread of the infectious process; and it was pointed out that in Russia chest physiotherapy is not started in pneumonia patients until the fever has subsided, and it is then thought to give prompter and more complete healing.[34] Similarly, there is also little evidence to suggest benefit of its prophylactic use for preoperative or postoperative management or for any of the wide variety of clinical situations in which it is used. Thus although secretions may be mobilized by chest physiotherapy and there is increased sputum production, it has not been shown to translate into affecting the clinical course or the development of pneumonia.

The uncontrolled mobilization of secretions has the theoretic hazard of spreading the infection to otherwise uninvolved areas of the lung. In the absence of large volumes of secretions in the patient with a normal cough, there is no support for even the teleologic argument for the benefit of physiotherapy. In such situations, physiotherapy may well be expected to result in deterioration of lung function in patients with airway hyperreactivity, such as asthmatic bronchitis, presumably by inducing bronchospasm such as suction catheters are known to do. Moreover, as with lung inflation devices, several studies have shown that there may be worsening of the hypoxemia. Therefore chest physiotherapy should only be done with oxygen treatment in patients with concurrent arterial desaturation.

Arterial oxygenation has been observed to remain unchanged after chest physiotherapy in patients on mechanical ventilation[35] and to increase immediately after treatment with a mechanical vibrator in critically ill patients with pneumonia.[36] It is postulated that sputum that is thixotropic becomes more liquid upon constant disruption, and increased clearance results if there is an expiratory flow bias (two-phase flow) allowing for its mobilization and the opening of peripheral lung units. Vibrations are also thought to excite the walls of large airways, so secretions detach from the mucosa and are carried away by the oscillatory air flow. It has been suggested that the standard duration of the physiotherapy sessions are inadequate. During this era of resource rationing, such claims require substantial support by objective data to show the value of physiotherapy—not obtained during the nearly 100 years of its documented use—before this mode of therapy, on the wane, is restored to modern therapeutic protocols.

A similar question of dose has been raised most recently for continuous lateral rotational therapy, which has been introduced as a kinetic form of prophylactic therapy against nosocomial pneumonia for use in immobile patients. It involves continuous slow rotation in the longitudinal axis over 124 degrees. Studies have suggested that effective prophylaxis can be achieved, with pneumonia occurring in fewer stroke and trauma patients compared to the standard hospital bed, but the mortality among stroke patients was unchanged. Patients with sepsis and pneumonia had a shorter intensive care unit (ICU) stay compared with controls; but again overall mortality was no different.[37] The prospective medical and economic benefits of prophylactic physical therapy creates pressure for premature acceptance of yet another unproved modality for which pulmonary medicine as other subspecialty areas have a well recognized heritage.

Lung Expansion Devices

The concept of early ambulation classically utilized during the postoperative period to mobilize peripheral blood flow (and thereby prevent phlebitis due to venous stasis) is similarly applied to the bedridden pneumonia patient. Provided this concept in reality is not corrupted into becoming, as it has in phlebology, a state of early angulation, it is probably as effective as any of the growing number of devices available to alleviate microatelectasis and promote sputum mobilization. Sitting in a chair with the proximal and distal portions of the lower extremities at right angles is not the goal, but the deep breaths that occur as a result of the exertion of getting to the chair and returning to the bed is the presumed therapeutic segment of this maneuver, which is further enhanced by walking. The use of simple devices, such as the classic Dale-Schwartz tube, blow battle, IPPB instrument, and incentive spirometer, has been shown to add little if any therapeutic advantage. Moreover, these devices present potential dangers of worsening hypoxia or barotrauma, or of being the source of nosocomial infection.

Enlarging the physiologic deadspace with a hollow breathing tube without supplemental oxygen may cause dramatic lowering of the alveolar PO_2 in the predisposed patient, despite an autoregulatory attempt by the central respiratory center and peripheral chemoreceptors to maintain the effective alveolar ventilation by hyperventilation. Thus the Dale-Schwartz tube fell into disuse to be replaced by mechanical devices to induce hyperventilation other than by "purposeful" deep breathing. When the ineffectiveness of blow bottles was subsequently demonstrated, it was attributed to the expiratory mode of action, which was suggested to worsen the existing atelectasis by promoting further small airway collapse. A potential beneficial effect results or predominates in some patients from the deep inspiration preceding the blow that is performed to generate a greater expiratory force.

The IPPB instruments were initially introduced not only to expand the lung in the debilitated patient but to deliver medication such as bronchodilators, mucolytics, and antibiotics as well. On the basis of available clinical studies, IPPB remains an accepted valid intervention only in the patient with a chest deformity, such as kyphoscoliosis. The "therapeutic" pressure bolus has been shown to worsen hypoxemia, bronchospasm, and gas exchange with the life-threatening danger of barotrauma as well.

Incentive spirometry remains the most popular and a much utilized mode of therapy, primarily in the postoperative patient. Documentation of its benefits is poor, and most studies have failed to show that it has value. It has been shown to be as "effective" as the previously discredited prophylactic measure of IPPB postoperatively in coronary bypass patients.[38] Its cost aside, patients are frequently given the instructions for its use without being given nasal oxygen during the inspiratory exercise despite being maintained on oxygen by mask.

Continuous positive airway pressure (CPAP) masks have been more consistently shown to result in the desired expansion of lung volume. However, its efficacy as a prophylactic or therapeutic measure for managing microatelectasis does not speak for its role, much less its benefit, in decreasing the incidence or the treatment of established airway collapse or pneumonia. None of these techniques has been shown to alter the severity, duration, or course of an established pneumonia.

Mucology: Expectorants and Mucolytic Drugs

The Bible, the earliest pharmacopoeia that emphasized mucokinetic drugs, was in reality only continuing to give them the prominence already endowed by the preceding ancient Eastern civilizations.[39] The goal regarding pneumonia was, as stated by Hippocrates, to soothe the cough and promote expectoration. The prescription of Maimonides for "highly spiced chicken soup" was for the same purpose: to promote a "gustatory reflex" and productive cough, which because of the vapors (if served appropriately steaming) acts as a mucorrheic agent. Since the nineteenth century therapeutic doses of iodide have been prescribed to make sputum less tenacious; thus iodide has been thought to be of value in refractory cases of pneumonia. These are but two common examples not only of our customary practices without scientific basis that are widespread in mucokinetic therapy but that fail to differentiate between expectorants, antitussives, demulcents, and so on. All of these agents are aggregated under the banner of mucoactive drugs, implying their common endpoint of promoting mucociliary clearance. Many of the most traditional expectorants (e.g., potassium iodide) in therapeutic doses may act on the gastric mucosa, evoking a "gastropulmonary mucokinetic reflex" through the vagus nerve, whereas in toxic doses nausea results via the central vomiting center.

Mucin Structure

Airway mucins are synthesized by both goblet cells of the epithelium and mucous cells in the submucosal glands. Although control is probably complex, these glands appear normally to be under autonomic regulation. The mucins are hydrated on the mucosal surface, forming the mucous gel. Just as a liquid and its gas vapor phase coexist at the boiling point, polymer gels can exist in one of two phases: a condensed phase or an expanded hydrated phase.[40] The transition from the condensed polymer (released by the cells) to its hydrated phase on the surface of the mucosa is reversible and is associated with a several hundredfold volume change.

Rheologically, bronchial mucus forms a complex nonnewtonian viscoelastic polymer gel layer flowing over an underlying serous sol layer, allowing the cilia's oscillatory movements. The rheologic and viscoelastic properties of mucus that enable ciliary transport are primarily conferred by the glycoprotein mucin component. Polymerization creates the high molecular weight (HMW) mucous glycoprotein and gel matrix. The basic unit of the glycoprotein macromolecule is a linear polypeptide backbone from which side chains of carbohydrate extend. The "oligosaccharide clusters" (o-glycans) are joined by o-glycoside bonds to the core protein or apomucin. These side chains are responsible for the high carbohydrate content (80%) of mucin, as well as its density, hydrodynamic volume, and viscosity.

The bronchial mucus, which is a heterogeneous mixture of HMW glycoproteins, has a tertiary structure of flexible, tortuously coiled, entangled threads. These threads are polydispersed in size from a minute 300 nm to "immense" chains up to 5 μm in length; they have a "bottle brush" structure of amino acid cores with glycoprotein branches.[41] The rheologic properties of the mucous gel are determined by what is termed its tangle density, which rapidly decreases with increasing hydration. Thus the capacity and degree of mucous hydration (swelling) is the main determinant of mucous rheology. The absence of interchain bonds allows dispersion of the tangled polymer network in solution.[40]

The flexible, long, "coiled thread" model proposes one long peptide containing highly protease-resistant glycosylated regions covered by hundreds of heterogeneous glycan chains that are interspersed with poorly glycosylated (naked), protease-sensitive regions.[41] The conformation of mucin macromolecules were formerly thought to be dependent on branched, covalently cross-linked disulfide bridges, but it is their quaternary structure that is now being emphasized as being responsible for the linear conformation of mucin strands tangled in the mucus matrix.

The architecture of the mucin peptide moiety shows extreme polydispersity, and the quaternary structure of carbohydrate chains are heterogeneous. The diversity of carbohydrate chains may undergo subtle but specific modifications during inflammatory processes, possibly reflecting differences in cell origins or disease-induced alterations. The carbohydrate chains are recognized by surface adhesins of microorganisms and represent potential sites for their attachment. This trait allows their trapping on the mucous blanket, their removal by mucociliary elevation, and under normal circumstances swallowing of the raised mucus. Thus the carbohydrate chains play an important role in the pulmonary defense system.[41]

Mucokinesis

The hundreds of oligosaccharide clusters or chains on a single mucin molecule may vary in length between 1 and 20 sugars and may be neutral, sialylated, or sulfated. Mucolytics generally contain a free thiol group thought necessary to interact with the cysteine-SH group, thus breaking the disulfide bond, reducing the viscosity (mucolysis) of the mucous structure, and enhancing mucokinesis. Such an agent, acetylcysteine, has been reported to be an effective mucokinetic agent despite its irritative properties in making pulmonary secretions more easily removed by ciliary action or cough, thereby reducing pulmonary complications and the need for endotracheal aspiration.

Mast cells and neutrophils are sources of inflammatory mediators, especially proteases, such as chymase, elastase, and cathepsin G, which have been found to be the most potent secretagogues of airway submucosal gland secretion ever described.[42] It has been proposed that the release of these enzymes near glands in inflammatory diseases plays an important role in the pathogenesis of the accompanying hypersecretion. An important strategy for intervention may eventually involve inhibitors of these enzymes. Similar roles have been suggested for several neuropeptides, including substance P, neurokinin A, and the parasympathetic neuropeptide vasoactive intestinal peptide; the therapeutic use of neuropeptidases has also been proposed.

Hypertonic saline given by ultrasonic aerosol has been used to induce sputum; this technique has been adapted for routine use in acquired immunodeficiency syndrome (AIDS) patients to diagnose *Pneumocystis carinii* pneumonia. Impaired mucokinesis in some instances is presumed to be related to a deficiency in depth or an increase in viscosity of the sol layer, preventing the cilia from maintaining an effective coordinated beat with their tips extending into the overlying mucous gel layer. Water and saline solutions have long been used ineffectually in efforts to modify the sol layer and for the hydration of mucus. Similarly, efforts to correct imagined or real systemic dehydration in order to hydrate an often viscous desiccated mucous layer has proved futile, as respiratory tract fluid appears to be resistant to dehydration. Primary mist treatments, encouraged by manufactures rather than suggested on a scientific basis supported by clinical data, is also without benefit in lower respiratory tract infections. Cold humidification of oxygen administered by mask, nasal cannula, or venturi apparatus does not achieve a real increase in humidification. Such adult "cold steamers" palliate the senses, not the bronchial mucosa. Normal saline has no specific mucokinetic action when given orally, intravenously, or by aerosol; although topical administration can induce coughing, its main value in aerosol form is as a vehicle for drug administration rather than as a mucokinetic agent.[43]

In summary, much emphasis has been placed on the therapeutic benefits of enhancing elimination of the purulent material that results from the inflammation of pneumonia, just as it is characteristically pursued for inflammatory airway disease. Although many of the mucologic drugs currently available are ineffectual products of, or direct descendants from, ancient preparations, the current growth spurt in the understanding of mucus—its physiochemical properties, control, and mechanisms of secretion—promises revised therapeutics in the near future.

Steroidal and Nonsteroidal Antiinflammatory Agents

Bacterial Pneumonia

Much discussion if not controversy has been focused on the mechanisms of hypoxemia and diminished perfusion of the consolidated lung associated with bacterial lobar pneumonia. There are various postulates for the apparent increase in vascular resistance redirecting blood flow to uninvolved lung: intravascular occlusion by active thrombotic or cell aggregative processes; extrinsic vascular compression from the weight of surrounding alveolar and interstitial tissues due to exudative edema-forming processes; necrosis or destruction of parenchymal tissue or vasculature; and vasoactive hypoxic vasoconstriction.[44] Emphasis for therapeutic purposes has been placed on impairing the synthesis of vasoactive prostanoids such as the vasodilators prostaglandin E_1 (PGE_1) and prostacyclin (PGI_2), which have been shown to be capable of increasing the venous admixture of experimental lobar pneumonia.

It has been demonstrated in a dog model that infusion of PGE_1 results in disappearance of the selective perfusion deficit and the redistribution of blood flow to consolidated lung tissue in lobar pneumonia.[44] Thus rather than mechanical control, a pharmacologic "imbalance" of vasoactive dilator and constrictor mediators were postulated, specifically the prostanoids. Subsequently, efforts were initiated to abort the arachidonic acid cascade proximally with inhibition of phospholipase A or more distally at the cyclooxygenase level in order to restore or augment the normal autoregulatory hypoxic pulmonary vasoconstriction mechanisms and homeostasis.

It has been demonstrated that administration of acetylsalicylic acid or indomethacin, potent inhibitors of cyclooxygenase, reduce blood flow to the consolidated lung in dogs with experimental pneumococcal pneumonia, thereby improving oxygenation.[45] It has become apparent that, because of the varying type and intensity of the inflammatory process, the degree of impairment of the responsiveness of vascular elements to vasoconstrictor drugs is unpredictable. Moreover, even if complete blockade can be accomplished, vasoactive mediators other than prostanoids are involved in the inflammatory process, and "appropriate" hypoxic vasoconstriction appears to remain an unachievable goal. Such pharmacologic manipulation therefore may favor not only redirection of the arachidonic acid cascade to the lipoxygenase pathway with the net synthesis of excess leukotriene vasoconstrictors[45] but other, as yet unknown metabolic effects that affect mediators capable of altering vaso-motor responses. Subsequent studies in humans with respiratory failure due to bacterial pneumonia supported the failed hypoxic vasoconstrictor hypothesis by showing clinically significant increases in arterial oxygenation in five patients immediately following oral administration of indomethacin.[46] Efficacy may be expected to be negilgible in diffuse processes and enhanced in localized processes of interstitial or bronchopneumonia because the extent to which blood flow is diverted away from a hypoxic segment (i.e., the strength of the hypoxic vasoconstrictor response) is inversely proportional to the size of the segment.

Acute Lung Injury Syndrome

Because CPAP was shown to be an ineffective means of prophylactic therapy for ARDS, despite favorable early reports, other therapeutic interventions, particularly antiinflammatory agents, steroidal and nonsteroidal, have been proposed. Early reports of PMN-aggregation-induced ARDS preceded by complement activation and successful prophylaxis with corticosteroid treatment, presumably acting to inhibit complement activation, led to their use in clinical trials. In such studies of patients with septic shock, corticosteroids did not affect the development of ARDS,[47,48] and no correlation was found with complement levels and the development of ARDS.[47] Moreover, corticosteroid treatment seemed to be associated with an increased incidence and severity of ARDS with a greater mortality, which may be attributed to a higher incidence of secondary infections.[48] It has also been shown that once ARDS is established corticosteroid administration has no beneficial effect on outcome when it is considered in terms of reversal of the respiratory failure of ARDS (characterized by chest roentgenoram, lung mechanics, arterial oxygenation, or associated mortality).[49]

Animal studies suggest that for corticosteroids to effectively ameliorate increases in pulmonary microvascular permeability they must be given prior to or within 30 minutes of the induction of endotoxemia. Therefore it was suggested that once ARDS is present it is too late; previous studies did not carefully assess the effect of corticosteroids, when given early, on parenchymal lung injury associated with sepsis short of ARDS. Once again, even when the immediacy of administration was stressed, it was found that neither mortality nor even lesser degrees of parenchymal lung injury were ameliorated by corticosteroid treatment.[50] Thus corticosteroids were again not found to decrease the incidence of ARDS in the presence of sepsis. Additionally, a high dose of corticosteroid was not found to affect the time interval between the clinical suspicion of septic shock and the onset of ARDS or the time to resolution of ARDS from its onset. However, it is difficult to diagnose septic shock readily enough for truly early intervention; and the process of parenchymal lung damage leading to respiratory insufficiency has already been initiated during the initial interval of time devoid of the critical clinical manifestations of sepsis that would allow early diagnosis. In contrast to these negative results, others have reported benefit from a sustained (3 weeks), rather than short (24–48 hours), course of corticosteroid treatment in patients with established ARDS in whom the primary process that produced ARDS was controlled.[51]

Finally, several studies have suggested that corticosteroids might be of benefit in human immunodeficiency virus (HIV)-positive patients with *Pneumocystis* pneumonia. It was concluded that the early use of such adjunctive therapy in patients with moderate to severe pneumonia decreases the magnitude of the Herxheimer type of initial deterioration in oxygenation, progressive respiratory failure, and death associated with antimicrobial treatment.[52,53] These conclusions and recommendations, noted in a consensus statement, have created a number of questions, including the role of shorter pulse therapy, the risk of superinfection especially with tuberculosis, the pathophysiology of deterioration in oxygenation, and the apparent unique mechanism for therapeutic efficacy with this type of pneumonia. Additionally, all studies have not found benefits for survival. Because of the lack of initial response and the early recurrence of complicating secondary infection, corticosteroids as "rescue therapy" in a clinical state perhaps more synonymous with "true" ARDS has not been shown to be of value.[53] Similar apparent benefit from such adjuvant therapy has also been reported for the treatment of severe tuberculosis infection in both HIV-positive and HIV-negative patients.

Because of the eventual disappointments for which steroids have been historically responsible when definitive studies have followed up on the initial positive accounts of therapeutic responses, it is difficult to become a strong believer in the current favorable reports regarding *Pneumocystis* pneumonia. It does seem reasonable, however, that higher dosage and longer durations of treatment at different stages of disease for different etiologic agents, pathogenesis, and pathophysiology might well produce different results.

Fluid

The long recognized relation and coexistence of pulmonary edema and pneumonia, seen both clinically and at autopsy, led to warnings nearly 40 years ago regarding the potential adverse consequences of parenteral fluid therapy.[54] Terms such as serous pneumonia, satellite and localized pulmonary edema, and congestive atelectasis were subsequently assimilated into the semantics of the acute lung injury syndrome. The synergistic interactions between hydrostatic pressure, vascular permeability, oncotic pressure, and impaired lymphatic fluid resorption are largely ignored in attempts to "hydrate" the pneumonia patient. These attempts at "early hydration" are in fact due to the clinician's innocent acts of "early drowning."

Numerous studies utilizing animal models of noncardiogenic pulmonary edema have demonstrated that changes in left ventricular filling pressure within the normal range affected the rate and amount of lung water accumulation. Vasodilator and diuretic treatment of aspiration pneumonia in dogs was observed to decrease lung water accumulation and reduce venous admixture while maintaining cardiac output despite a decrease in left ventricular filling pressure.[55] In contrast, volume expansion in a

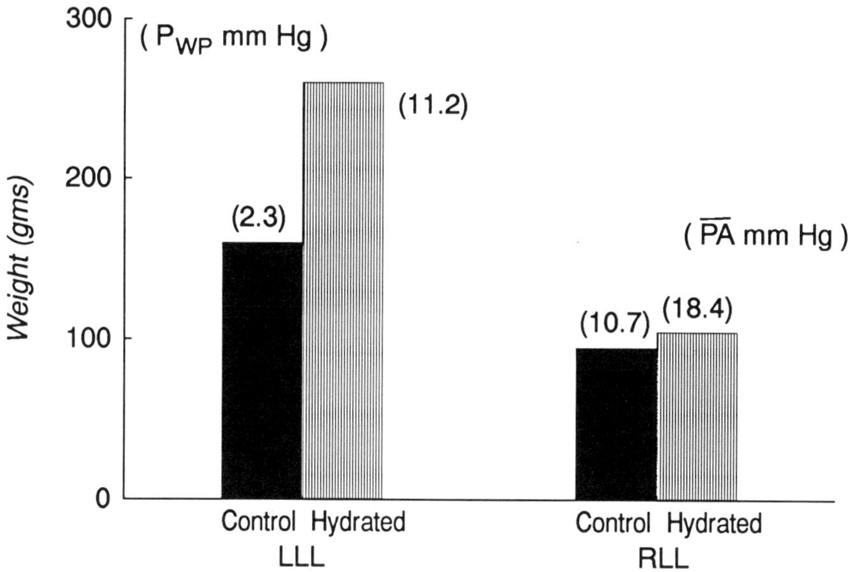

FIGURE 8.8. Mean values of lung weight 48 hours after the induction of pneumococcal pneumonia in the left lower lobe (LLL) of 14 dogs (RLL = right lower lobe). The hydrated group (n = 7) were made hypervolemic for 3 hours prior to being sacrificed and were compared with the control animals (n = 7) who were not volume-loaded. The mean values of pulmonary capillary wedge pressure and mean pulmonary artery pressure in both groups are indicated. (Data from Cooligan et al.[56])

canine model of pneumococcal pneumonia has been shown not only to increase lung water (Fig. 8.8) but to enhance spread of the infection to the contralateral lung as well.[56]

Approximately one-third of patients with bacterial pneumonia have evidence of ventricular dysfunction and demonstrate a hypodynamic circulatory response to the acute infection and its metabolic stress. It has been attributed to ventricular interdependence as well as to a circulating myocardial depressant factor such as reported for sepsis.[57] The response of pneumonia patients to volume infusion is thus diminished (Fig. 8.9). Therefore unless there is evidence of impaired regional blood flow to a level inappropriate for metabolic needs, volume expansion is poorly handled hemodynamically and serves to enhance fluid accumulation in the lung.

In a canine experimental model of pneumococcal pneumonia, the clinical concept that dehydration delays the appearance or decreases the extent of radiologic infiltrates has also been assessed. It was found that dehydration did not alter the radiologic picture or time of appearance of infiltrates.[58] Similarly, a retrospective study of dehydrated patients with

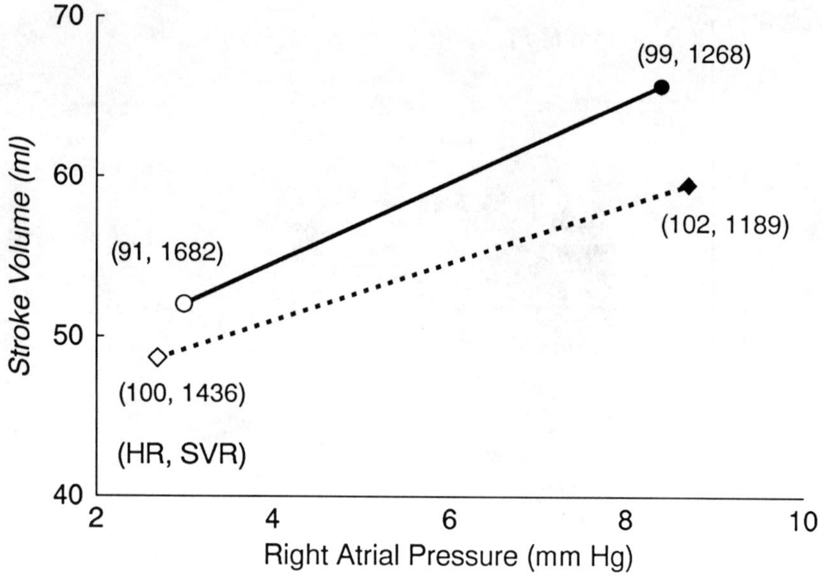

FIGURE 8.9. Ventricular function curves in acute pneumonia (diamonds) and the immediate convalescent period (circles). Mean values in 5 patients (4 pneumococcal, 1 *Klebsiella*) prior to (open figures) and following (solid figures) volume expansion with dextran or saline (hematocrit decreasing 5.7%). The metabolic rate (VO_2) decreased from 290 to 236 ml/minute with recovery and was unaffected by volume infusion. The mean values of heart rate (HR) and calculated systemic vascular resistance (SVR) in both groups are indicated. (Data from Kumar et al.[57])

pneumonia did not support the concept of delayed or diminished radiologic manifestations.[58] The effects of hypohydration in normal subjects has been studied,[59] and improved lung function (hyperinflation and increased flow rates with change in the DLCO) was found to be associated with volume contraction (Fig. 8.10). It was related to a decrease in airway resistance due to loss of interstitial lung water (bronchovascular sheath) or pulmonary vascular volume in contrast to the peribronchial fluid collection or mucosal edema observed with pulmonary edema. Lung volumes may also increase as a result of the associated increase in lung compliance. Thus perhaps dehydration should be a therapeutic goal in pneumonia patients.

Weight loss and favorable fluid balances[60] and a strategy aimed at decreasing lung water[61] have been reported to be correlated with improved survival in patients with ARDS. This balance may not be easy, as the kidneys of patients with mechanical ventilation and pneumonia have difficulty clearing free water. Acute infectious pneumonia appears to cause a resetting of the vasopressin osmostat, impairing renal water excretion.[62] This defect varies in proportion to the severity of the pneu-

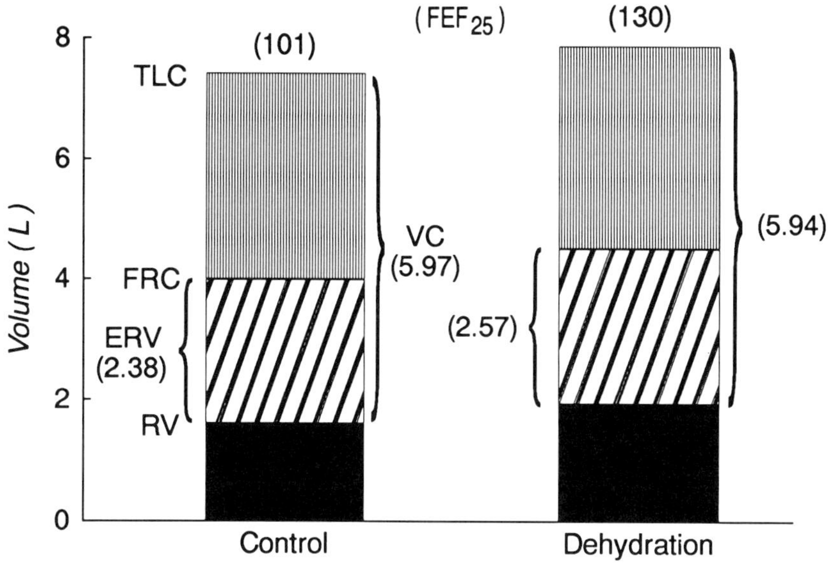

FIGURE 8.10. Effects of acute dehydration (hemoglobin 15.7–18.2 g/dl) after 48 hours of diuretic administration to 6 normal male subjects. Changes in mean values of lung volumes are shown with weight loss of 2 kg. TLC = total lung capacity; RV = residual volume; FRC = functional residual capacity, ERV = expiratory reserve volume, VC = vital capacity; FEF_{25} = flow rate in terminal 25% of vital capacity. (Data from Javaheri et al.[59])

monia and persists until the pneumonia resolves. In a report of a dog model of acid aspiration, plasmapheresis has been suggested as a particularly effective therapeutic alternative to effect a negative fluid balance in order to reduce pulmonary vascular pressures.[63] On the basis of the linear correlation between lung water and the measured pressures, it was concluded that the "leak" occurs predominantly from extraalveolar vessels, and the reduction of pulmonary pressures allows vascular derecruitment, thereby decreasing the number as well as the size of the pulmonary vascular leak sites.[63]

In summary, the cumulative clinical experience suggests that outcome after severe pulmonary edema can be affected by judicious fluid management. When pulmonary artery catheterization is used to maximize diuresis and fluid restriction in patients with nonhydrostatic (permeability) pulmonary edema, extravascular lung water significantly decreases as do ventilator and ICU days.[64] There is an ever-increasing database in support of increasing and perhaps maintaining cardiac output and oxygen delivery by the use of inotropic and vasoactive drugs, rather than by intravascular volume expansion.

Prophylaxis and Prevention

Pneumococcal Vaccine

The pneumococcus is still the major cause of community-acquired bacterial pneumonia. Moreover, the limited epidemiologic evidence available suggests that although mortality from pneumococcal infection has declined during the antibiotic era attack rates have not. Current estimates are that 15–30% of pneumonia cases requiring admission to the hospital are caused by *Streptococcus pneumoniae*. Morbidity data on pneumococcal disease are sparse and mortality figures often unreliable. Among bacteremic patients, mortality is approximately 20%, with 60% of deaths occurring within 5 days of "onset" despite antibiotic treatment. These early deaths are presumably due to irreversible physiologic injury in the face of an antibiotic infectious "cure." The presence of chronic systemic illness and age over 50 years, increases mortality to almost 30%. Therefore prophylaxis appears to be the only alternative in high risk groups to lower the unacceptable high mortality rates (Table 8.7).

The immunogenicity of the pneumococcal capsular polysaccharides provide a vaccine efficacious in preventing type-specific pneumonia. Such vaccines have been available for about 50 years. The continued morbidity and mortality even in the face of effective antibiotic therapy led to the revival of interest in pneumococcal vaccines. Polyvalent vaccines of purified capsular polysaccharides were developed and have been in general use since their licensing in 1977. Pneumococcal vaccine currently contains the capsular carbohydrate antigens of the serotypes (polyvalent, $n = 23$) most commonly found in bacteremic infections (88%) in the United States. A single injection usually induces an antibody response in adults (poor response in infants) that lasts at least 3 years and probably more than 8 years. There is little or no secondary response to a later injection. The efficacy of the vaccine remains controversial, particularly in the elderly. The cumulative weight of evidence indicates that the vaccine is safe and approximately 60% effective against bacteremic disease in immunocompetent persons.[65] The vaccine is significantly less effective in immunocompromised patients, with increasing age, and with increasing time since vaccination.[65] Because of the difficulty of determin-

TABLE 8.7. Recommendations for pneumococcal vaccination in adults.

Individuals 64 years of age
Immunocompetence with chronic disease: heart, lungs, diabetes, alcoholism, cirrhosis, cerebrospinal fluid leak
Immunocompromised: Hodgkin's disease, lymphoma, multiple myeloma, chronic renal failure, nephrotic syndrome, organ transplantation with immunosuppressive therapy, splenic dysfunction (including sickle cell disease)
HIV infection
Residents of institutional care facilities

ing causative organisms in pneumonia patients, efficacy studies are limited to bacteremic cases; the efficacy of the vaccine against non-bacteremic pneumonia is unknown. Even though there appears to be reduced efficacy in men, there is still a substantial cost savings supporting the cost-effectiveness of a vaccination for patients predisposed to developing pneumonia or those over 50 years of age.[66]

Pneumococcal polysaccharide vaccine has been recommended for use in all people 65 years of age and older. Although lowering the age for universal vaccination has been suggested, only about 10% of this already recognized high-risk population has been immunized.[67] Achieving the national goal of vaccinating 60% of the noninstitutionalized elderly and 80% of the institutionalized elderly is far off.

Influenza Vaccination

Influenza and AIDS are the most significant pandemic killers worldwide. Influenza-related illnessess in the United States causes 10,000–40,000 deaths annually and in excess of as many as 100,000 during pandemic years. Mortality due to epidemic influenza is, as with other pneumonias, increased in the elderly; and vaccination is thus advised for their protection. Presumably due to immunologic senescence, the serologic response to vaccination is decreased with advanced age, but protection against bronchopneumonia is conferred and infection successfully restricted to the "upper" respiratory tract. As a result of annual antigenic drift, susceptibility returns to a strain with a new antigenic subtype. Heterotypic immunity does not prevent infection but may speed recovery and decrease severity. Thus vaccination offers only short-term protection with no definite long-term advantage. How to bring patients at risk in contact with the medical care system for annual prewinter revaccination with reformulated vaccine remains uncertain. Much the same population, with the important addition of pregnant women who have high-risk medical conditions, should be vaccinated for both influenza and pneumococcal infection as there is no viremia induced by the inactivated vaccine (Table 8.8).

Vaccination reduces clinical infection by only about 30% in elderly institutionalized patients, but serious morbidity and mortality from

TABLE 8.8. Recommendations for influenza vaccination in adults.

Individuals >64 years of age
Those who are immunocompetent with chronic disease: diabetes, renal, pulmonary cardiac, anemia
Immunoincompetent persons
Residents of institutional care facilities
Persons in contact with those at high risk
Pregnant women with a high risk medical condition

respiratory infections are probably cut by about 50% and 70%, respectively. Pneumococcus and influenza vaccines can be given at the same time if injected at different sites. As with pneumococcal vaccine, the chief problem with the influenza virus vaccine is the failure to use it. Each year fewer than 30% of the target population of 45 million to 50 million persons receive the vaccine.[68] As with other preventive medicine programs, physicians' recommendations for vaccination have been strongly associated with receipt of the vaccine. Vaccination rates up to only 39% have been achieved among enrollees in a large health maintenance organization and a slightly higher rate of 55% among patients older than 65 years in a private practice setting. In one study, the major reason for nonvaccination was patient refusal.[69] Almost one-half of patients refusing vaccination when it is offered do so for fear of a reaction despite the evidence available showing no increased incidence of side effects other than a sore arm with the highly purified vaccines now available. Others refuse on the basis that they think it does not work or that it was not suggested the previous year; finally, there is the mistaken perception that the medical provider had not recommended it.[69]

A strategy for inpatient "flu shots" have been increasingly advocated, and one such program utilizing ward nurses, patient-oriented educational intervention, and emphasis on other administrative and organizational components, such as a walk-in clinic for inpatients, has proved successful.[70] Despite the fact that since 1984 the Centers for Disease Control has recommended influenza immunization of physicians treating high risk patients, compliance among this group has been estimated to be among the lowest.[71] As a result of the growing awareness of the need to regard each contact with health care providers as an opportunity for vaccination, a particularly successful effort using a mobile vaccine cart has been reported by offering vaccine to medical house staff and students in clinics and conferences, as had been done with other hospital personnel.[71]

Chemoprophylaxis

The use of antiviral agents as a supplemental strategy in the prevention of viral pneumonia in susceptible patients has focused primarily on influenza. Nonimmunized or suboptimal immune responses in immunocompromised individuals including the elderly has been generating growing interest in the potential use of additional drug-related prophylactic measures. Amantadine and its closely related analog rimantadine are approximately as effective as influenza virus vaccine in preventing influenza A. Simultaneous administration with the vaccine does not suppress the antibody response and can afford protection during the 2- to 3-week interval required for a serologic response. Influenza B or other respiratory viruses are not affected by either drug. Prophylactic use of amantadine has been advised for certain high risk groups, such as residents of institutional care facilities where there is an outbreak of influenza A infections. It may be used as an adjunct to immunization in unvaccinated residents and for seasonal chemoprophylaxis for high risk (immunocompromised) groups.

Transplantation patients have presented challenging problems for the development of strategies to prevent lower respiratory tract infection. Pneumonia is a major cause of morbidity after transplantation with an incidence as high as 40–60% and a comparably high mortality rate. Viruses have been suspected; and specific agents, such as cytomegalovirus (CMV), respiratory syncytial virus (RSV), and uncommonly adenovirus and influenza, have been subsequently identified as causative agents in previously diagnosed idiopathic pneumonias. Parainfluenza has also been identified as a cause of serious lower respiratory tract involvement in bone marrow transplant recipients, illustrating the relation between the expanding spectrum of causative agents and advances in laboratory technology.[72] Treatment for parainfluenza is relatively unsatisfactory, the diagnosis elusive, and nosocomial transmission the most probable mode of infection. Aerosolized ribavirin, a broad-spectrum antiviral agent that has been approved for the management of severe RSV infection in children and reported to be successful in adults as well, has been suggested as a potentially useful agent, similar to amantidine for influenza, if initiated within the first 48 hours of the onset of symptoms. This approach to management clearly rides the line between prophylactic preventive versus empiric treatment.

Cytomegalovirus pneumonia is one of the most serious infections in transplant patients. Ganciclovir has been found to reduce the incidence of CMV pneumonia in asymptomatic bone marrow transplantation recipients with evidence of viral shedding, seen by bronchoalverlar lavage (BAL). Prophylactic ganciclovir administration after heart transplantation in CMV-seropositive patients also is effective in reducing the incidence of pneumonia and in suppressing CMV shedding as observed in bone marrow transplant patients.[73] Also with respect to bone marrow transplant patients, fluconazole, in contrast to ketoconazole, has been found to effectively reduce the incidence of systemic candidiasis and the number of deaths due to fungal infection.

In patient populations predisposed to *Pneumocystis* pneumonia (PCP), both trimethoprim-sulfamethoxazole (TMP-SMX) or dapsone orally and pentamidine by aerosol have been used for prophylaxis. The agents are used for both primary prophylaxis (those with significantly enhanced probability of infection) and secondary prophylaxis (after a course of therapy for an episode of PCP). There are few studies comparing PCP prophylactic regimens in HIV-infected patients, though experience suggests that TMP-SMX is superior to dapsone or pentamidine.

An intravenous form of concentrated immune globulin is now available for therapeutic purposes as a result of chemists learning how to prevent its aggregation and denaturation while undergoing processing for purification and stabilization. The use of intravenous immune globulin as an adjuvant agent in patients with secondary, compared to primary, immunodeficiency disorders does not appear to be indicated with the possible exception of HIV-infected children. There is controversy regarding its benefit, which appears limited to invasive pneumococcal infections in patients with depressed CD4 counts (but more than 0.2×10^9/L) and IgG levels (<2 g/L). Immune globulin has been anecdotally reported to have prophylactic benefit against fatal CMV infection in transplant (especially bone marrow) patients. Neither the value nor the cost-effectiveness of this expensive therapeutic tool has been demonstrated for other pneumonias in immunosuppressed hosts.

Selective Decontamination

Aerosolized antibiotics have been shown to decrease the incidence of gram-negative oropharyngeal colonization and nosocomial pneumonia. Mortality, however, is not reduced, attributed in part to finding resistant organisms in those infected. Other topical regimens of antimicrobial prophylaxis, including oral mucosal antibiotic pastes, have been proposed to affect the oropharyngeal colonization of critically ill patients, especially those being mechanically ventilated. Effective pneumonia prophylaxis has been demonstrated in an animal model of ARDS, but the value of this stratagem in patients remains controversial.

In addition, poorly absorbed enterically administered drugs are also used as part of this protective intervention in order to selectively decontaminate the lower digestive tract as well. Because the indigenous anaerobic flora of the gut are thought to play an important role in the protection against gram-negative bacillary (and perhaps fungal) colonization at these sites, agents are used that leave this flora intact. Beneficial effects have been reported to be variable, and some regimens have therefore included the use of antifungal agents and systemic antibiotics to prevent primary pneumonia due to indigenous flora.[74] Although colonization and infections with gram-negative bacilli are reduced in patients undergoing selective decontamination, altered survival is uncertain. Metaanalysis of studies comparing patients treated by such regimens with untreated controls show at best a limited protective effect.[75] Mortality benefit was less clear, in part attributable to the problems involved in making the diagnosis of pneumonia in ventilated patients.

Comparisons between trials are difficult because of differing regimens, the small number of patients involved in each study, and the unblinded nature of the studies.[76] A multicenter, randomized, blinded, placebo-controlled European study was carried out in 445 mechanically ventilated patients (>48 hours) utilizing prophylactic topical antifungals and non-absorbable antibiotics effective against gram-negative organisms in nasooropharyngeal preparations and through a nasogastric tube. The overall incidence of pneumonia was not affected by treatment, but there were more staphylococcal and fewer gram-negative infections in the treated group. Survival was similar in the treatment and placebo groups, with no significant difference in any specific subgroups, as determined by physiologic scores.[76] Most of these patients had preexisting disease, in contrast to other studies involving surgical or trauma patients; the incidence of pneumonia in the placebo group was low, only 15%, presumably reflecting the strict diagnostic criteria utilized.

It has been suggested that failure to demonstrate that a reduction in respiratory tract infections has an effect on overall mortality is due to the severity of the underlying diseases which are responsible for mortality rather than nosocomial pneumonia. It was further suggested that patients acquire pneumonia only as a marker of terminal illness.[75]

Morbidity and Mortality

Community-Acquired Pneumonia

Although mortality due to pneumonia decreased dramatically with the introduction of antibacterial agents, during the 1980s pneumonia and influenza regained some of their lost public health stature and became the fifth leading cause of death in the United States. Moreover, between 1979 and 1987 the death rate in the United States attributable to these two diseases increased by 19.3%, one of only 4 of the 15 leading causes of death to increase. Pneumonia-induced mortality is not uncommon and, along with hospitalization rates, increased in the elderly. A population-based study showed a mortality of 6.7% in the 65- to 69-year-old group, with an increase to 20.5% in the age 85+ group.[77] The mortality rate increases further and survival is greatly diminished with age in patients requiring mechanical ventilation.

Clinical characteristics with prognostic significance with respect to both mortality and morbidity that have been demonstrated for pneumococcal pneumonia are bacteremia, multilobar involvement, concomitant disease (especially alcoholism), and leukopenia.[78] Moreover, the day of the disease on which effective antibiotic therapy was started shows no significant correlation with mortality or complications.[78] In a prospective study, however, none of the 37 patients with pneumococcal pneumonia who received antibiotics prior to admission died, whereas 7 of 114 not treated with antibiotics before admission died ($p = 0.13$).[79] Thus although antibiotic therapy greatly improves the outcome of pneumococcal pneumonia, it does not eliminate the significance of adverse clinical parameters or their additive effect on both mortality and morbidity.[78]

Other studies have shown that the only prognostic factors of predictive value for death due to primary community-acquired pneumonia is an admission respiratory rate of 30 breaths/minute or more, a diastolic blood pressure of 60 mm Hg or less, and a BUN of more than 7 mmol/L (19.6 mg/dl).[79,80] No deaths occurred among patients without tachypnea at admission (respiratory rate < 20 breaths/minute) or with a BUN of less than 7 mmol/L at admission.[79]

The presence of any two of these three criteria of physiologic derangement is associated with a 21-fold greater risk for death.[79,81] In addition, although mortality has not been related to the etiologic agent, the combination of influenza A virus and *Staphylococcus aureus* infection appears particularly lethal.[79]

It has been reported that mortality due to pneumococcal pneumonia is not influenced acutely by antibiotic therapy or admission to the ICU in those with bacteremia. This report has led to the suggetion that death due to pneumonia is predetermined and that intensive care merely prolongs the interval before death. Mortality rates associated with pneumococcal pneumonia continue to be reported as 45% in adults with bacteremia and about 5% in adults without bacteremia during the antibiotic era. However, identification of these high risk patients on admission influences immediate triage to the ICU, which has been suggested to enhance prognosis in a population that has otherwise accounted for 70% of the deaths that occurred within 24 hours of admission.[82] This high risk group requires more aggressive monitoring, as well as diagnostic and life support strategies, including arterial and pulmonary artery catheterization, percutaneous lung aspiration, bronchoscopy, and "routine" ventilator management or vasopressor therapy in an effort to "forestall" death and allow time for the antibiotics to take effect.

The hospital stay of survivors in a British study averaged 10.8 days; after 6 weeks, 79% were able to participate in normal activities.[79] Hypoalbuminemia and age were associated with prolonged hospital stay and delayed returns to fitness. At the time of discharge, only 15% of chest films had cleared (Table 8.9); and although resolution was delayed in the elderly (Table 8.10), there was complete resolution in 55% of patients at 6 weeks.

Nosocomial Pneumonia

Nosocomial pneumonia is the second most frequent hospital-acquired infection, but among the various types of nosocomial infection it is the leading cause of mortality. Various factors have been associated with adverse prognosis[83] (Table 8.11), which significantly worsens in patients being mechanically ventilated.[83,84] The mortality rate is variable but in general is reported to be higher than 30%. Additional adverse prognostic factors in mechanically ventilated patients are a longer than 5-day interval of mechanical ventilation preceding the pneumonia and being a non-

TABLE 8.9. Resolution of chest radiograph with community-acquired pneumonia.

Time from admission (days)	Patients with normal radiograph (%)
Discharge	15
42	55
100	75
157	83

Source: Research Committee of the British Thoracic Society and the Public Health Laboratory Service.[79]

TABLE 8.10. Community-acquired pneumonia: time to baseline radiograph in 50% of patients, by age group.

Age group (years)	Normal chest radiograph (days)
15–32	22
33–53	29[a]
54–64	44
64–74	68

a = also the mean for all ages.
Source: Research Committee of the British Thoracic Society and the Public Health Laboratory Service.[79]

TABLE 8.11. Adverse prognostic factors for nosocomial pneumonia.

Fatal underlying disease
Inappropriate antibiotic therapy
Noncardiac surgery patient, i.e., ICU or medical patient
Presence of shock
Preceding mechanical ventilation of more than 5 day's duration
Age >60 years
"High risk" organism (i.e., *Pseudomonas*)
Polymicrobial infection
Bilateral involvement
Development, or worsening, of respiratory failure

cardiac surgery patient, both factors suggesting the importance of an absence of severe underlying disease.[84]

Although underlying disease is important, there are significant differences for specific diseases, such as between types or severity of immunosuppression. The virulence of different pathologic agents, be they gram-positive or gram-negative, also varies independent of their antibiotic resistance. *Pseudomonas* and *Staphylococcus aureus*, which are generally considered to be associated with the highest mortalities, are also associated with more frequent bacteremias, seeming to combine the factors of virulence with bacterial load in the lung. Mortality is variable and may be increased to as much as 60% in selected populations (e.g., the elderly, patients whose pneumonia is complicated by bacteremia, and those who acquire their infection in the ICU). Numerous scoring systems to determine severity of illness have been used with varying success for predicting mortality. They include the Acute Physiologic and Chronic Health Evaluations (APACHE II), the Simplified Acute Physiologic Score (SAPS), Mortality Prediction Model (MPM), and the Therapeutic Intervention Scoring System (TISS), among others.

Pneumocystis carinii *Pneumonia*

Pneumocystic carinii pneumonia (PCP) is the most common pulmonary manifestation of AIDS, with 50–80% of patients surviving their initial episode. Although the duration of presenting symptoms (fever, dyspnea, cough), physical findings (rales), and initial mean leukocyte and lymphocyte counts do not have prognostic significance, the severity of respiratory distress on presentation does. The more severe the impairment in gas exchange (low initial PaO_2) and the higher the respiratory rate, the worse is the prognosis. The adverse prognostic implication of an elevated serum lactate dehydrogenase level (LDH) may reflect the severity of lung parenchymal damage.[85] Those patients with PCP requiring mechanical ventilatory support have a mortality rate of 60–80%.

Factors predictive of hospital survival are the initial presence of metabolic acidosis, a continued need for more than 10 cm H_2O PEEP after 96 hours of ventilator management, and the requirement of an escalating FIO_2.[86] In those patients who require mechanical ventilatory support there is no prognostic significance to the initial severity of impairment of oxygenation, nor are there significant differences in radiographic grades between survivors and nonsurvivors at the time of hospital admission. The mean duration of survival after discharge from the hospital is just over 1 year.[86] Additionally, patients requiring ICU admission demonstrate an inverse relation between length of ICU stay and survival.[87] It has been observed to drop continuously from 39% at the time of ICU admission to 17% at the end of 1 week, with survival not observed after 2 weeks of intensive care.

Adult Respiratory Distress Syndrome

The underlying disease, if not the cause and pathogenesis of the insult leading to the episode of ARDS, and the age of the patient have been reported to be important prognostic factors. Thus an acute lung injury syndrome associated with bone marrow transplantation for patients with malignancy carries 95% mortality.[88] Risk stratification for the development of respiratory failure and mortality in these patients is the same. Such factors include receptor of an HLA-nonidentical donor marrow, an active phase of malignancy, and older age (>21 years).[88] Even if the patients survive the initial episode of respiratory failure, recurrence is common, and no patient who requires repeat mechanical ventilatory support survives to hospital discharge.[88] None of the long-term survivors in the largest cohort of marrow recipients reported for respiratory failure required ventilatory support for longer than 9 days or had a respiratory infection documented as the precipitating event.[88] Survival rates are thus lower in infected patients than in patients with other conditions predisposing to ARDS.

To enhance quantification of lung injury and to assess prognosis, standardized scoring systems for assessment of pulmonary and nonpulmonary organ dysfunction have been created. These select indicators of severity include (1) acute lung injury: radiologic involvement (quadrants), impairment of oxygenation (PaO_2/FIO_2), lung compliance, and magnitude of PEEP required; (2) parameters of extrapulmonary organ dysfunction; and (3) pathogenesis. It is hoped that more careful stratification utilizing these considerations may clarify the observed varying mortality and morbidity. How one differentiates dysfunction from failure of a particular organ (i.e., lung in the presence of sepsis versus multiorgan failure) is frequently unclear. When systematically and prospectively evaluated, however, only pesistent metabolic acidosis and the presence of fewer than 10% band forms on the initial peripheral blood smear have been demonstrated to have a significant association with increased mortality.[89] The poor prognostic outlook of acidemia is common to sepsis-like syndromes, including pneumonia, and reflect the associated multiorgan dysfunction. The diminished number of band forms mobilized from the bone marrow implies failure of at least that organ to have an appropriate response. Of interest is the difficulty showing prognostic significance of the initial severity of impairment of gas exchange, pulmonary mechanics, and systemic hemodynamics.

There is ongoing debate on the significance—and the existence—of supply-dependent oxygen uptake on survival of ARDS patients. Various groups have reported that delivery and utilization of oxygen is greater in survivors than nonsurvivors. This factor is thought by some investigators to be critically facilitated by an increased stroke volume due to increased ventricular compliance allowing for an increased ventricular end-diastolic volume or preload in the presence of a normal or decreased afterload, which in turn is dependent on the presence of a sepsis-like myocardial depressant factor.[90] The intuitive relation implied between such hemodynamic and derived "oxygen profile" indices and the development of a metabolic acidosis is more apparent than real. The classic association of an increased lactate concentration secondary to the presumed anaerobic tissue environment has been only inconsistently demonstrated at best.

Death of patients with ARDS is characteristically a septic picture with nonpulmonary organ system failure, the lungs having achieved a chronic, stable degree of dysfunction. The development of a complicating infection, which is most commonly pneumonia, in contrast to the precipitating

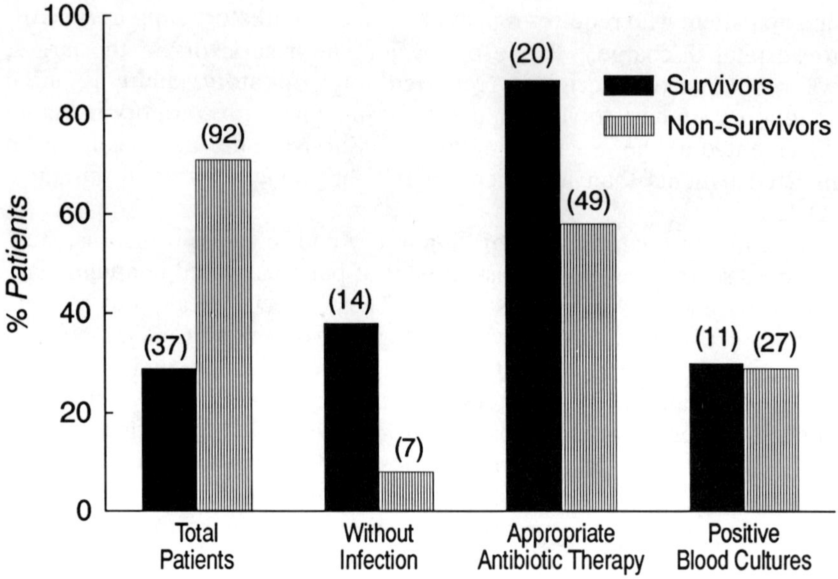

FIGURE 8.11. Clinical and autopsy diagnosis of infection in patients with ARDS (n = 129) who survived (n = 37), of whom 14 were without evidence of infection. The use of adequate antibiotic therapy is also shown (n = 69) in all patients with infection with site unknown (n = 82). Appropriate antibiotic therapy was more frequent in survivors; and although the incidence of documented bacteremia was the same in survivors and nonsurvivors, the site of the infection was identified in all of the survivors but in only 18 of 27 nonsurvivors. The numbers in parentheses indicate the number of patients in each group. (Data from Seidenfeld et al.[91])

infection, is the most apparent adverse prognostic factor. The importance of proper treatment of the infection is most clearly illustrated by an observed 100% mortality in patients with a positive blood culture if the site of the primary infection cannot be identified.[91] When infection is a complicating factor, adequate antibiotic therapy, if not a critical factor for determining survival, is associated with a greater survival rate. Although only 29% of infected patients treated with appropriate antibiotics survived, of the 23 survivors with infection 20 (87%) were treated appropriately[91] (Fig. 8.11). This situation is reminiscent of the apparent lack of effect of antibiotics on the immediate mortality due to primary pneumonia, where the degree of initial physiologic injury appears to predetermine response to therapy and survival.

Survivors of ARDS have varying degrees of impaired pulmonary function that in general has been reported to be of little clinical significance (Fig. 8.12). It has proved difficult to maintain adequate follow-up of patients, which would allow relating pulmonary sequelae to the course or severity of the episode of ARDS. As with survival, there is no evidence

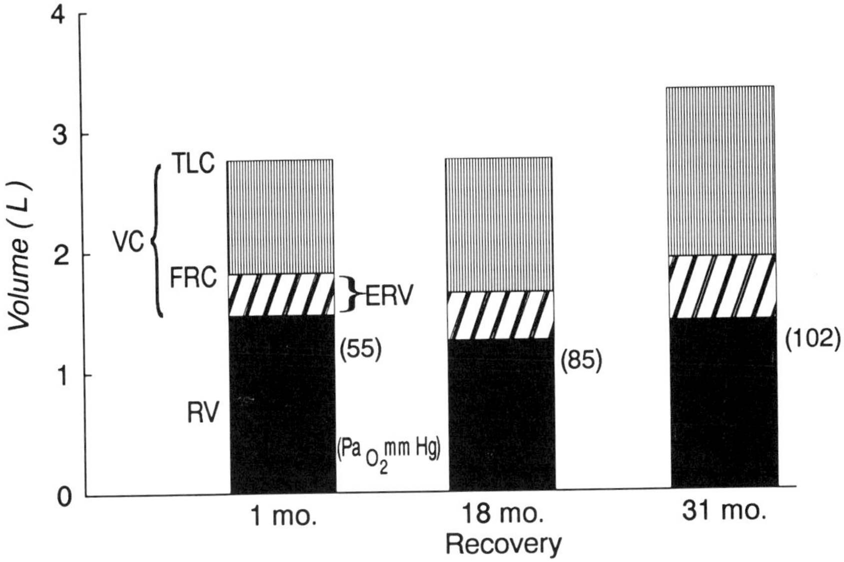

FIGURE 8.12. Pulmonary function tests after a peripartum episode of noncardiogenic pulmonary edema (ARDS) in a 23-year-old woman without a history of previous lung disease. (See Table 8.12) TLC = total lung capacity; VC = vital capacity; FRC = functional residual capacity; RV = residual volume; ERV = expiratory reserve volume.

TABLE 8.12. Exercise values after 18 months recovery.[a]

Index	Rest	W_{MAX} (40 watts)
V_E (L/min)	12.0	34.2
f (b/min)	26	41
V_T (ml)	462	834
V_E/MVV (%)	29	81
V_T/VC (%)	27	48
$\dot{V}O_2$ (ml/min)	230	830
$\dot{V}CO_2$ (ml/min)	180	680
R	0.78	0.82
D_LCO (% pred)	45	

Endurance at 25 watts (2.5 minutes)

Index	Rest	2 minutes
Q (L/min)	3.9	7.8
CI (L/min/m^2)	3.3	4.0
SV (ml)	71	64
SVI (ml/m^2)	48	43
PA (mean mm Hg)	14	23
PAWP (mm Hg)	7	12
PvO_2 (mm Hg)	44[b]	30

[a] The measurement were done in a 23-year-old woman with a peripartum episode of ARDS.
[b] Mixed venous PO_2.

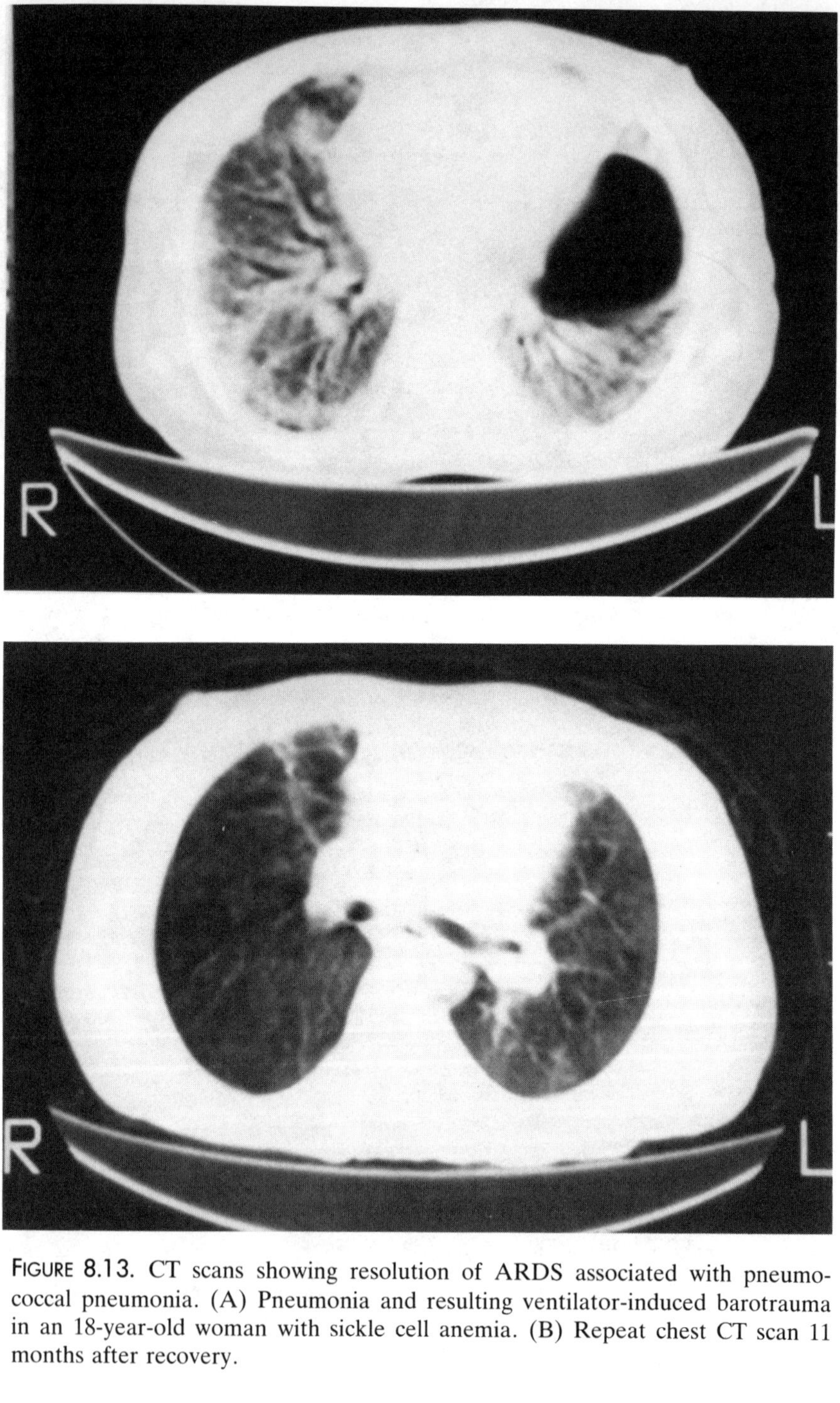

FIGURE 8.13. CT scans showing resolution of ARDS associated with pneumococcal pneumonia. (A) Pneumonia and resulting ventilator-induced barotrauma in an 18-year-old woman with sickle cell anemia. (B) Repeat chest CT scan 11 months after recovery.

that long-term pulmonary function differs according to the precipitating cause, apparent severity of the episode, or (as shown in animal studies) the occurrence of secondary pneumonia. Lung function continues to recover during the months following the acute episode but "classically" plateaus by 6–12 months with little apparent reversibility thereafter (Fig. 8.13). Glottal damage from long-term intubation may also resolve with time. A reduced diffusing capacity is the most commonly observed persistent abnormality, and it has been attributed to destruction of the pulmonary vascular bed. Survivors generally do not complain of dyspnea but have a restrictive ventilatory defect, a decrease in exercise capacity (Wmax), and exercise-induced arterial desaturation (Table 8.12). Therapeutic residua have been suggested for the level of PEEP, the duration of ventilation support, and the degree of enhancement of the inspired oxygen concentration ($F_{IO_2} > 0.6$), but correlation with pulmonary function values in ARDS survivors has been variable.[92] Finally, the importance of minimizing barotrauma during mechanical ventilation has been supported by reports correlating high inflation pressures, rather than initial PaO_2 and Q_S/Q_T, with long-term morbidity, thus emphasizing the value of therapeutic strategies of low PEEP to minimize long-term pulmonary sequelae.

References

1. Stadie WC: The oxygen of the arterial and venous blood in pneumonia and its relation to cyanosis. J Exp Med 1919;30:215–240.
2. Barach AL, Woodell M: Studies in oxygen therapy. II. In pneumonia and its complications. Arch Intern Med 1921;28:394–420.
3. Meakins J: Observations on the gases in human arterial blood in certain pathological pulmonary conditions and their treatment with oxygen. J Pathol Bacteriol 1921;24:79–90.
4. Stadie WC: The treatment of anoxemia in pneumonia in an oxygen chamber. J Exp Med 1922;35:337–360.
5. Barach AL: Methods and results of oxygen treatment in pneumonia. Arch Intern Med 1926;37:186–211.
6. Barach AL, Richards DW: Oxygen therapy in pulmonary tuberculosis. Am Rev Tuberc 1932;26:241–252.
7. Karetzky M: Current concepts of oxygen therapy in COPD. N J Med 1986; 83:587–590.
8. Mithoefer JC, Karetzky M, Mead GD: Oxygen therapy in respiratory failure. N Engl J Med 1967;277:947–949.
9. Karpman J, McDonough M, Karetzky M: The effects of oxygen administration in critical care. Am Rev Respir Dis 1992;145(Suppl):A793.
10. Winslow RM, Samaja M, West JB: Red cell function at extreme altitude on Mount Everest. J Appl Physiol 1984;56:109–116.
11. Tenney SM: Tissue oxygenation. Curr Pulmonol 1987;8:299–328.
12. Light RB: Intrapulmonary oxygen consumption in experimental pneumococcal pneumonia. J Appl Physiol 1988;64:2490–2495.

13. Ward ME, Magder SA, Hussain SNA: Oxygen delivery-independent effect of blood flow on diaphragm fatigue. Am Rev Respir Dis 1992;145:1058–1063.
14. McMahon SM, Halprin GM, Sieker HO: Positive end-expiratory pressure in severe arterial hypoxemia. Am Rev Respir Dis 1973;108:526–535.
15. Kaplan JD, Schuster DP: Physiologic consequences of tracheal intubation. Clin Chest Med 1991;12:425–432.
16. Mitzner W, Wagner EM: Pulmonary and bronchial vascular resistance. In Scharf SM, Cassidy SS (eds): Heart-Lung Interactions in Health and Disease. Lung Biology in Health and Disease, Vol. 42. New York: Marcel Dekker, 1989, pp. 45–75.
17. Biondi JW, Schulman DS, Wiedemann HP, Matthay RA: Mechanical heart-lung interaction in the adult respiratory distress syndrome. Clin Chest Med 1990;11:691–714.
18. Robotham JL, Scharf SM: Effects of positive and negative pressure ventilation on cardiac performance. Clin Chest Med 1983;4:161–187.
19. Cassidy SS, Schwiep F: Cardiovascular effects of positive end-expiratory pressure. In Scharf SM, Cassidy SS (eds): Heart-Lung Interactions in Health and Disease. Lung Biology in Health and Disease, Vol. 42. New York: Marcel Dekker, 1989, pp. 463–506.
20. Hedley-Whyte J, Burgess GE III, Feeley TW, Miller MG: Applied Physiology of Respiratory Care. Boston: Little Brown, 1976.
21. Zaman I, McDonough M, Karetzky M, Sikdar A: Transcutaneous blood gas measurements and their relationship to tissue oxygenation. Chest 1991; 100:122S.
22. Zaman I, Anandarangam T, Karetzky M: "T"-bar with a deflated cuff: usefulness as a weaning aid. Chest 1992;102:126S.
23. Mithoefer JC, Bossman OG, Thibeault DW, Mead GD: The clinical estimation of alveolar ventilation. Am Rev Respir Dis 1968;98:868–871.
24. Tobin MJ, Perez W, Guenther SM, et al: The pattern of breathing during successful and unsuccessful trials of weaning from mechanical ventilation. Am Rev Respir Dis 1986;134:1111–1118.
25. Rochester DF: Malnutrition and the respiratory muscles. Clin Chest Med 1986;7:91–99.
26. Thurlbeck WM: Diaphragm and body weight in emphysema. Thorax 1978; 33:483–487.
27. Arora NS, Rochester DF: Respiratory muscle strength and maximal voluntary ventilation in undernourished patients. Am Rev Respir Dis 1982; 126:5–8.
28. Doekel RC Jr, Zwillich CW, Scoggin CH, et al: Clinical semistarvation: depression of hypoxic ventilatory response. N Engl J Med 1976;295:358–361.
29. Baier H, Somani P: Ventilatory drive in normal man during semistarvation. Chest 1984;85:222–225.
30. Zwillich CW, Sahn SA, Weil JV: Effects of hypermetabolism on ventilation and chemosensitivity. J Clin Invest 1977;60:900–906.
31. Herve P, Simonneau G, Girard P, et al: Hypercapnic acidosis induced by nutrition in mechanically ventilated patients: glucose vs fat. Crit Care Med 1985;13:537–540.
32. Veterans Affairs Total Parenteral Nutrition Cooperative Study Group: Perioperative total parenteral nutrition in surgical patients. N Engl J Med 1991; 325:525–532.

33. Graham WGB, Bradley DA: Efficacy of chest physiotherapy and intermittent positive-pressure breathing in the resolution of pneumonia. N Engl J Med 1978;299:624–627.
34. Britton S, Bejstedt M, Vedin L: Chest physiotherapy in primary pneumonia. BMJ 1985;290:1703–1704.
35. Machenzie CF, Shin B, McAslan TC: Chest physiotherapy: the effect on arterial oxygenation in acutely ill patients with atelectasis or pneumonia. Anesth Analg 1978;57:28–30.
36. Holody B, Goldberg HS: The effect of mechanical vibration physiotherapy on arterial oxygenation in acutely ill patients with atelectasis or pneumonia. Am Rev Respir Dis 1981;124:372–375.
37. Sahn SA: Continuous lateral rotational therapy and nosocomial pneumonia. Chest 1991;99:1263–1267.
38. Oikkonen M, Karjalainen K, Kahara V, et al: Comparison of incentive spirometry and intermittent positive pressure breathing after coronary artery bypass graft. Chest 1991;99:60–65.
39. Ziment I: Historic overview of mucoactive druges. In Braga PC, Allegra L (eds): Drugs in Bronchial Mucology. New York: Raven Press, 1989, pp. 1–33.
40. Verdugo P: Mucin exocytosis. Am Rev Respir Dis 1991;144(part 2):S33–S37.
41. Lamblin G, Lhermitte M, Klein A, et al: The carbohydrate diversity of human respiratory mucins: a protection of the underlying mucosa. Am Rev Respir Dis 1991;144(part 2):S19–S24.
42. Nadel JA: Role of mast cell and neutrophil proteases in airway secretion. Am Rev Respir Dis 1991;144(part 2):S48–S51.
43. Rossing TH: Supportive measures in the treatment of pneumonia. In Pennington JE (ed): Respiratory Infections: Diagnosis and Management, 2nd ed. New York: Raven Press, 1988, pp. 601–607.
44. Goldzimer EI, Konopka R, Moser KM: Reversal of the perfusion defect in experimental canine lobar pneumococcal pneumonia. J Appl Physiol 1974; 37:85–91.
45. Light RB: Indomethacin and acetylsalicylic acid reduce intrapulmonary shunt in experimental pneumococcal pneumonia. Am Rev Respir Dis 1986; 134:520–525.
46. Hanly PJ, Dobson K, Roberts D, Light RB: Effect of indomethacin on arterial oxygenation in critically ill patients with severe bacterial pneumonia. Lancet 1987;1:351–354.
47. Schein RMH, Bergman R, Marcial EH, et al: Complement activation and corticosteroid therapy in the development of the adult respiratory distress syndrome. Chest 1987;91:850–853.
48. Bone RC, Fisher CJ Jr, Clemmer TP, et al: Early methylprednisolone treatment for septic syndrome and the adult respiratory distress syndrome. Chest 1987;92:1032–1036.
49. Bernard GR, Luce JM, Sprung CL, et al: High-dose corticosteroids in patients with the adult respiratory distress syndrome. N Engl J Med 1987; 317:1565–1570.
50. Luce JM, Montgomery B, Marks JD, et al: Ineffectiveness of high-dose methylprednisolone in preventing parenchymal lung injury and improving mortality in patients with septic shock. Am Rev Respir Dis 1988;138:62–68.

51. Hooper RG, Kearl RA: Established ARDS treated with a sustained course of adrenocortical steroids. Chest 1990;97:138–143.
52. Bozzette SA, Sattler FR, Chiu J, et al: A controlled trial of early adjunctive treatment with corticosteroids for Pneumocystic carinii pneumonia in the acquired immunodeficiency syndrome. N Engl J Med 1990;323:1451–1457.
53. National Institutes of Health–University of California Expert Panel for Corticosteroids as Adjunctive Therapy for Pneumocystis Pneumonia: Consensus statement on the use of corticosteroids as adjunctive therapy for Pneumocystis pneumonia in the acquired immunodeficiency syndrome. N Engl J Med 1990;323:1500–1504.
54. Robin ED, Thomas ED: Some relations between pulmonary edema and pulmonary inflammation (pneumonia). Arch Intern Med 1954;93:713–724.
55. Prewitt R, Ducas J: Hemodynamic management of acute respiratory failure. In Scharf SM, Cassidy SS (eds): Heart-Lung Interactions in Health and Disease. Lung Biology in Health and Disease, Vol. 42. New York: Marcel Dekker, 1989, pp. 879–914.
56. Colligan T, Light RB, Wood LDH, Mink SN: Plasma volume expansion in canine pneumococcal pneumonia: its effects on respiratory gas exchange and pneumonia size. Am Rev Respir Dis 1982;126:86–91.
57. Kumar R, Wallace WA, Ramirez A, et al: Hemodynamic effects of pneumonia. II. Expansion of plasma volume. J Clin Invest 1970;49:799–805.
58. Caldwell A, Glauser FL, Smith WR, et al: The effects of dehydration on the radiologic and pathologic appearance of experimental canine segmental pneumonia. Am Rev Respir Dis 1975;112:651–656.
59. Javaheri S, Bosken CH, Lim S, et al: Effects of hypohydration on lung functions in humans. Am Rev Respir Dis 1987;135:597–599.
60. Simmons RS, Berdine GG, Seidenfeld JJ, et al: Fluid balance and the adult respiratory distress syndrome. Am Rev Respir Dis 1987;135:924–929.
61. Eisenberg PR, Hansbrough JR, Anderson D, Schuster DP: A prospective study of lung water measurements during patient management in an intensive care unit. Am Rev Respir Dis 1987;136:622–668.
62. Dreyfuss D, Leviel F, Paillard M, et al: Acute infectious pneumonia is accompanied by a latent vasopressin-independent impairment of renal water excretion. Am Rev Respir Dis 1988;138:583–589.
63. Long R, Breen PH, Mayers I, Wood LDH: Treatment of canine aspiration pneumonitis: fluid volume reduction vs fluid volume expansion. J Appl Physiol 1988;65:1736–1744.
64. Mitchell JP, Schuller D, Calandrino FS, Schuster DP: Improved outcome based on fluid management in critically ill patients requiring pulmonary artery catheterization. Am Rev Respir Dis 1992;145:990–998.
65. Shapiro ED, Berg AT, Austrian R, et al: The protective efficacy of polyvalent pneumococcal polysaccharide vaccine. N Engl J Med 1991;325:1453–1460.
66. Gable CB, Holzer SS, Engelhart L, et al: Pneumococcal vaccine: efficacy and associated cost savings. JAMA 1990;264:1910–1915.
67. McBean AM, Babish JD: The utilization of pneumococcal polysaccharide vaccine among elderly Medicare beneficiaries, 1985 through 1988. Arch Intern Med 1991;151:2009–2016.

68. Douglas RG Jr: Prophylaxis and treatment of influenza. N Engl J Med 1990;322:443–450.
69. Fiebach NH, Viscoli CM: Patient acceptance of influenza vaccination. Am J Med 1991;91:393–400.
70. Nichol KL: Improving influenza vaccination rates for high-risk inpatients. Am J Med 1991;91:584–588.
71. Ohrt CK, McKinney WP: Achieving compliance with influenza immunization of medical house staff and students: a randomized controlled trial. JAMA 1992;267:1377–1380.
72. Wendt CH, Weisdorf DJ, Jordan C, et al: Parainfluenza virus respiratory infection after bone marrow transplantation. N Engl J Med 1992;326: 921–926.
73. Merigan TC, Renlung DG, Keay S, et al: A controlled trial of ganciclovir to prevent cytomegalovirus disease after heart transplant. N Engl J Med 1992; 326:1182–1186.
74. Aerdts SJA, Van Dalen R, Clasener HAL, et al: Antibiotic prophylaxis of respiratory tract infection in mechanically ventilated patients: a prospective, blinded, randomized trial of the effect of a novel regimen. Chest 1991; 100:783–791.
75. Vanderbroucke-Grauls CMJE, Vanderbroucke JP: Effect of selective decontamination of the digestive tract on respiratory tract infections and mortality in the intensive care unit. Lancet 1991;338:859–862.
76. Gastinne H, Wolff M, Delatour F, et al: A controlled trial in intensive care units of selective decontamination of the digestive tract with nonabsorbable antibiotics. N Engl J Med 1992;326:594–599.
77. Houston MS, Ballard DJ, Silverstein MD: Mortality in the elderly from lower respiratory tract illness: a population-based study. Clin Res 1991;39: 792A.
78. Van Metre TE Jr: Pneumococcal pneumonia treated with antibiotics: the prognostic significance of certain clinical findings. N Engl J Med 1954; 251:1048–1052.
79. Research Committee of the British Thoracic Society and the Public Health Laboratory Service: Community-acquired pneumonia in adults in British hospitals in 1982–1983: a survey of aetiology, mortality, prognostic factors and outcome. Q J Med 1987;62:195–220.
80. Farr BM, Sloman AJ, Fisch MJ: Predicting death in patients hospitalized for community acquired pneumonia. Ann Intern Med 1991;115:428–436.
81. Karalus NC, Cursons RT, Leng RA, et al: Community acquired pneumonia: aetiology and prognostic index evaluation. Thorax 1991;46:413–418.
82. Franklin C, Henrickson K, Weil MH: Reduced mortality of pneumococcal bacteremia after early intensive care. J Intens Care Med 1991;6:302–307.
83. Celis R, Torres A, Gatell JM, et al: Nosocomial pneumonia: a multivariate analysis of risk and prognosis. Chest 1988;93:318–324.
84. Torres A, Aznar R, Gatell JM, et al: Incidence, risk, and prognosis factors of nosocomial pneumonia in mechanically ventilated patients. Am Rev Respir Dis 1990;142:523–528.
85. Garay SM, Greene J: Prognostic indicators in the initial presentation of Pneumocystis carinii pneumonia. Chest 1989;95:769–772.

86. Peruzzi WT, Skoutelis A, Shapiro BA, et al: Intensive care unit patients with acquired immunodeficiency syndrome and Pnemocystis carinii pneumonia: suggested predictors of hospital outcome. Crit Care Med 1991;19:892–900.
87. Bozzette SA, Feigal D, Chiu J, et al: Length of stay and survival after intensive care for severe Pneumocystis carinii pneumonia. Chest 1992; 101:1404–1406.
88. Crawford SW, Petersen FB: Long-term survival from respiratory failure after marrow transplantation for malignancy. Am Rev Respir Dis 1992;145: 510–514.
89. Fowler AA, Hamman RT, Zerbe GO, et al: Adult respiratory distress syndrome: prognosis after onset. Am Rev Respir Dis 1985;132:472–478.
90. Russell JA, Ronco JJ, Lockhart D, et al: Oxygen delivery and consumption and ventricular preload are greater in survivors than in nonsurvivors of the adult respiratory distress syndrome. Am Rev Respir Dis 1990;141:659–665.
91. Seidenfeld JJ, Pohl DF, Bell RC, et al: Incidence, site and outcome of infections in patients with the adult respiratory distress syndrome. Am Rev Respir Dis 1986;134:12–16.
92. Elliot CG: Pulmonary sequelae in survivors of the adult respiratory distress syndrome. Clin Chest Med 1990;11:789–800.

9
Antibiotic Therapy of Pulmonary Infections

BURKE A. CUNHA

Early, appropriate antimicrobial therapy determines the outcome with life-threatening pulmonary infections. Therefore it is imperative that the clinician correctly diagnose the type of infectious pulmonary process and determine the most likely organisms associated with the patient's clinical presentation or relevant epidemiology and appropriate laboratory tests. All of these factors determine the appropriateness of empiric antimicrobial therapy against the presumed pathogens in patients with bacterial pneumonias. The working diagnosis should include a differential diagnosis that takes into account the most likely pathogens given the aforementioned factors. After the appropriate spectrum has been determined, the clinician must consider the pharmacokinetic factors that determine the dose, dosing regimen, and method of administration of the antibiotic. Hepatic and renal functions must also be determined, as they affect antibiotic selection and dosing modifications. The patient's allergic history must be taken into account as well as the safety profile of the antibiotic. An important factor when selecting an antimicrobial is its resistance potential. When an organism is finally identified as the primary pathogen in a pneumonic process, attention may be given to specific antimicrobial therapy. The duration of antimicrobial therapy is empiric, and the duration of treatment for most pulmonary infections is based on arbitrary limits.[1–7]

Appropriate Spectrum

Because early antimicrobial therapy is especially important for treating bacterial pneumonias, it is important that empiric antimicrobial therapy be started as soon as possible after the diagnosis. Therapy initially is usually empiric, so selection of an antimicrobial agent must be based on the presumed pathogens given the patient's clinical presentation, local epidemiology, and selected laboratory tests.

The location of the pathologic process determines the usual pathogenic flora. The respiratory tract is contiguous with the oropharynx, and it is not surprising that upper and lower respiratory tract pathogens are identical. Although many organisms may colonize the oropharynx, only a relatively few (e.g., pneumococcus, *Hemophilus influenzae*, *Branhamella catarrhalis*) are capable of causing infection of the upper and lower respiratory tracts. Group A streptococci are the exception and may colonize or invade the oropharynx as well as the upper or lower respiratory tract. Therefore the usual organisms involved in upper respiratory tract infections (i.e., *Streptococcus pneumoniae*, *H. influenzae*, group A streptococci, *B. catarrhalis*) are the most common pathogens encountered in both upper and lower respiratory tract infections. Some organisms have a predilection for the lower respiratory tract while occasionally causing pharyngitis or otitis (e.g., *Mycoplasma pneumoniae*). Other pathogens such as *Legionella* appear to cause only lower respiratory tract infections when legionellosis is not extrapulmonary. Similarly, *Staphylococcus aureus* and *Klebsiella pneumoniae* are pathogens that primarily cause lower respiratory tract disease but may colonize, though ordinarily do not invade, the upper respiratory tract.[1–3]

The clinician should be able, on the basis of clinical presentation, roentgenographic findings, and minimal laboratory tests, to differentiate easily typical from atypical pneumonias. This distinction is clinically important because up to the present time therapy for typical bacterial pathogens is essentially ineffective against atypical organisms (e.g., *M. pneumoniae*, *Legionella pneumophila*, *Chlamydia* pneumoniae—TWAR agent). If it can be established that the pneumonic process is due to an atypical organism, clinical differentiation among the atypical pathogens is usually fairly straightforward based on differences in epidemiology, chest film findings, and liver function tests.[6] Fortunately, appropriate antimicrobial therapy directed against any of the agents causing atypical pneumonia is usually effective against all of the agents causing atypical pneumonia (e.g., doxycycline therapy).[8,9]

The organisms responsible for chronic bronchitis are exactly the same as those responsible for otitis and sinusitis, as they are all derived from the same oropharyngeal flora.[1] The organisms in anaerobic pleural pulmonary infections, whether aspiration pneumonia, anaerobic necrotizing pneumonitis, or lung abscess, have in common the same pathogens (e.g., the anaerobic oropharyngeal flora). The oropharyngeal flora of aspiration pneumonia acquired in the community setting is mixed, consisting primarily of "pigmented" *Bacteroides* (e.g., *Bacteroides melaninogenicus*) and a variety of other anaerobic mouth floras, e.g., *Veillonella*, *Peptococcus*). All of these organisms are usually sensitive to β-lactam antibiotics, but some strains, particularly *B. melaninogenicus*, may be avid producers of β-lactamase, which may inactivate therapy with β-lactam antibiotics. The decision to treat anaerobic pleural pulmonary infections with β-lactam antibiotics depends on the incidence of β-lactamase-producing pigmented *Bacteroides* species in any given location. If β-lactamase production is a local issue, therapy should be started with β-lactamase-resistant agents (e.g., clindamycin) or β-lactamase inhibitors (e.g., clavulinic acid, sulbactam).[10]

With the exception of *Pneumocystis carinii* pneumonia (PCP) in patients with human immunodeficiency virus (HIV) disease, empiric treatment of pneumonias due to unusual organisms is usually not possible. Specific therapy depends on demonstrating a pathogen by any one of a variety of ways and then selecting appropriate specific therapy. PCP occurs in a distinctive clinical setting, which permits one to suspect the diagnosis and begin empiric therapy pending a definitive diagnostic procedure. *P. carinii* occurs in patients with severe T-lymphocyte defects, particularly HIV patients and organ transplant patients. Although the chest roentgenogram is not specific, the clinical presentation of a diffuse bilateral interstitial process in an organ transplant patient or in someone suspected of having HIV makes empiric anti-*Pneumocystis* therapy clinically justifiable.[11–13]

Viral pneumonias may be more common than bacterial pneumonias; but they are not usually as severe and therefore are less frequently seen in the hospital setting. It is generally possible to differentiate a viral respiratory infection from a bacterial infection in the community setting in immunocompetent hosts, but it is difficult to differentiate one viral pneumonia from another in normal patients unless there are extrapulmonary findings that suggest the diagnosis; for example, conjunctivitis and pharyngitis in a patient with pneumonia suggest adenoviral pneumonia. Because antiviral therapy is limited and specific viral identification is usually not possible on clinical grounds, empiric antiviral therapy is not a clinical consideration. Viral pneumonitis should be specifically diagnosed; and therapy, though limited, may be applied to selected situations (e.g., viral influenza, cytomegalovirus pneumonitis, respiratory syncytial viral pneumonia). Therefore the limited antiviral armamentarium should be used only when a specific viral agent can be identified for which appropriate antiviral therapy exists.[14]

The nosocomial pneumonias also require early empiric antimicrobial therapy to minimize mortality and morbidity due to these serious and common infections. Nosocomial pneumonias are usually associated with ventilator assistance devices, and the pathogens most frequently encountered are those of the hospital or intensive care setting. Although community-acquired pathogens occur in patients with nosocomial pneumonias, it is the hospital-acquired organisms that are more common and more invasive.[15] *Pseudomonas aeruginosa* is the most common organism associated with hospital-acquired pneumonias. Furthermore, it is associated with the highest mortality and is trophic for the respiratory epithelium. Its predilection for the respiratory tract epithelium and its virulence factors combine to make it the primary pathogen toward which therapy should be directed in patients with hospital-acquired pneumonias.[16] Atypical pneumonias may also occur in the hospital setting, but fortunately such patients have features in common with community-acquired atypical pneumonias. In the hospital setting, atypical pneumonias are limited to *Legionella*, *Mycoplasma*, *or Chlamydia pneumoniae* (TWAR agent), as the other zoonotic pathogens are not transmitted or harbored within the hospital setting. Tuberculosis in normal hosts and *Mycobacterium tuberculosis* and *M. avium intracellulare* in HIV patients are ordinarily treated after demonstration/identification of the organism in the appropriate body site.

Empiric therapy also has no place in the treatment of pneumonias in immunocompromised or organ transplant patients. The time course after organ transplantation can be used as a rough guide to predict the usual pathogens, but there is much overlap and every effort should be made to diagnose specific pathogens before therapy is begun. In contrast, the febrile leukopenic compromised hosts with pneumonia may be treated as hospital-acquired pneumonias, as these patients have the same bacterial pathogens as patients with hospital-acquired pneumonias.

Except for *Aspergillus* pneumonia in immunosuppressed patients with prolonged leukopenia or prolonged antibiotic/steroid therapy, fungal pneumonias are not common in the nosocomial setting.[17] In contrast, community-acquired fungal pneumonias have a varying incidence depending on the epidemiology of the fungal organisms (e.g., coccidioidomycosis is common in the Southwest, histoplasmosis in the Mississippi and Ohio valleys, and blastomycosis in northern New England).

In summary, the usual problem faced by the clinician is treatment of bacterial pneumonias, either community- or hospital-acquired. The main difficulty is to differentiate infectious from noninfectious pulmonary infiltrates. If one can be reasonably sure the process is infectious, the next step is to differentiate between typical and atypical bacterial pneumonias and begin appropriate empiric therapy. Viral pneumonias, tuberculous pneumonia, and exotic pneumonias must be diagnosed and a specific organism demonstrated; in these situations empiric therapy is ordinarily not recommended. When bacterial pneumonia is acquired in the community, the aim is to select a single agent that is adequate against the expected bacterial pathogens; the same approach is volid for atypical pneumonias. Combination therapy is usually necessary to treat bacterial nosocomial pneumonias because *P. aeruginosa* is the primary pathogen and combination therapy is required to treat serious infections caused by this organism.

Pharmacokinetic Considerations

Once the proper spectrum has been determined based on the presumed pathogens, pharmacokinetic concerns are the next most important clinical consideration. The clinician must keep in mind that the most important thing is adequate concentration of the antibiotic at the site of infection to achieve tissue penetration. Dosing regimens are frequently based on achieving adequate serum concentrations, which may or may not be relevant to treating infections in various respiratory tract locations. The concentration of the antibiotic at the site of infection should be two to four times the minimal inhibitory concentration (MIC) needed to inhibit MIC 90 of the presumed pathogens. The ratio of the achievable blood or tissue level to the MIC 90 of the organism is the "kill ratio" and may be used as an index or predictor of antimicrobial efficacy. To compare the predicted efficacy of dissimilar antibiotics in pulmonary or any other infections, the "kill ratio" is the best comparative parameter to use. One should never select an antibiotic with a lower MIC against a given pathogen without taking into consideration the blood (or preferably tissue) concentration. These two factors taken together as a "kill ratio" more correctly reflect the in vivo situation as opposed to MIC 90s, which are strictly an in vitro parameter[18] (Table 9.1).

Tissue penetration data are difficult to obtain and even more difficult to interpret. The concentration of an antibiotic in a tissue depends on many factors, including the serum level, the number and nature of membrane barriers that must be traversed by the antibiotic to reach the site of

TABLE 9.1. "Kill ratios" of selected antibiotics against common pulmonary pathogens.

Antibiotic	Serum conc. (μg/ml)	Lung conc. (μg/g)	MICs of respiratory pathogens[a]				Antib. "kill ratios"; lung conc. MIC[b]			
			Pn	Hf[c]	K	Ps	Pn	Hf[c]	K	Ps
Penicillin G	2–61	2	0.01	0.8	>400	>500	E	I	I	I
Ampicillin	4–12	2	0.02	0.5	>200	>500	E	E	I	I
Amoxicillin	5.6	2	0.02	0.5	200		E	E	I	I
Bacampicillin	8.8	0.5–0.9	0.02	0.5	>200	>500	E	E	I	I
Ticarcillin	469	30–45	<1	0.5	>400	50	E	E	I	E
Mezlocillin	140	25–35	0.02	0.1	16	16	E	E	A	E
Piperacillin	196	55	0.02	0.1	16	16	E	E	A	E
Cefotaxime	40	10	≤1	0.03	0.25	>32	A	E	E	I
Ceftizoxime	18	18	≤1	0.01	0.25	>32	A	E	E	I
Cefoperazone	97	45	≤1	0.06	4.0	16	A	E	A	A
Ceftazidime	43	16	≤1	0.1	0.5	8	A	E	E	A
Ceftriaxone	127	57	≤1	0.1	0.1	>32	A	E	E	I

Source: Adapted from Cunha.[18] With permission.
[a] Pn = *Streptococcus pneumoniae*; Hf = *Hemophilus influenzae*; K = *Klebsiella*; Ps = *Pseudomonas* aeruginosa.
[b] E = more than adequate antibiotic concentrations (≥4 × MIC); A = adequate antibiotic concentrations (2–4 × MIC); I = inadequate antibiotic concentrations (≤2 × MIC).
[c] β-Lactamase-negative strains.

infection, the physiochemical characteristics of the antibiotic, the physiochemical characteristics of the intra- and extracellular milieu on the way to and including the site of infection, and the concentration of antibiotic in special sites (e.g., in abscesses or within the alveolar macrophage).

First, the drug must be absorbed or introduced into the vascular system. It does not matter how the drug is given so long as adequate serum concentrations are achieved in a timely and appropriate fashion. For example, if the patient can tolerate oral trimethoprim-sulfamethoxazole (TMP-SMX) or ciprofloxacin, blood levels are commensurate with equivalent doses when given by the intravenous route. Intramuscular therapy should be discouraged in general, but oral therapy under the proper circumstances is equivalent to intravenous therapy if the blood and tissue levels are similar. Oral therapy is not an option if the patient cannot tolerate medications orally or if there are barriers or impediments to oral absorption of the drug.[19,20] There are few or no data on giving oral medications to critically ill patients; and until such data are available initial intravenous therapy is preferred. With chronic infectious processes such as lung abscesses, oral therapy is equivalent and preferred after initial patient stabilization, as such patients ordinarily need to be treated for extended periods. The key point is to achieve adequate blood and tissue levels regardless of the mode of administration.

Once the antibiotic is within the blood compartment, the antibiotic is reversibly bound to serum albumin depending on its protein binding. As albumin binding sites are saturated with the antibiotic, the excess unbound or free antibiotic then moves along a concentration gradient across membrane barriers to areas of lower concentration (e.g., the site of infection). Antibiotic is "consumed" in moving along the concentration gradient from the serum compartment to the tissue site of infection (Fig. 9.1). Therefore the amount of antibiotic available at the site of infection is a percentage of the achievable serum level, and this measurement is the best way to estimate what the concentration will be in a particular tissue. The estimated tissue concentration can then be compared to the MIC 90 of the presumed pathogens to construct the kill ratios mentioned previously. The antibiotic at the site of infection in tissue also exists in a reversibly bound form and an unbound form. The factors determining the relative concentration of free and unbound antibiotic at the tissue level are complex and difficult to determine. For clinical purposes, it is sufficient to know that approximately 25% of the simultaneous serum level of most cephalosporins are present in lung tissue, for example. This approximation is an oversimplification and does not take into account a bewildering complexity of other factors that affect the movement of antibiotics in the various bodily compartments at any given time. It should be remembered that the antibiotic is constantly being metabolized, inactivated, or excreted, which is changing its concentration in the serum and the tissues. For practical purposes, however, the serum level represents the net result of all of

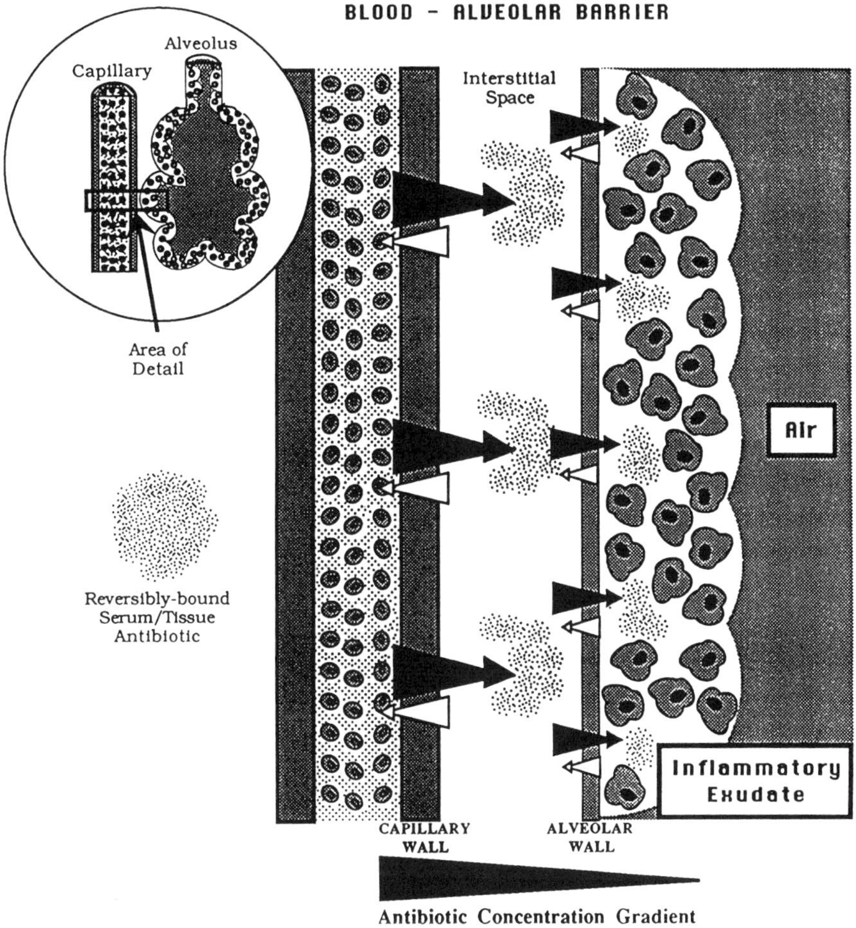

FIGURE 9.1. Blood-alveolar antibiotic barrier showing decreasing antibiotic levels along the concentration gradient from the serum compartment.

these factors acting simultaneously and thus is a reasonable and useful clinical guideline.[18]

Different degrees of tissue permeability exist in different locations of the respiratory tract. Tenacious mucus and alveolar macrophages make the lower respiratory tract different from the upper respiratory tract in terms of tissue penetration, even though the pathogens are in large part identical. An antibiotic that may be inadequate to treat otitis media may be perfectly adequate to treat *L. pneumophila* in the lung if the alveolar macrophage concentrates the antibiotic to high levels, as with clarithromycin or azithromycin. The effect of capillary permeability or tissue membrane permeability explains the relative ineffectiveness of most penicillins for treating infections through membrane or mucous barriers; for example, penicillin fails to eradicate group A streptococcal pharyngitis in approximately 15% of cases. The superiority of amoxicillin over ampicillin given at the same dose explains the superiority of amoxicillin for treating otitis and bronchitis.

Inflammation tissue penetration is a characteristic of the β-lactam antibiotics, aminoglycosides, monobactams, and carbopenems. In general, inflammation-independent antibiotics include the tetracyclines, quinolones, clarithromycin, and azithromycin[21] (Table 9.2). There are many factors that influence the penetration of antibiotics, but the most important are the serum tissue concentration gradient, lipid solubility, and degree of local inflammation at the membrane level. In addition, there are a variety of minor factors such as the number and thickness of the biologic membranes to be traversed, the pK_a of the antibiotic, and the molecular size of the antibiotic. It is also important to appreciate that the activity of antibiotics may be modified by a variety of local factors (e.g., volume of secretions, pH of the inflammatory exudate, local β-lactamase production by microorganisms) (Table 9.3). For example, aminoglycosides achieve good levels within the pulmonary parenchyma but are less active at the site of infection, where local conditions of acidosis, hypoxemia, and WBC debris decrease the activity of this class of drugs. Aztreonam, which has a similar spectrum of activity, is not affected by these factors. It should be appreciated that the concentration of an antibiotic at any given dose is usually different in the sputum, bronchial fluid, or lung tissue, and data such as those in Table 9.4 can be used to predict the adequacy of antibiotic concentration at the site of infection under usual circumstances (Fig. 9.2). Therefore the clinician should select for community-acquired

TABLE 9.2. Inflammation-dependent antibiotic penetration.

Inflammation-dependent penetration
Penicillins
Cephalosporins
Erythromycin
Clindamycin
Monobactams
Carbapenems
Aminoglycosides
Inflammation-independent penetration
Chloramphenicol
Oxytetracycline
Minocycline
Doxycycline
IMP-SMX
Quinolones

Source: Adapted from Cunha.[18] With permission.

TABLE 9.3. Factors influencing antibiotic penetration/activity.

- Antibiotic tissue penetration
  - Major factors
    - Serum-tissue concentration gradient
    - Lipid solubility
    - Degree of local inflammation
    - Protein binding (serum/interstitial/tissue)
    - Pulmonary vascular status
  - Minor factors
    - Number/thickness of biologic membranes
    - Area of pulmonary capillary bed
    - Antibiotic pKa
    - Antibiotic molecular size
    - Antibiotic molecular weight
    - Concentration in alveolar macrophages[a]
    - Volume of secretions
- Antibiotic activity
    - Chemical content of local exudate (enzyme bioactivation)
    - pH of inflammatory exudate
    - Local hypoxemia (decreased PO_2)
    - Microbial enzyme production (β-lactamases)

Source: Adapted from Cunha.[18] With permission.
[a] Important in intracellular infections, e.g., *Legionella*.

TABLE 9.4. Concentration ratios of antibiotics in sputum/lung tissue.

Antibiotic	Serum/sputum ratio (%)	Serum bronchial ratios (%)	Serum/lung ratios (%)
Penicillin	2	3	
Ampicillin	3	3	
Amoxicillin/clavulanate		3/15	0.4/0.2
Bacampicillin	13–20	6.7	
Amoxicillin	6	3.5	43
Ticarcillin	2		
Mezlocillin	4	9.6	
Azlocillin	4		
Piperacillin	4–15		28
Cefaclor	8–10	15	
Cefadroxil			64
Cephalothin	20–25		
Cefuroxime	18	18	90
Cefazolin	25	25	
Cefoxitin	20–25	24	33
Cefamandole			78
Cefotaxime	25	25	26

Source: Adapted from Cunha.[18] With permission.

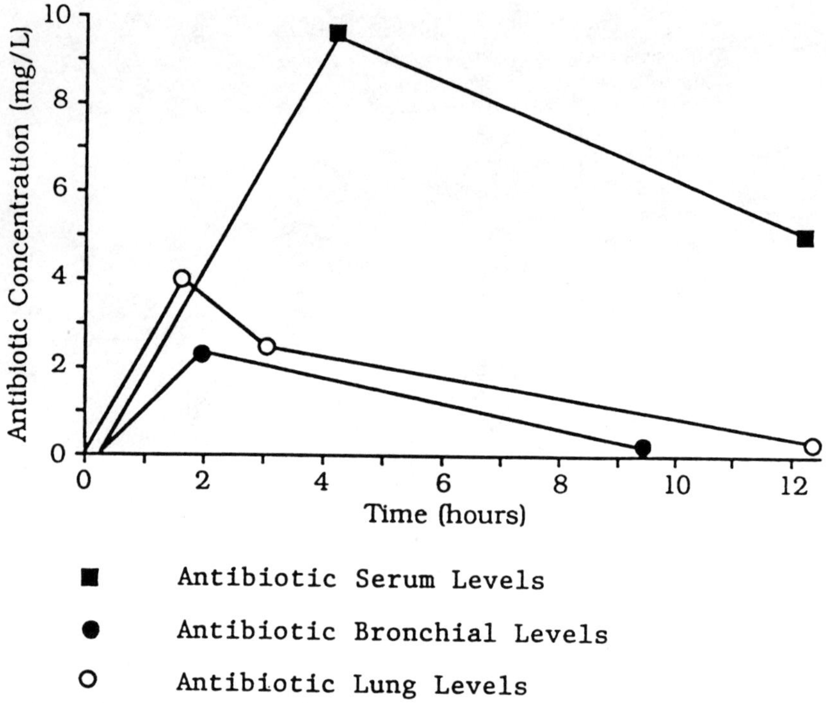

FIGURE 9.2. Tissue penetration characteristics of cefadroxil after a 1 g oral dose.

pneumonias preferably a single antibiotic, dosed appropriately, that provides a pharmacokinetic profile that ensures adequate concentration at the site of the respiratory tract infection. The relevant tissue penetration data of antibiotics commonly used for pulmonary infections are presented in Table 9.5.

Whether an antibiotic is being given by continuous or intermittent infusion, the antibiotic is being inactivated or eliminated by the liver or the kidneys as a function of time. It is well to keep in mind the drugs that are eliminated via the hepatic versus the renal route, as this information is a useful factor when selecting a drug in patients with hepatic or renal insufficiency. If the patient has severe renal insufficiency, most clinicians prefer to substitute a drug with the appropriate spectrum and tissue penetration characteristics but that is eliminated by the liver. Conversely, with severe hepatic insufficiency, drugs eliminated primarily via the renal route are usually preferred. Alternately, if an antibiotic is renally eliminated and renal insufficiency exists, the dose may be decreased according to the creatinine clearance results. For example, cefotaxime 2 g IV q6h is the usual dose for serious infection given to a patient with intact renal function. If renal insufficiency is present and the creatinine clearance is approxi-

TABLE 9.5. Antibiotic levels in the respiratory tract.

Antibiotic/dose/route	Serum level (μg/ml)	Sputum conc. (μg/ml)	Bronchial fluid (μg/ml)	Pleural fluid (μg/ml)	Lung tissue level (μg/g)
Penicillin 1 MU (IV)	2–61		2.5	1–56	2.4
Ampicillin 500 mg (IV)	4–12	0.2–0.4		4	2
Sulbactam/ampicillin					
1 g (IV)	3.2/30	0.1/5–7		0.2/4–11	
Bacampicillin					
400 mg PO	6.5	0.42		4.7–7.8	
800 mg PO	8.8	2.6		6–7	0.5–0.9
Amoxicillin					
1 g PO	5.6	0.4–0.6			2
500 mg IV	11.0	3.5	0.48		
Ticarcillin 5 g IV	469	4		57.4	30–45
Mezlocillin 5 g IV	140		10–20		25–35
Piperacillin 4 g IV	196				55
Erythromycin					
1 g PO	4	0.2			3
500 mg PO		0.2		3	4
Erythromycin ethylsuccinate					
1 g PO	0.7				4
Erythromycin lactobionate					
0.5 g IV	1.5				6.5
Erythromycin stearate					
0.5 g PO	3.1				4.7
Clindamycin					
300 mg PO		4.7		1.4	
150 mg PO		1.4		4.9	3–9
Vancomycin 1 g IV	5.3				13

TABLE 9.5. *Continued*

Antibiotic/dose/route	Serum level (μg/ml)	Sputum conc. (μg/ml)	Bronchial fluid (μg/ml)	Pleural fluid (μg/ml)	Lung tissue level (μg/g)
Tetracycline					
500 mg PO	2.0	0.2			
1 g PO		1–2		3–4	3–4
Minocycline					
200 mg PO	4–6	1.7			5–6
1 g PO	5–6	1.4			
Gentamicin 5/mg/day	5	1		0.6	6
Tobramycin 1.7 mg/kg	6	3		3	6–9
Cephalexin 500 mg PO	3	0.8	1.2		
Cephradine					
1 g PO	48	4.2	1.3	3.6–5.6	
500 mg PO	7				2.6
Cefaclor 500 mg PO		0.5			
Cefadroxil 1 g PO	5.2				7.6
	11.5	1.5		5.0	7.4
Cephalothin 1 g IV	50				15
Cefazolin				5	35–65
500 mg IV	7.6	3.0	10	10	
1 g IV	200		25		9.6
Cefuroxime 750 mg IV	28			50	
Cefonicid 1 g IM	71			29	23
Cefoxitin 2 g IV	10	3	3		
Cefamandole 2 g IV	20	5		6	10–15
	23				40

Cefotaxime					18
2 g IV	40	0.5			10
1 g IM	5			4	
1 g IV	37.8				19
			1.4		4.8
Amikacin 500 mg IV	20	2.7	2–3		8
Ciprofloxacin					
500 mg PO		1.4			1.2–1.7
750 mg PO		1–2	5		
Enoxacin 600 mg PO		3.7			7
Ofloxacin					
400 mg PO		5			
200 mg PO		3			7
Imipenem 1 g IV		20			12
Aztreonam 2 g IV			5–15		
TMP-SMX 0.2 g PO		2.7			10.9
Ceftizoxime 200 mg IV	18				18
Cefoperazone 2 g IV	97				45
Ceftazidime 2 g IV	43				16
Ceftriaxone					
1 g IV	67		2.3		10.7
2 g IV	127				57

Source: Adapted from Cunha.[18] With permission.

mately 50 ml/minute, the dose should be halved and the appropriate dose is 1 g IV q6h. If renal insufficiency is severe, with a creatinine clearance of approximately 10–20 ml/minute, the dose must be further modified such that 1 g given q12h would be an appropriate dose and still maintain the desired concentration of the antibiotic in the respiratory tract. The kinetics of antiviral, antiparasitic, or antimycobacterial drugs are not discussed here, and reference texts should be consulted for specific recommendations and pharmacokinetic considerations concerning these agents.

Empiric Therapy

Empiric therapy is optimally employed when a differential diagnosis is sufficiently narrowed to permit directed antibiotic therapy. The clinician should try and use a single agent to treat virtually all pulmonary infections with the exception of nosocomial pneumonias. For community-acquired pneumonias, whether they are typical or atypical pneumonias, single-agent therapy is preferred. Combination therapy offers no advantage in the treatment of community-acquired pneumonias for most patients.[22,23] For example, it makes no sense to add aztreonam for enhanced gram-negative coverage to a drug such as sulbactam-ampicillin or a second-generation cephalosporin. Similarly, adding an aminoglycoside to a cephalosporin adds pseudomonal coverage, which is unnecessary.[6] Unnecessary duplication—using two antibiotics with a similar spectrum of activity—does not produce better clinical results; it only increases the chances of drug interactions, drug side effects, and the possibility of superinfection with resistant organisms of *Candida*. There are relatively few drugs where antimicrobial synergy can be used as the rationale for combination therapy. It is certainly true for empiric therapy of nosocomial pneumonias where *Pseudomonas* is a prime consideration, and double-drug antipseudomonal therapy is mandatory.[17,24] Currently, antibiotics have such a high degree of activity against all the community and nosocomial pathogens that, except for the serious *Pseudomonas* infections, combination therapy is unnecessary and adds nothing. In the past, double-drug therapy had been necessary to treat *Klebsiella pneumoniae* pulmonary infections, but today it is no longer frequently done. Antibiotics such as third-generation cephalosporins have such a high degree of anti-*Klebsiella* activity that monotherapy with these potent anti-*Klebsiella* antibiotics are all that is necessary. Similarly, the addition of rifampin to erythromycin- or a tetracycline-containing regimen for legionnaires' disease is usually unnecessary.

A frequent clinical error is to increase the antibiotic spectrum of a drug or add another antibiotic if the patient is anything but a normal host. For example, if a patient with chronic obstructive pulmonary disease or alcohol abuse is very ill with pneumonia, additional drugs are given to somehow "make up" for the severity of the patient's illness. Empiric therapy should be based on the appropriate spectrum; the antibiotic selected must be appropriate for normal as well as abnormal hosts, and the dosing should be on the high end of the dosing range. The alcoholic patient with pneumonia has the same pathogens as an otherwise normal host and in a technical sense is "compromised" on the basis of somewhat impaired chemotactic function; but the empiric choice of antibiotic remains the same, and the addition of other antibiotics does not enhance outcome. The outcome of any infectious disease process, including pneumonias, depends ultimately on the host, not on the antimicrobial therapy. Empiric therapy has little if any role in treating organ transplant patients or HIV patients with pneumonia, with the exception of *P. carinii* pneumonia[13,17] (Table 9.6).

Specific Therapy

Specific therapy of pulmonary infections presupposes that the pathologic organism has been recovered from a properly collected and processed specimen of fluid from the lower respiratory tract or from blood cultures. Specific therapy is possible in many, but by no means all, patients with pulmonary infections. The clinical question frequently arises about whether one should change drugs from the initial empiric choice to an antibiotic with a narrower spectrum once the putative organism has been identified. There is little rationale for such a change. If the initial empiric therapy was appropriate, cost-effective, and pharmacokinetically sound, there is no reason to switch to a narrower spectrum antibiotic unless there are compelling reasons to do so or it is less expensive. For example, if a community-acquired bacterial pneumonia is initiated with a long-acting second-generation cephalosporin such as cefonicid, and the organism responsible is shown to be *S. pneumoniae*, switching to penicillin G will not produce better clinical results. The clinical outcome will be the same, and the cost of administering penicillin G in the hospital setting compared to cefonicid is usually more expensive.[6] As with empiric therapy, the switch to an oral equivalent antibiotic with the same spectrum and kinetic characteristics should be done as soon as the patient clinically defervesces and is stabilized[10,18,25] (Table 9.7).

Duration of Therapy

For bacterial pneumonias, ordinarily therapy is continued for 7–14 days. Traditionally, 1–2 weeks of therapy has been employed, but there are few data available to support this practice. There is a trend to decrease both the length of hospitalization and the total length of therapy for

TABLE 9.6. Empiric treatment of pneumonias.

Pneumonia syndrome	Usual pathogens	Appropriate IV therapy	Appropriate PO therapy
Community-acquired penumonia (typical)			
Normal host (all ages)	*Streptococcus pneumoniae* *Hemophilus influenzae* *Blanhamella catarrhalis* Group A streptococcus *Klebsiella*	2nd Generation cephalosporin Sulbactam/ampicillin Doxycycline	Clarithromycin Doxycycline Azithromycin Temafloxacin Cefadroxil
Abnormal host (DM, SLE, steroids)	*S. pneumoniae* *H. influenzae* Group A streptococcus *Klebsiella*	3rd Generation cephalosporin Sulbactam/ampicillin	Clarithromycin Azithromycin Cefadroxil
Special host (COPD, ETOH, nursing home)	*H. influenzae* *Klebsiella* *S. pneumoniae*	3rd Generation cephalosporins Sulbactam/ampicillin	Clarithromycin Azithromycin Temafloxacin Cefadroxil
Asplenic host	*S. pneumoniae* *H. influenzae* *N. meningitidis*	3rd Generation cephalosporin Sulbactam/ampicillin	Clarithromycin Azithromycin Cefadroxil
Community-acquired pneumonia (atypical)			
Normal/abnormal host	*Legionella* *Mycoplasma* TWAR *Chlamydia* Q fever Tularemia Psittacosis	Doxycycline Erythromycin	Doxycycline Erythromycin Clarithromycin Azithromycin Temafloxacin 3rd Generation cephalospiron

Nosocomial pneumonia (typical)			
Normal/abnormal host	*Pseudomonas aeruginosa* *Klebsiella* *Serratia* *E. coli*	Anti-pseudomonal 3rd Generation cephalosporin *plus* Aminoglycoside or Aztreonam or Antipseudomonal quinolone or Antipseudomonal penicillin	NA
Nosocomial pneumonia (atypical)			
Normal/abnormal host	*Legionella* *Mycophasma*	Doxycycline Erythromycin Azithromycin	Clarithromycin Doxycycline
Pneumonias in abnormal hosts (atypical)			
Leukopenic	*Legionella* *Mycoplasma*	NA	NA
HIV	*Legionella* *Mycoplasma* *Salmonella*	TMP-SMX Doxycycline Temafloxacin	Clarithromycin Azithromycin TMP-SMX Doxycycline
Transplant	*Pneumocystis carinii*	TMP-SMX	TMP-SMX

NA = not available; HIV = human immunodeficiency virus; TMP-SMX = trimethoprim-sulfamethoxazole.

TABLE 9.7. Specific therapy of pneumonias.

Pneumonia syndrome	Usual pathogens	Appropriate IV therapy[a]	Appropriate PO therapy[a]
Bacterial (typical)	*S. pneumoniae*	Same as empiric therapy	Same as empiric therapy
	S. aureus	Nafcillin	Clindamycin
		Vancomycin	1st Generation oral cephalosporin
	Group A streptococci	Same as empiric therapy	Same as empiric therapy
	E. coli	Same as empiric therapy	Same as empiric therapy
	Klebsiella	3rd Generation cephalosporin	3rd Generation oral cephalosporin
		Aztreonam	*or* quinolone
	Acinetobacter	Imipenem	Quinolone
		TMP-SMX	TMP-SMX
	Serratia	3rd Generation cephalosporin	TMP-SMX
		Quinolone	Quinolone
		Aztreonam	
	P. aeruginosa	Same as empiric therapy	Same as empiric therapy
	H. influenzae	Same as empiric therapy	Same as empiric therapy
	B. catarrhalis	Same as empiric therpay	Same as empiric therapy
Bacterial (atypical)	*Legionella*	Same as empiric therapy	Same as empiric therapy
	Mycoplasma	Same as empiric therapy	Same as empiric therapy
	Nocardia	TMP-SMX	Minocycline
		Minocycline	
	Actinomyces	Penicillin G	Penicillin V
		Doxycycline	Doxycycline
	Francisella tularensis	Streptomycin/gentamicin	Tetracycline *or* chloramphenicol
	C. burnetii (Q fever)	Doxycycline	Doxycycline
		Quinolone	Quinolone

Viral			
RSV		Riboviran	NA
Influenza		Amantadine	Amantidine
Varicella-zoster		Acyclovir	Acyclovir
Cytomegalovirus		DDI/DDC + IVIG	NA
Chlamydia	*C. trachomatis*	Doxycycline	Doxycycline
	C. pneumoniae	Erythromycin	Erythromycin
			Clarithromycin
			Azithromycin
Parasitic			
	Pneumocystis carinii	TMP-SMX	TMP-SMX
		Pentamidine	
Mycobacterial	*Mycobacterium tuberculosis*	Rifampicin	INH
		Streptomycin	Rifampin
			Ethambutol
	Mycobacterium avium intracellulare	Rifampicin	Azithromycin
		Ciprafloxacin	Clarithromycin
		Amikacin	
		Doxycycline	
Fungal	*Cryptococcus*	Amphotericin B	
		Fluconazole	Fluconazole
	Aspergillus	Amphotericin B	NA

TMP-SMX = trimethoprim-sulfamethoxazole; RSV = respiratory syncytial virus; DDI/DDC + IVIG = dideoxygenosine/dideoxycytidine plus intravenous immunoglobulin; NA = not available; INH = isoniozid.

[a] Consult standard reference works in suggested readings for antibiotic doses and dosing regimens.

patients with bacterial pneumonias. Whereas 14 days was the previous standard, 7–10 days is now preferred if the patient's clinical condition permits. Also in the past, the full course of therapy has been given by the intravenous or parenteral route. At the present time, initial therapy usually via the intravenous route, with change to an oral antibiotic that has an equivalent spectrum and a commensurate pharmacokinetic profile, is the preferred approach. The rapid switch to oral agents decreases the hospitalization time and minimizes the cost and complications associated with intravenous antibiotic therapy. So long as the blood and tissue levels are the same with the oral antibiotic and the spectrum is similar, there is no difference in clinical outcome in terms of how the drug is administered once the patient has stabilized, defervesced, and is able to take oral medications. With the newer antibiotics that are available (e.g., clarithromycin, azithromycin, oral quinolones), great changes are taking place regarding the way we treat most infectious diseases including pulmonary infections.[26,27]

The duration of therapy varies also according to the host defense status of the patient; that is, it is reasonable to treat a diabetic with pneumonia for a longer period than a nondiabetic. Some pathogens are more difficult; for example, *Staphylococcus aureus* pneumonia would normally be treated for at least 2 weeks (if not longer), whereas uncomplicated pneumococcal pneumonia might be treated for 7–10 days. Patients with systemic lupus erythematosus on steroids or alcoholics frequently require longer rather than shorter courses of therapy. The disease process also influences the duration of therapy. For example, an anaerobic lung abscess may require months of therapy until the disease process is resolved. Obviously, tuberculous pneumonia must be treated for months rather than days to be effective because of the slow replication cycle of the tubercle bacillus. Other organisms that are difficult to eradicate because of their location, e.g., *Mycoplasma*, *Chlamydia pneumoniae* (TWAR agent), or *Legionella*, usually require prolonged therapy either for cure or to prevent early relapse. *L. pneumophila* may be treated for 4 weeks rather than the customary 2 weeks with the usual typical bacterial pneumonias.

In summary, the duration of therapy depends on the pathogen, the site of infection, and the nature of the pulmonary infection; hence all these factors must be taken into account when selecting an appropriate antimicrobial agent. The clinician also must consider the cost of antimicrobial therapy, agent versus agent, intraverous versus oral administration, short-term versus long-term therapy, hospital versus home, and so on to provide cost-effective, optimal antibiotic therapy of pulmonary infections. In addition, the clinician must consider the resistance potential to the antibiotic being used as well as the side effect profile of the antibiotic. The longer the patient is to be given an antibiotic, the more careful is the consideration that must be given to resistance potential, side effects, and cost to the patient.

References

1. Berman S: Acute respiratory infections. Infect Dis Clin North Am 1991;5: 319–336.
2. Donowitz GR, Mandell GL: Empiric therapy for pneumonia. Rev Infect Dis 1983;5:40–54.
3. Ellner JJ: Management of acute and chronic respiratory tract infections. Am J Med 1988;85(3A):2–5.
4. Macfarlane JT: Treatment of lower respiratory infections. Lancet 1987;2: 1446–1449.
5. Rodnick JE, Gude JK: Diagnosis and antibiotic treatment of community-acquired pneumonia. West J Med 1991;154:405–409.
6. Cunha BA: Pneumonia acquired from others. I and II. Postgrad Med 1987; 82:126–156.
7. Tan JS, File TM Jr, Thomson RB Jr: Ambulatory management of lower respiratory tract infections. Am Fam Physician 1991;44(5):73–77, 80.
8. Cunha BA: Atypical pneumonias. Postgrad Med 1991;90:89–101.
9. Nguyen MH, Stout JE, Yu VL: Legionellosis. Infect Dis Clin North Am 1991;5:561–584.
10. Hampson NB, Woolf RA, Springmeyer SC: Oral antibiotics for pneumonia. Clin Chest Med 1991;12:395–407.
11. Magnenat JL, Nicod LP, Aukenthaler R, Junod AF: Mode of presentation and diagnosis of bacterial pneumonia in human immunodeficiency virus-infected patients. Am Rev Respir Dis 1991;144:917–922.
12. Smith D, Gazzard B: Treatment and prophylaxis of Pneumocystis carinii pneumonia in AIDS patients. Drugs 1991;101:451–457.
13. Sattler FR, Feinberg J: New developments in the treatment of Pneumocystis carinii. Chest 1992;101:451–457.
14. Betts RF: Antiviral agents in respiratory infections. Semin Respir Infect 1991;6:147–157.
15. Levine SA, Niederman MS: The impact of tracheal intubation on host defenses and risks for nosocomial pneumonia. Clin Chest Med 1991;12:523–543.
16. Matthay RA, Moritz ED: Invasive procedures for diagnosing pulmonary infection: a critical review. Clin Chest Med 1981;2:3.
17. Rubin RH, Greene R: Etiology and management of the compromised patient with fever and pulmonary infiltrates. In Rubin RH, Young LS (eds): Clinical Approach to Infection in the Compromised Host. New York: Plenum, 1981, p. 123.
18. Cunha BA: Antibiotic pharmacokinetic considerations in pulmonary infections. Semin Respir Infect 1991;6:168–182.
19. Wollschlager CM, Raoof S, Khan FA, et al: Controlled, comparative study of ciprofloxacin versus ampicillin in treatment of bacterial respiratory tract infection. Am J Med 1987;82(4A):164.
20. Vogel F, Lode H: The use of oral temafloxacin compared with a parenteral cephalosporin in hospitalized patients with pneumonia. J Antimicrob Chemother 1991;28:81–86.
21. Kinasewitz G, Wood RG: Azithromycin versus cefaclor in the treatment of acute bacterial pneumonia. Eur J Clin Microbiol Infect Dis 1991;10:872–877.

22. Mangi RJ, Ryan J, Berenson C, Greco T, Simms M, Thorton G, Andriole VT: Cefoperazone versus ceftazidime monotherapy of nosocomial pneumonia. Am J Med 1988;85(1A):44–48.
23. Chelluri L: Cefoperazone versus combination antibiotic therapy of hospital-acquired pneumonia [letter]. Am J Med 1988;84:1091–1092.
24. Collins T, Gerding DN: Aminoglycosides versus beta-lactams in gram-negative pneumonia. Semin Respir Infect 1991;6:136–146.
25. Klein NC: Fluoroquinolones in respiratory infections. Semin Respir Infect 1991;6:131–135.
26. Schonwald S, Skerk V, Petricevic I, et al: Comparison of three-day and five-day courses of azithromycin in the treatment of atypical pneumonia. Eur J Clin Microbiol Infect Dis 1991;10:877–880.
27. Anderson G, Esmonde TS, Coles S, et al: A comparative safety and efficacy study of clarithromycin and erythromycin stearate in community-acquired pneumonia. J Antimicrob Chemother 1991;27:117–124.

Suggested Reading

American Medical Association: Drug Evaluations Annual 1992, pp. 1139–1677. Chicago: AMA, 1992.

Bartlett J: Pocketbook of Infectious Disease Therapy, 1989–1990. Baltimore: Williams & Wilkins, 1990.

Conte JE Jr, Barriere SL: Manual of Antibiotics and Infectious Diseases, 6th ed. Philadelphia: Lea & Febiger, 1988.

Cunha BA (ed): Antimicrobial therapy. Med Clin North Am 1982;66(1):1–316.

Cunha BA, Gerding DA: Antimicrobial penetration into respiratory secretions. Parts I and II. Semin Respir Infect 1991;6(3).

Kucers A, Bennett NMcK: The Use of Antibiotics, 4th ed. Philadelphia: Lippincott, 1987.

Peterson PK, Verhoef J (eds): The Antimicrobial Agents. Annual 3. New York: Elsevier, 1988.

Cunha BA, Ristuccia AM (eds): Antimicrobial Therapy. New York: Raven Press, 1984.

Sanford JP: Guide to Antimicrobial Therapy 1992. Bethesda: Antimicrobial Therapy, Inc., 1992.

10
Pulmonary Disorders Mimicking Infectious Pneumonia

Robert D. Brandstetter

The initial insult to the respiratory tract and the manner in which a response occurs are reflected in a patient's clinical presentation and supporting laboratory data.[1] A person presenting with a productive cough of green sputum, fever and chills, and a peribronchial infiltrate on chest radiograph probably has bronchopneumonia. Because the pulmonary parenchyma has similar responses to a wide variety of insults, however, the radiographic findings in many infectious and noninfectious disorders are the same. A chest radiograph therefore should not be interpreted in a void. Accordingly, clinical setting and pertinent laboratory data are essential for establishing the correct diagnosis.

This chapter describes the common respiratory illnesses that may mimic an infection. The spectrum of disorders range roentgenographically from a normal picture to diffuse bilateral infiltrates. Patients may have few symptoms (e.g, a dry, nonproductive cough or profound shortness of breath). Supporting laboratory data may be minimal or overwhelming. Finally, the importance of recognizing these noninfectious disorders obviously lies in the difference in management and therapy.

Normal Chest Radiograph

A normal chest radiograph in a patient with cough or shortness of breath often poses a difficult diagnostic problem. Because the cough reflex is one of the major defense mechanism of the body against any particulate matter aspirated, it may be a symptom of a wide variety of disorders. Such problems include the obvious infectious bronchitis as well as allergic rhinitis, asthma, and gastroesophageal reflux (GER). If the cough is productive of sputum and the Gram stain demonstrates leukocytes and bacteria, a diagnosis of infectious bronchitis may be established.[2] On the other hand, a productive cough with a negative sputum examination, a normal chest radiograph, and a history of post-nasal drip, allergies, or sinusitis suggests the diagnosis of allergic rhinitis.

In this case, a trial of antihistamines and nasal corticosteroids may be indicated.

The presence of cough with exercise, change in temperature, or inhalation of noxious fumes in a patient with a normal chest radiograph should raise the suspicion of irritable airways disease or asthma. Pulmonary function tests, which may be normal during asymptomatic periods, help to support this diagnosis. A low forced expiratory flow rate in 1 second (FEV_1), high residual volume, normal or high total lung capacity, and a flow rate that improves after administration of aerosol bronchodilators are consistent with the diagnosis of asthma. Indeed certain patients may require bronchoprovocation with an inhaled airway irritant such as methacholine to demonstrate bronchoconstriction. A trial of inhaled bronchodilators is justified in any of these patients.

A cough that intensifies when the patient is recumbent may be due to postnasal drip.[3] In the presence of the appropriate history, however, the possibility of GER with aspiration must also be considered. If aspiration is suspected, a barium swallow may help to confirm the diagnosis. It has been shown that cough and wheezing associated with GER may be due to entities other than aspiration. Increased parasympathetic tone in the esophagus from GER can result in narrowing of the airways and consequent wheezing. Elevating the head of the patient's bed and avoiding pharmacologic substances that relax the gastroesphageal junction prior to retiring may be helpful in these patients. In addition, a trial of histamine type 2 (H2) blockers (e.g., cimetidine or ranitidine) may be indicated in this group of patients or those with documented asthma who are not responding to conventional therapy.

A patient presenting with shortness of breath, chest pain, and a normal chest radiograph may have pulmonary emboli. If this diagnosis is suspected, an arterial blood gas assay and a perfusion lung scan should be obtained as the initial procedures to establish a diagnosis.

Table 10.1 lists clues to the causes of cough in the presence of a normal chest film, and Table 10.2 presents some of the accepted modes of management.

Focal Infiltrates

In the appropriate clinical setting, a focal infiltrate on chest radiograph usually suggests an inflammatory pneumonia. In these patients, air in the alveoli and alveolar ducts is replaced by an inflammatory exudate or inflammatory cells (or both), resulting in the radiographic findings of consolidation. However, several noninfectious disorders may have similar radiographic and clinical findings. For example, a patient with a history of heavy smoking who presents with cough, sputum production, and an infiltrate on chest radiograph is often thought to have tracheobronchitis

TABLE 10.1. Clues to causes of cough.

Cause	Position or activities precipitating or aggravating cough
Postnasal drip	Supine
Gastroesophageal reflux	Supine
Nocturnal asthma	Supine
Congestive heart failure	Supine
Occupational asthma	Worse at work
Asthma	Exercise, cold air, smoke

TABLE 10.2. Accepted modes of therapy for common causes of cough.

Cause of cough	Therapy
Postnasal drip	Cessation of smoking Remove from other offending inhaled agents Antihistamine-decognestant therapy
Asthma	Cessation of smoking Remove from other offending inhaled agents Cromolyn sodium
Gastroessophageal reflux	Diet Do not eat or drink 4 hours before bedtime Do not wear tight clothing around waist Bed blocks Antacids H2 antagonists

due to smoke inhalation or an infectious pneumonia. Nevertheless, the absence of systemic evidence of infection and incomplete clearing of the infiltrate after treatment with appropriate antibiotics should lead the clinician to suspect the possibility of a bronchogenic carcinoma. In such cases, the infiltrate is usually the result of partial or complete obstruction of the bronchus affected by the neoplasm.

Less commonly, bronchogenic carcinoma involves an entire segment or lobe, which in itself may cause bulging of the fissures. Alveolar cell carcinoma may closely mimic a pyogenic pneumonia radiographically. Systemic signs of infection are usually absent, however, and the patient produces large amounts of watery, clear sputum. Bronchoscopic examination with transbronchial biopsy is often diagnostic of neoplasm.

Other common entities that should be considered in the differential diagnosis of noninfectious focal pulmonary infiltrates are listed in Table 10.3. Of special note is asymmetric cardiac pulmonary edema in which the distribution of edema fluid is often related to the underlying architectural distortion of the lung parenchyma. It results in focal infiltrates, which clear spontaneously as congestive heart failure is treated. Pulmonary

TABLE 10.3. Noninfectious focal pulmonary infiltrates: differential diagnosis.

Bronchogenic carcinoma
Chemical pneumonitis following aspiration of gastric contents
Asymmetric cardiac pulmonary edema
Drug-induced pneumonitis
Radiation pneumonitis
Pulmonary infarct
Pseudolymphoma
Cholesterol pneumonia

infarction also may be a cause of focal consolidation in the lung secondary to hemorrhage. These patients often complain of pleuritic pain, shortness of breath, and hemoptysis. Clinical evidence of deep venous thrombosis may also be present, supported by noninvasive vascular studies of the lower extremities. If this diagnosis is suspected, a ventilation-perfusion lung scan may be helpful for clarifying the diagnosis.

Bilateral Infiltrates: Interstitial and Alveolar

A wide variety of noninflammatory pulmonary disorders may manifest as shortness of breath with or without sputum production and bilateral or diffuse parenchymal infiltrates on chest radiograph. The infiltrates may be alveolar, interstitial, or a combination of the two. Table 10.4 lists some of the entities that should be considered in the differential diagnosis of bilateral or diffuse parenchymal infiltrates in the absence of systemic evidence of infection. Many of these disorders are progressive, and prompt diagnosis and treatment are important.

The combination of a history of occupational exposure to inhaled inorganic dusts and an interstitial infiltrate on the chest radiograph should raise the suspicion of pneumoconiosis. Silicosis causes a nodular interstitial infiltrate most commonly involving the upper lung fields. Often there are associated eggshell calcifications bilaterally in the hilar lymph nodes. These patients may develop insidious progressive massive fibrosis, which can mimic infectious alveolar infiltrates. They also have an increased incidence of superimposed tuberculosis.

Exposure to asbestos may result in asbestosis after several decades of working in the vicinity of this material. Roentgenographic changes may not occur until many years later, long after exposure has ceased. Lower lobe infiltrates may be found, as may an increased incidence of mesothelioma and parenchymal neoplasia. The relation of asbestos to smoking is particularly striking with regard to malignancy.

Chemotherapeutic drugs (e.g., bleomycin, chlorambucil, cyclophosphamide, melphalan, carmustine, mitomycin C) also can cause interstitial

TABLE 10.4. Bilateral or diffuse parenchymal infiltrates: differential diagnosis.

- Known etiology (25%)
  - Occupational and environmental inhalants
    - Inorganic dusts: silica, aluminum, beryllium, asbestos
    - Organic dusts: chemical (polyester), living sources (moldy hay)
  - Drugs
    - Chemotherapeutic drugs
    - Antibiotics
    - Others (gold salts)
  - Poisons; paraquat
  - Radiation
  - Uremia
  - Lymphangitic metastases
  - Hemosiderosis
  - Adult respiratory distress syndrome
  - Transfusion reactions
  - Pulmonary hematoma
  - Near-drowning
  - Intravenous drug abuse
  - Pulmonary contusion
- Unknown etiology
  - Granulomatous disease
    - Sarcoidosis
    - Eosinophilic granuloma
  - Idiopathic pulmonary fibrosis
  - Chronic interstitial disease associated with collagen-vascular disease
  - Wegener's granulomatosis
  - Lymphangitic infiltrative disorders
  - Pulmonary vasculitis
  - Goodpasture syndrome
  - Alveolar proteinosis
  - Pulmonary alveolar microlithiasis

pulmonary infiltrates. Both alveolar and interstitial infiltrates can be seen after exposure to methotrexate. Other drugs that have been reported to cause pulmonary infiltrates include nitrofurantoin, gold salts, and methysergide. The infiltrates seen with nitrofurantoin may be either interstitial or alveolar and usually disappear when the drug is withdrawn.

Radiation pneumonitis can masquerade as an inflammatory infectious process. Cough, fever, and parenchymal infiltrates may appearing 6–12 weeks after exposure, particularly if the total radiation dose exceeds 4000 rads. In addition to infection, progressive or recurrent carcinoma should be ruled out. Bronchoscopy may be required to establish a diagnosis of radiation pneumonitis, which is usually made on the basis of excluding these other entities. Although steroids have not been shown conclusively to improve the course or outcome of radiation pneumonitis, they are frequently administered.

Pulmonary edema appears as a bilateral butterfly infiltrate resulting from the transudation of fluid into the interstitial and alveolar spaces. Congestive heart failure is probably the most common cause of this pattern, but it may also be seen with the adult respiratory distress syndrome (ARDS), elevated intracranial pressure, blood product transfusion reactions, intravenous fluid volume overload, and renal failure. A similar pattern may be seen in near-drowning victims and intravenous heroin abusers. An accurate history and supporting laboratory data are again essential for establishing the correct diagnosis of these illnesses.

Many of the noninfectious disorders that can cause bilateral parenchymal infiltrates have no known etiology. For example, sarcoidosis, which may manifest as constitutional symptoms suggestive of infection or may be completely asymptomatic, appears radiographically as bilateral hilar adenopathy, mediastinal adenopathy, reticulonodular interstitial infiltrates, or any combination thereof.[4] Occasionally, multiple areas of consolidation (alveolar sarcoid) are seen. On biopsy, these apparent areas of alveolar consolidation actually represent areas of interstitial disease. Noncaseating granulomas on histology solidify the diagnosis when acid-fast and fungal organisms fail to grow in culture 6–8 weeks later. Corticosteroids are the treatment of choice for patients with biopsy-proved sarcoid.

Collagen-vascular disorders (e.g., systemic lupus erythematosus, rheumatoid arthritis, scleroderma) can also affect the lungs.[5] Fever, cough (which may be productive), shortness of breath, and pleuritic pain may be present. Systemic lupus erythematosus most commonly manifests as painful pleural disease when the chest is involved. Other radiographic findings can include basilar atelectasis secondary to splinting, acute lupus pneumonitis, and a diffuse reticulonodular basilar interstitial infiltrate. In patients with rheumatoid arthritis, pulmonary changes include basilar interstitial infiltrates, cavitating (necrobiotic) nodules, and pleural disease. A basilar reticular interstitial pattern may be present in patients with scleroderma. Esophageal motility problems may be present in these patients, predisposing them to chronic aspiration and the roentgenographic finding of bilateral lower lobe infiltrates. Clinical history and laboratory studies are needed to help distinguish between these collagen-vascular diseases. Infectious processes must be carefully ruled out prior to treatment, as corticosteroids and cytotoxic drugs (agents of choice in collagen vascular diseases) can mask the signs and symptoms of infection.

Solitarity and Multiple Parenchymal Nodules

About half of the solitary nodules (<3 cm) found on a chest radiograph in an asymptomatic patient are granulomas secondary to previous infection or exposure to fungal or tuberculous diseases (or both).[6] Other causes of

TABLE 10.5. Solitary nodules of the lung: differential diagnosis.

Malignant tumors
Primary bronchogenic carcinoma
Bronchial adenoma
Metastatic carcinoma
Benign tumors
Infectious granulomas
Noninfectious granulomas—sarcoidosis
Hamartoma
Miscellaneous lesions
Amyloid
Arteriovenous fistulas
Pulmonary varix
Hematoma
Pulmonary infarction

solitary pulmonary nodules (Table 10.5) that must be included in the differential diagnosis include hamartoma (40% contain calcification); bronchogenic cyst; mucoid impaction; pulmonary infarct; pseudotumors (fluid loculated in a fissure, chest-wall tumors, skin tumors, nipple shadows); pulmonary varix; pulmonary arteriovenous fistula; intra-pulmonary lymph node; and pulmonary hematoma.

A patient with a solitary pulmonary nodule may also have bronchogenic carcinoma.[7,8] Often there is a long history of smoking, and on careful questioning the patient may report symptoms of increasing cough and hemoptysis. Bronchoscopy with transbronchial biopsy or transthoracic aspiration biopsy may help to establish the diagnosis in these patients.

Bronchial adenomas (most of which are carcinoid) can also appear as solitary pulmonary nodules on a chest radiograph, with most being located centrally. These patients may be asymptomatic, but cough or hemoptysis (or both) is often present.

Table 10.5 outlines some of the noninflammatory causes of a solitary pulmonary nodule. When evaluating these patients, it is important to search for an old chest radiograph. A lesion that remains unchanged radiographically for 2 years or more is considered to be stable and may be simply observed. More aggressive management is indicated if the nodule is either new or changing in appearance, and in particular if the patient is or was a smoker.

It is more difficult to distinguish noninfectious disorders from infectious ones in the presence of multiple pulmonary nodules (Table 10.6). For example, tuberculosis, histoplasmosis, and coccidioidomycosis may cause multiple pulmonary nodules with or without calcification. In an asymptomatic patient the clinical history and skin testing are helpful for narrowing the diagnosis.

TABLE 10.6. Multiple pulmonary nodules: differential diagnosis.

Malignant nodules
Metastatic lesions
Lymphoma
Benign nodules
Infectious granulomas
Noninfectious granulomas
Sarcoidosis
Rheumatoid nodules
Wegener's granulomatosis
Benign tumors
Hamartoma
Amyloid
Septic emboli
Parasites
Arteriovenous malformations

Septic pulmonary emboli may appear on a chest radiograph as multiple cavitating pulmonary nodules. The clinical history, systemic evidence of infection, and the presence of risk factors for septic pulmonary emboli help to establish the diagnosis.

Multiple, noncalcified pulmonary nodules in a patient with minimal complaints of shortness of breath or cough (or both) are often secondary to early metastatic disease. Bronchoscopy with transbronchial biopsy may be diagnostic in these patients. In patients with pronounced symptoms of weight loss, dyspnea, and a known malignancy, the presence of multiple pulmonary nodules is strongly suggestive of pulmonary metastases.

Cavitary Disease

Although cavitation of pulmonary nodules or infiltrates is often seen in inflammatory disorders such as mycobacterial and fungal infections, lung abscesses, and septic emboli, the possibility of a noninfectious cavitary process must be considered when no systemic or laboratory signs of infection exist.

For example, squamous cell carcinoma of the lung (primary or secondary) may cavitate.[8] Multiple cavitary nodules due to metastatic squamous carcinoma usually appear in the head and neck region or, in women, the uterine cervix. In the appropriate clinical setting, biopsy is indicated to establish the diagnosis.

Bland pulmonary emboli with infarction may also cavitate. The presence of risk factors for pulmonary emboli and a positive ventilation-perfusion scan suggest the diagnosis.

Cavitary sarcoidosis also may be overlooked in the differential diagnosis of cavitary lesions of the lung. Patients with long-standing, extensive sarcoid involvement of the pulmonary parenchyma may develop extensive fibrosis and thin-walled cavities. Often these cavities become superinfected by fungi; and occasionally they cause life-threatening hemoptysis, requiring emergency thoracotomy with resection of the offending lung parenchyma.

Cavitary disease is not infrequent in Wegener's granulomatosis. Intranasal lesions should be sought and biopsied to possibly avoid more invasive pulmonary procedures (usually open lung biopsy). In patients with rheumatoid arthritis, preexisting nodules may undergo cavitation (necrobiotic lesions). This change usually occurs with long-standing disease and rarely presents diagnostic difficulties, especially when previous radiographs are available.

Mediastinal Disease

Most disorders of the mediastinum are inflammatory in nature.[9] It must be remembered that primary tuberculosis, especially in children, can initially manifest as mediastinal adenopathy (a rare manifestation of tuberculosis in adults). Other inflammatory conditions that may cause mediastinal adenopathy include primary coccidioidomycosis and histoplasmosis. Clinical history and supporting laboratory data are essential to establish the diagnosis. The differential diagnosis of mediastinal disease is broad. Anatomic localization of the disorder is important for narrowing the differential diagnosis. Some of the common mediastinal disorders are listed in Table 10.7.

Pleural Disease

Pleural reaction (thickening or fluid) is an important response to many infectious and noninfectious insults to the pleura. If the pleural reaction is secondary to an infection, a pleural effusion usually occurs. Pleural fluid may be a transudate, exudate, empyema, or chyle.

The history and laboratory data are often helpful for determining the etiology of pleural fluid. For example, a patient with a history of a recent myocardial infarction who develops a pleural effusion may have Dressler syndrome. Pleural fluid in a patient with pulmonary emboli suggests the diagnosis of pulmonary infarction, and pleural fluid in a patient with recent trauma suggests the presence of a hemothorax.

To evaluate the cause of the pleural fluid, diagnostic thoracentesis is often required. Careful examination of the fluid is essential. A transudate is usually clear, has a specific gravity of less than 1.016, and contains

TABLE 10.7. Mediastinal masses: differential diagnosis.

Anterior site
Thymoma
Thyroid gland
Teratoma
Lymphoma
Middle site
Lymphadenopathy
Bronchogenic cyst
Aneurysm
Enteric cyst
Hiatus hernia
Posterior site
Neurogenic tumor
Lymphoma
Enteric cyst
Lymphadenopathy
Hernia of the foramen of Bochdelak
Aneurysm
Extramedullary hematopoiesis

TABLE 10.8. Pleural effusion: differential diagnosis.

Transudative pleural effusions
Congestive heart failure
Cirrhosis of the liver
Nephrotic syndrome
Hypoproteinemia
Exudative pleural effusions
Infectious diseases
Neoplastic diseases
Collagen-vascular diseases
Pulmonary embolization
Trauma
Drug hypersensitivity

protein at a concentration of less than 3 g/dl.[10] Noninfected exudates are often clear yellow fluid, have a specific gravity higher than 1.016, and contain protein at a concentration of more than 3 g/dl. Furthermore, exudates may have lactate dehydrogenase levels greater than 200 IU. Exudates may be bloody or have a high white blood cell count. Table 10.8 lists some of the common causes of pleural fluid transudates and exudates.

When an effusion is secondary to pancreatitis, the fluid may contain a high level of amylase. A high amylase level may also be found with a ruptured esophagus, where salivary amylase is present in the pleural space in large amounts. Effusions secondary to rheumatoid arthritis contain low pH and low glucose levels and may have a positive rheumatoid factor and a low complement level.

Cytologic evaluation of pleural fluid may be obtained if a malignancy is suspected. The fever, chills, and sweats, so common with infectious pleural effusions, may indeed be due to lymphoma. An abundance of lymphocytes found in the pleural fluid may make a clinician initially consider this entity.

Conclusion

Rapid identification of the causes of infectious lung disease is essential to reduce morbidity and improve survival of all patients. Signs, symptoms, and the radiographic appearances of noninfectious disorders can mimic those of infectious illnesses and may go unrecognized. The differential diagnosis of chest diseases can be divided into basic patterns in order to help organize a diagnostic approach.

References

1. Reynolds HY: Lung host defenses—a status report. Chest 1979;75(s):239.
2. Bates DV: Chronic bronchitis and emphysema. N Engl J Med 1968;278:546.
3. Irwin RS, Rosen MJ, Bramon SS: Cough: a comprehensive review. Arch Intern Med 1977;62:361.
4. Littner MR, Schachter EN, Putnam CE, et al: The clinical assessment of roentgenographically atypical pulmonary sarcoidosis. Am J Med 1987;62:361.
5. Hunnighake GW, Fauci AS: Pulmonary involvement in collagen vascular diseases. Am Rev Respir Dis 1979;119:471.
6. Steele JD: Solitaire pulmonary nodule. J Thorac Cardiovasc Surg 1963;46:21.
7. Byrd RB, Carr DT, Miller WE, et al: Radiographic abnormalities in carcinoma of the lung as related to histological cell type. Thorax 1969;24:573.
8. Geddes DM: Hypothesis: the natural history of lung cancer: review based on rates of tumor growth. Br J Dis Chest 1979;73:1.
9. Lyons HA, Calvy GL, Samson BP: The diagnosis and classification of mediastinal masses. I. A study of 782 cases. Ann Intern Med 1959;51:897.
10. Light RW, MacGregor MI, Luchsinger PC, Ball WC: Pleural effusions: the diagnostic separations of transudates and exudates. Ann Intern Med 1972;77:507.

11
Pitfalls in the Diagnosis of Pneumonia

Burke A. Cunha

As the diagnosis of pneumonia depends on a careful analysis of historical information, the physical examination, the chest roentgenogram, and selective laboratory values, the "pitfalls in the diagnosis of pneumonia" are concerned with noninfectious entities that may mimic bacterial pneumonia. There are two major areas of diagnostic difficulty facing the clinician who approaches the patient with presumed pneumonia. First, it must be determined if the patient in fact has an infectious explanation for the pulmonary symptomatology and findings, or if the process is noninfectious but has features that mimic an infectious pneumonia (Table 11.1). Second, if the process is infectious, the presentation may be atypical and mimic a noninfectious disorder in certain subpopulations (e.g., compromised hosts, the elderly, children). The essential diagnostic task is to differentiate infectious from noninfectious processes. The most common diagnostic confusion is caused by malignant diseases and, to a lesser extent, collagen-vascular diseases, drug reactions, and radiation pneumonitis.[1–6] The clue to diagnostic pitfalls exists among the historical clues, physical findings, chest film abnormalities, and key laboratory tests. Such pitfalls should be kept in mind to avoid over- or underdiagnosing the infectious pneumonias.

History

When obtaining a history, keep in mind the noninfectious conditions that can mimic an infection so additional information may be found to corroborate the diagnostic impression during the physical examination and subsequent laboratory tests. For example, hemoptysis is a cardinal sign of many diseases but most frequently suggests bronchitis, bronchiectasis, bronchogenic carcinoma, or pulmonary embolus. It is important not to forget that these noninfectious etiologies may mimic an infectious pneumonia presenting with hemoptysis (e.g., *Klebsiella*, *Streptococcus pneu-*

TABLE 11.1. Noninfectious mimics of pneumonia.

Common	Uncommon
Acute	
Left ventricular failure	Eosinophilic pneumonias
Adult respiratory distress syndrome	Leukoagglutinin reactions
Hypersensitivity pneumonitis	Noncardiogenic pulmonary edema
Systemic lupus erythematosus	
Pulmonary emboli/infarction	
Chronic	
Bronchogenic carcinomas	Eosinophilic pneumonias
Sarcoidosis	Rheumatoid lung
Wegener's granulomatosis	Radiation pneumonitis

moniae, viral influenza, or *Mycobacterium tuberculosis*). Mitral stenosis is an often forgotten cause of hemoptysis, and its presence is suggested by characteristic findings on auscultation of the heart during the physical examination. Similarly, pleuritic chest pain may be infectious or noninfectious. Without an associated pulmonary infiltrate, one should always think of costochondritis due to coxsackie B viruses, pulmonary embolism, or metastatic carcinoma to a rib before considering the diagnosis of a bacterial pneumonia.[2]

Usually there are historical features that suggest the diagnosis before the chest film or other tests confirm it. It is important to obtain a careful history in terms of previous radiation therapy or medications that may result in a variety of pulmonary reactions that mimic pneumonia. Cough may be an early symptom of pneumonia, but do not forget to consider bronchitis, congestive heart failure, asthma, or bronchogenic carcinoma in such patients before a chest film is ordered. Careful inquiries should be made in terms of a travel history and contact with sick individuals. A history of animal or bird contact is also important especially with respect to the atypical pneumonias (e.g., tularemia, Q fever, psittacosis). The age of the patient suggests age-related diagnostic possibilities.[3,4] For example, malignancy is common in the elderly population but is an unusual cause of pulmonary infiltrates in those under age 40. Using the same line of reasoning, it would be unusual to have the first manifestation of systemic lupus erythematosus (SLE), pneumonitis, in an elderly individual, whereas that is an appropriate diagnostic consideration in a younger patient with the appropriate clinical presentation.[2] Age should not be used to exclude certain diagnoses solely on the basis of low probability, however. Viral influenza and legionnaires' disease are common in elderly patients, but one cannot exclude *Chlamydia pneumoniae* or *Mycoplasma pneumoniae* solely on the basis of advanced age. There are many pitfalls when obtaining a history of conditions that may mimic infectious disorders or vice versa. Such information is best presented in aphoristic form.

Pitfalls

1. Do not forget to inquire about animal contact in a patient with an atypical pneumonia. For example, it is easy to miss the significance of a cat next door having kittens, with airborne *Coxiella* being transmitted via the airborne route to individuals nearby.

2. Histoplasmosis is commonly associated with hilar lymph node calcifications without lymph node enlargement.

3. A coin lesion in a patient with dog contact suggests *Dirofilaria immitis*.

4. In children with a sore throat and pneumonia, be careful not to diagnose bacterial pneumonia, as this picture is a common presentation of adenoviral pneumonitis.

5. Do not overlook the seasonal importance of certain infections; for example, legionnaires' pneumonitis is most common during early fall, whereas viral influenza is most common during late winter or early spring. Influenza in the fall is considered legionnaires' disease until proved otherwise.

6. Alcoholics with cirrhosis suggests *M. tuberculosis* or malignancy.

7. In elderly populations, do not exclude *Mycoplasma* pneumonia or *Chlamydia* pneumoniae (TWAR agent) pneumonia solely on the basis of advanced age. These pneumonias are less common than *Hemophilus influenzae*, *Klebsiella*, or legionnaires' pneumonia in this age group but nevertheless do occur.

8. Be careful not to overlook a history of mild, transient pulmonary hemorrhage in a patient with gastroenteritis and guaiac-positive stool; it suggests *Strongyloides*.

9. Cytomegalovirus (CMV) pneumonitis occurs within the first 6 months after renal transplantation but is uncommon after this time.

10. Radiation pneumonitis develops 2 months after the course of radiation therapy in the fields of irradiated lung.

11. If there is a history of travel to Southeast Asia, one should not overlook the possibility of tuberculosis, melioidosis, or paragonamiasis. Hemoptysis is an important clue to each of these disorders.

12. Do not forget that a history of sinusitis does not necessarily suggest a bacterial process and may be the clue to Wegener's granulomatosis.

13. A nonproductive cough suggests bronchogenic carcinoma, heart failure, or infectious etiologies.

14. Hemoptysis may occur with bronchiectasis, bronchitis, lung abscess, necrotizing bacterial pneumonias, fungal pneumonias,, and neoplasms. In addition, Goodpasture syndrome, Wegener's granulomatosis, and idiopathic hemosiderosis should be considered in the differential diagnosis of hemoptysis. Mitral stenosis is often forgotten as a cause of mild hemoptysis.

15. Acute hoarseness is usually caused by viruses rather than bacteria. However, be careful not to miss *Candida*, which may present with hoarseness and dysphasia.

16. Hoarseness may be the presenting symptom of a pancoast lesion (superior sulcus tumor/squamous cell carcinoma) or a dissecting aortic aneurysm.

17. Community-acquired pneumonia in normal hosts does not present with septic shock.

18. A patient with pneumonia and a sore throat is not likely to have *H. influenzae* or *S. pneumoniae* pneumonia.

19. Hoarseness in a patient with pneumonia suggests *C. pneumoniae* acutely and *M. tuberculosis* if the hoarseness is chronic.

20. Someone who develops shortness of breath acutely may have developed a spontaneous pneumothorax. If pneumothorax is not due to bullous disease, consider legionnaires' disease, eosinophilic granuloma, or osteogenic sarcoma.

21. A history of nightsweats suggests not only *M. tuberculosis* or histoplasmosis but lymphoma as well.

22. Mental confusion may be present with a severe systemic infection, but it may also be the clue to *Legionella* pneumonia. Pneumonia and abdominal pain points to a diagnosis of legionnaires' disease.

23. Do not forget that *Neisseria meningitidis* is a cause of pneumonia in asplenic individuals in addition to the pneumococcus and *H. influenzae*.

24. A drug history is all-important when sorting out pulmonary drug reactions. Acute pulmonary drug reactions may present as pulmonary hemorrhage or noncardiac pulmonary edema. Subacute pulmonary drug reactions manifest as drug-induced lupus or hypersensitivity pneumonitis, whereas chronic pulmonary infiltrates are characteristic of illicit drug abuse and certain drug reactions (e.g., gold or nitrofurantoin).

25. Hemoptysis may occur with tuberculous, *Klebsiella*, pneumococcal, or viral influenza, but do not overlook the more common noninfectious etiologies of hemoptysis (i.e., mitral stenosis, pulmonary embolism, bronchogenic carcinoma, bronchiectasis).

26. Dyspnea out of proportion to clinical findings or the chest film appearance suggests an interstitial disease such as sarcoidosis or interstitial fibrosis. Only relatively few infections present with disproportionate dyspnea (e.g., viral influenza or *Pneumocystis carinii* in a compromised host).

27. Obscure chest pain may be due to a preeruptive phase of herpes zoster, costochondritis (Tietze syndrome), or postpericardiotomy syndrome (Dressler syndrome), but these disease entities are not usually associated with pulmonary infiltrates.

28. Pleuritic chest pain argues against the diagnosis of atypical pneumonia (except *Legionella*) and viral pneumonia (except viral influenza).

29. Be careful not to miss a history of medications (e.g., nitrofurantoin, sulfonamides, bleomycin, gold salts, nitrosoureas, chlorthiazide, busulfan,

methotrexate) or radiation therapy, which may suggest a drug-induced injury or radiation pneumonitis mimicking pneumonia.

30. Always inquire about environmental exposure to inhaled fumes/dusts (e.g., silica, asbestos, talc, sugar cane, beryllium, chlorine, sulfur dioxide), which could explain an undiagnosed pulmonary infiltrate.

31. A history of cough with a negative chest film suggests congestive heart failure, asthma, bronchitis, bronchogenic carcinoma, or bronchial adenoma.

32. The absence of fever in a patient with pneumonia is unusual in the nonelderly, immunocompetent adult.

33. Wheezing by an adult patient with a pulmonary infiltrate almost never indicates an infectious process; the exceptions include endobronchial tuberculosis and postobstructive bacterial pneumonia. Multiple small pulmonary emboli and congestive heart failure are common causes and may be the clue to Churg-Strauss granulomatosis.

Physical Diagnosis

Avoiding pitfalls during the physical examination involves correct interpretation of physical findings and their association with the appropriate clinical entity. A good example is found in the case of clubbing, which is usually associated with cyanotic heart disease, suppurative lung disease, tuberculosis, or bronchogenic carcinoma. Although clubbing occurs with primary biliary cirrhosis and inflammatory bowel disease, these entities are not associated with pulmonary infiltrates and therefore cause no diagnostic difficulty. Painful clubbing immediately suggests bronchogenic carcinoma as the etiology, and a careful search for unidigital clubbing would point to the diagnosis of sarcoidosis.[2,3] The physical findings are best interpreted in light of the history, and when these date or considered together certain diseases are immediately eliminated as diagnostic possibilities (e.g., cyanotic heart disease).

The finding of a pleural effusion on physical examination is of great diagnostic importance because it suggests a wide variety of infectious and noninfectious etiologies. It also provides an analyzable fluid that assists in determining the cause of the pleural effusion. The commonest pitfall associated with pleural effusions and bilateral diffuse infiltrates is to ascribe an infectious explanation to this common clinical problem. Bilateral pleural effusions are never due to infection, with or without associated pulmonary infiltrates. Keeping this aphorism in mind, one can eliminate needlessly treating patients with congestive heart failure (CHF) or adult respiratory distress syndrome (ARDS) with antibiotics for nonexistent but presumed pneumonia. Another example is a positive d'Espine's sign, which is usually due to the bilateral hilar adenopathy associated with sarcoidosis. However, a mass lesion strategically placed between the trachea and the spine would also result in d'Espine's sign being positive, but it would be due to malignancy rather than sarcoidosis.[7] In terms of misinterpreting information, it is a common clinical pitfall to fail to consider the diagnosis of *Mycoplasma* pneumonia in a patient with pharyngitis or otitis, especially if the characteristic but uncommon bullous myringitis is absent. The pitfalls possible with physical findings are presented in aphoristic form here.

Pitfalls

1. A patient with pneumonia and perforated nasal septum suggests Wegener's granulomatosis or disseminated histoplasmosis.
2. In a patient with pneumonitis and mouth ulcers, do not forget SLE or disseminated histoplasmosis.
3. Pneumonitis and conjunctivitis in a neonate suggests *C. trachomatis* pneumonia. An important clue is peripheral eosinophilia and low-grade fevers accompanied by diffuse perihilar interstitial markings on the chest film.
4. With *Mycoplasma* pneumonia, otitis is more common than bullous meningitis.
5. Splenomegaly in a patient with pneumonia suggests Q fever, disseminated tuberculosis, histoplasmosis, or lymphoma.
6. A pulse-temperature deficit (relative bradycardia) is an uncommon finding with pneumonias. If present, however, it suggests legionnaires' disease or pisttacosis.
7. Noninfectious causes of pulmonary infiltrates usually produce temperatures of 102°F or less (e.g., pulmonary embolism, CHF, ARDS). Pulmonary drug reactions are acutely associated with temperature elevations (e.g., nitrofurantoin), but chronic drug reactions are characteristically associated with little or no fever.
8. Clubbing argues against the diagnosis of pulmonary tuberculosis, and unidigital clubbing suggests sarcoidosis.
9. Bronchogenic carcinoma is the usual cause of painful clubbing.
10. Pulmonary edema without signs of heart failure may be due to drug-induced changes in pulmonary capillary permeability (noncardiopulmonary edema), including aspirin, heroin, nitrofurantoin, thiazides, phenylbutazone, and propoxyphene.

Chest Film

The greatest area for diagnostic error lies in misinterpreting the chest film. Many diseases present with similar findings that suggest a bacterial process, and therein lies the diagnostic dilemma. Because the chest film is key to diagnosing an infectious pneumonia, there are many roentgenographic findings that must be clarified before arriving at the diagnosis of a pneumonia or an infectious process in the chest or lungs. For example, an air bronchogram is correctly considered a sign of consolidation, usually indicative of a bacterial pneumonia; however, one must be wary not to overlook a bronchoalveolar carcinoma or a lymphoma, which occasionally presents in this fashion. Similarly, the bulging fissure sign is usually associated with *Klebsiella* pneumonia but may be found in volume-expanding bacterial pneumonias.[8] Once again, the "great imitator," bronchoalveolar carcinoma, may also present with this finding.[5] Pulmonary infiltrates should be analyzed in terms of their focality, speed of progression and regression, and associated findings (i.e., pulmonary effusions, hilar adenopathy, pulmonary nodules).

Pulmonary infiltrates are usually regarded as the sine qua non for the diagnosis of pneumonia. However, pneumonia without pulmonary infiltrates does occur in specific situations (e.g., very early pneumonia, in patients with endobroncheal tuberculosis, in leukopenic compromised hosts, and in patients with pulmonary emphysema).[8] However, the converse—pulmonary infiltrates without pneumonia—is the more common clinical dilemma. Nodules usually represent granulomatous disease or neoplasia and are rarely associated with pneumonias per se.[9]

In terms of the distribution of pulmonary infiltrates, much has been written with respect to central versus peripheral, upper lobe versus lower lobe, predisposition. This information is presented in asphoristic form below and is useful in a general sense when arriving at a differential diagnosis. For example, peripheral infiltrates except for *Nocardia* and actinomycosis are usually formed on a noninfectious basis. Perihilar infiltrates are characteristic of interstitial diseases (e.g., viral influenza), but one must be careful not to fail to consider radiation pneumonitis or bronchogenic carcinomas.

The rapidity of resolution of a pulmonary infiltrate is most helpful, albeit retrospectively, when determining the cause of the transient evanescent pulmonary infiltrate. Rapidly resolving lesions are virtually never infectious and are most commonly due to CHF, hypersensitivity, or pulmonary drug reactions.[10,11] Slowly resolving pulmonary infiltrates present a much more difficult problem, as many infectious and noninfectious conditions present in this fashion.[12,13] Once again, use of the aphoristic approach and analyzing the chest roentgenogram, in concert with the history and physical examination findings, solve most of the problems without resorting to additional invasive procedures. If there is clinical urgency or if malignancy is a consideration, however, clearly an invasive diagnostic procedure is indicated to arrive at a definitive diagnosis.

Pitfalls

1. In a patient with a "bulging fissure" sign, which usually suggests *Kelbsiella*, *S. pneumoniae*, or *H. influenzae*, do not forget bronchogenic carcinoma, especially bronchoalveolar carcinoma.

2. Solitary nodules are not commonly associated with pulmonary infiltrates. Therefore solitary nodules due to granulomatous diseases (tuberculosis, histoplasmosis), arteriovenous malformations (AVMs), mucoid plugs, *Dirofilaria*, or bronchial adenomas are not usually in cluded in the differential diagnosis of pneumonias.

3. Coccidioidomycosis and sporotrichosis may present with unilateral or bilateral hilar adenopathy.

4. Large bilateral effusions are not usually associated with an infectious etiology. Group A streptococci and primary tuberculosis are the only infectious diseases commonly associated with a large pleural effusion. Bilateral effusions argue strongly against an infectious etiology except in patients with PCP.

5. Consolidation is usually associated with the classic bacterial pneumonias but may be an uncommon feature of legionnaires' disease. The clinician should not forget that bronchoalveolar carcinoma and Wegener's granulomatosis frequently present with consolidative changes.

6. Pneumonia without infiltrates occurs in a few situations: leukopenic compromised host, chronic obstructive pulmonary disease (COPD), endobronchial tuberculosis, or very early pneumonias. Usually, some degree of pulmonary infiltrate is visible on the chest film within 24–48 hours of admission.

7. Minimal pulmonary infiltrates are characteristic of interstitial infection. Characteristically, *Pneumocystis carinii*, *Mycoplasma*, or viral pneumonias may have relatively unimpressive chest film findings.

8. Pulmonary edema is almost always bilateral and symmetric, but be wary of the unilateral pulmonary edema secondary to abnormal lung architecture mimicking pneumonia.

9. In an afebrile patient, peripheral infiltrates, except for actinomycosis and *Nocardia*, usually point to a noninfectious etiology (e.g., drug reaction, adenocarcinoma, large-cell carcinoma, vasculitis, Leoffler syndrome, SLE, or fat emboli).

10. It is unwise to ascribe pulmonary parenchymal involvement to lymphoma unless there is associated hilar adenopathy, which is nearly always bilateral and asymmetric.

11. The resolution of pulmonary infiltrates occurs at varying rates, but rapid resolution/diminution of an infiltrate strongly suggests interstitial fluid shifts (i.e., congestive heart failure).

12. It is unwise to consider sarcoidosis or lymphoma as the diagnosis in a patient with unilateral hilar adenopathy.

13. Be careful not to make the diagnosis of advanced sarcoidosis unless there is typical sparing of the apices.

14. "Eggshell calcification" of the hilar nodes is characteristic of silicosis but rarely is also seen in lymphomas (postradiation therapy) and sarcoidosis.

15. Be careful not to exclude a diagnosis of bronchogenic carcinoma in a patient with unilateral pleural effusion and a pulmonary infiltrate.

Although unilateral effusions are uncommon with most bronchogenic carcinomas, they are commonly found with bronchoalveolar cell carcinoma.

16. Small pleural effusions are common with rheumatoid lungs and SLE but are rare with sarcoidosis.

17. All causes of pulmonary fibrosis affect predominantly the lower lung fields except sarcoidosis, which most often affects the midzones and spares the apices.

18. Single or multiple pulmonary nodules peripherally located are usually neoplastic in origin, whereas centrally located nodes are usually benign (e.g., granulomas).

19. Pulmonary infarction with a pleural effusion is suggested by an elevated hemidiaphragm on the affected side.

Laboratory Tests

Laboratory tests should never be interpreted in a vacuum: They must always be considered in the clinical context of the history, physical examination, and chest film.

Sputum is the most readily available material that can provide either a diagnosis or misleading information for the unwary. First, the sputum must be properly collected and represent a lower respiratory tract specimen. Hence one should guard against overinterpretation of a specimen highly contaminated with epithelial cells, suggesting contamination by oropharyngeal flora. Sputum is not available or is uninterpretable in certain patients. For example, if patients are leukopenic compromised hosts, there are an insufficient number of white blood cells to produce a proper sputum specimen. Conversely, patients with chronic bronchitis produce copious amounts of sputum that is virtually always colonized with multiple organisms; sputum cultures from these patients almost invariably are reported as "normal flora." Sputum is also uninterpretable in the intensive care setting from patients who are intubated or have tracheostomy tubes. The sputum represents the ambient flora in the intensive care setting and does not necessarily represent the pulmonic process deep in the lung parenchyma. In contrast, with community-acquired pneumonias, a properly collected sputum specimen may provide the earliest clue to a definitive diagnosis of bacterial pneumonia, pulmonary tuberculosis, or malignancy.[14,15]

Other helpful laboratory tests are the complete blood count (CBC), platelet count, and erythrocyte sedimentation rate (ESR). The CBC may provide clues to the etiology of the pulmonary infiltrate. For example, typical lymphocytosis suggests a viral etiology, whereas eosinophilia may be the clue to a pulmonary hypersensitivity reaction. Basophilia immediately suggests malignancy, as do nucleated red blood cells. Thrombocytopenia suggests a drug reaction of a viral etiology, whereas thrombocytosis suggests tuberculosis or malignancy. Analogously, the ESR may be useful when properly combined with other clinical information. For example, if a patient presents with a pulmonary infiltrate, weight loss, fever, and night sweats, the differential diagnosis should include tuberculosis versus malignancy. Because the ESR does not usually exceed 70 mm/hour in uncomplicated pulmonary tuberculosis, finding an ESR of 100 mm/hour in such a patient favors the diagnosis of malignancy.[1,2]

Serum serologies provide another possible diagnostic pitfall for clinicians, especially in the diagnosis of viral pneumonias and atypical pneumonias. It is not commonly appreciated that a serologic response to viral infection takes weeks or months to fully develop. Therefore it is a common error to disregard a diagnosis because the initial acute titers are negative or positive or are minimally elevated. This result is to be expected initially, and the diagnosis is confirmed by a fourfold or greater titer rise with a subsequent sample abtained 6–8 weeks later. The convalescent titer is often forgotten and is not obtained after the patient has left the hospital or is well at home. In contrast, the initial positive titers are the problem in patients presenting with *Mycoplasma* pneumonia. If a patient has a pulmonary infiltrate or *Mycoplasma* is considered, usually an enzyme-linked immunosorbent assay (ELISA) is obtained. When the titer is moderately to highly elevated, the pulmonary infiltrate is ascribed to *Mycoplasma*. This diagnostic pitfall can be avoided if one remembers that the ELISA titer measures predominantly the immunoglobulin G (IgG) antibody response, indicating past exposure to the organism. Acute infection requires either a fourfold increase in IgG titers with paired specimens or, more usefully, a positive IgM *Mycoplasma* titer and a positive cold agglutinin titer at 1:64 or more. Obviously, serologic tests are useful for the diagnosis of collagen-vascular diseases as well as some of the fungal pneumonias.

Positive blood cultures rarely cause diagnostic confusion, as there are rarely false positive blood cultures found in association with a pulmonary infiltrate. Organisms that are common denizens of the skin (e.g., *S. aureus*, *S. epidermidis*, enterococcus, *S. viridans*) are uncommon causes of pulmonary infections. When *S. aureus* pneumonia is present, the patient is clinically ill with a readily recognizable syndrome complex, and the diagnosis does not depend on blood culture positivity.[3,4] The aphorisms associated with laboratory tests are presented here.

Pitfalls

1. Do not forget to obtain blood for cultures (×3) in all patients with pneumonia, as it may provide the only retrospective clue to the diagnosis of the patient who cannot produce sputum.

2. Urinary antigen tests for selected pathogens (e.g., pneumococcus, *H. influenzae*, *Legionella*) may be useful for patients unable to produce

sputum. Remember that these tests may not be positive initially, but they remain positive for a long time after the initial infection.

3. A transtracheal aspirate does not necessarily guarantee a lower respiratory tract specimen, as the catheter is often misdirected into the oropharynx.

4. Bronchoalveolar lavage (BAL), if positive, can confirm the diagnosis of *Pneumocytis carinii* pneumonia (PCP) in a human immunodeficiency virus (HIV)-infected patient; however, because PCP is an interstitial disease, a negative BAL does not rule out PCP.

5. Do not rely on sputum in the intensive care unit to diagnose nosocomial pneumonia, as it reflects the flora in the intensive care setting and not that of the lower respiratory tract. Therapy should not be based on sputum samples from endotracheal or tracheostomy site specimens).

6. Positive *Legionella* direct fluorescent antibody (DFA) sputum smears quickly become negative as appropriate antibiotic therapy is begun.

7. Negative *Legionella* titers in a patient presenting with possible *Legionella*, argues for rather than against the diagnosis. Remember, it takes 2–3 weeks for titers to begin to rise and 6–8 weeks for the titers to peak. Also remember that early therapy may delay, blunt, or eliminate the titer rise and eliminate proof of the diagnosis.

8. Be careful not to overinterpret an elevated *Mycoplasma* ELISA titer in a patient with an acute pulmonary infiltrate. *Mycoplasma* ELISA titers measure both IgM, and IgG (predominantly) antibodies and usually reflect prior exposure rather than acute disease. IgM *Mycoplasma* titers detect acute disease, as do elevated cold agglutinin titers of 1:64 or more.

9. The "agglutination association test" readily differentiates cold agglutinins on a viral or *Mycoplasma* basis if the cold agglutinin titer is 1:64 or more.

10. A sputum sample containing squamous epithelial cells suggests upper respiratory contamination and should not be processed or its results overinterpreted.

11. *Candida* does not cause pneumonia. Be careful not to diagnose *Candida* pneumonia on the basis of BAL or protected brush biopsy specimens, where oropharyngeal contamination is common with *Candida* and unavoidable when doing the procedure.

12. An elevated white blood cell (WBC) count or "shift to the left" does not always signify infection. Such shifts of the peripheral WBC count most commonly reflect stress rather than infection.

13. Certain organisms are frequent "colonizers" of sputum in the intensive care setting but are rarely pathogens. Be careful not to "chase" endotracheal aspirates that grow *Achromobacter*, *Enterobacter*, *Flavimonas*, non-*aeruginosa Pseudomonas*, or *Xanthomonas*.

14. Sputum samples from patients with aspiration pneumonia or COPD are notoriously misleading and should not be used to guide therapy. Coverage should be directed against the usual pathogens (e.g., *S. pneu-*

moniae, group A streptococci, *H. influenzae*) rather than relying on sputum data in COPD patients.

15. No polymorphonuclear neutrophils (PMNs) in the sputum in a patient with atypical pneumonia suggests Q fever.

16. Eosinophils in sputum suggest bronchopulmonary aspergillosis in a chronic asthmatic rather than a drug reaction.

17. Sputum assessment is usually misleading in nosocomial pneumonia or leukopenic patients. Empiric therapy should be based on the usual pathogen patterns rather than relying on sputum data.

Mimics

The most common "mimics" of an infectious pulmonary process are malignancies, collagen-vascular diseases, drug reactions, and radiation pneumonitis.[16–18] Therefore utilizing a history, physical examination, chest film, and selected laboratory tests, the clinician should analyze all the diagnostic data to arrive at a working differential diagnosis.

Patients with carcinoma usually present with a subacute course and on chest film show a mass lesion, pleural effusion, or some degree of nodal involvement.[2] The patients with collagen-vascular diseases (e.g., sarcoidosis) usually have extrapulmonary manifestations of these systemic illnesses. Rarely, pulmonary manifestations are the sole or initial finding in rheumatoid arthritis, sarcoidosis, or SLE.[18] This situation is the exception rather than the rule, however, and one must be careful to avoid ascribing these abnormalities to other disease processes. Pulmonary drug reactions depend largely on an adequate history of appropriate drug exposure and may present acutely with pulmonary hemorrhage or pulmonary edema, subacutely or chronically with chronic pulmonary infiltrates and fibrosis. Acute pulmonary reactions are associated with migratory pulmonary infiltrates and peripheral eosinophilia with variable degrees of fever, whereas, in general, chronic pulmonary reactions are characterized by a lack of peripheral eosinophilia, little or no fever, but chronic progressive bilateral and symmetric changes on the chest film[16] (Tables 11.2 and 11.3). The distribution of the lesions is not as important as the appropriate history and evolution in time of the infiltrates for arriving at a proper diagnosis. One should be familiar with the entities associated with noncardiac pulmonary edema, as well as drug-induced SLE. Radiation pneumonitis is suggested by the distribution on the chest film over the irradiated lung fields, as well as a history of irradiation of the chest.[2]

Once again, a diagnostic impression is gained from the "flavor" of the patient's presentation, taking into account all aspects of the history and physical and the proper interpretation of laboratory tests weighed against the appearance of the chest film. In some cases the diagnosis can

TABLE 11.2. Pneumonia: pulmonary drug reactions.

Acute pulmonary infiltrates		Subacute pulmonary infiltrates		Chronic pulmonary infiltrates
Noncardiac pulmonary edema	Pulmonary hemorrhage	Hypersensitivity pneumonitis	Drug-induced pneumonitis	Hypersensitivity: pneumonitis/ pulmonary fibrosis
Nitrofurantoin	Nitrofurantoin	Nitrofurantoin	Procainamide	Nitrofurantoin
Amphotericin B	Anticoagulants	Sulfasalzine	Hydralazine	Sulfasalazine
Acetylsalicylic acid		Isoniazid	Isoniazid	Gold
Opiates		*p*-Aminosalicylic acid	Diphenylhydantoin	Penicillamine
β-Sympathomimetics		Penicillin	Methydopa	Amiodarone
Hydrochlorothiazide			Penicillin	Tocainide
		Gold	Sulfonamides	Methysergide
		Diphenylhydantoin		Intravenous drug abuse
		Carbamazepine		
		Imipramine		
		Sulfonamides		
		Naproxen		
		Penicillamine		
		Hydrazaline		
		Chlorpropramide		
		Dantrolene		

TABLE 11.3. Pneumonias: cancer chemotherapy and drug-induced pulmonary infiltrates.

Drug	Clinical examination	Chest film	Course/outcome
Cyclophosphamide	Period between institution of drug and onset of symptoms variable: 2 weeks to 13 years; toxicity possible after drug is discontinued	Diffuse interstitial infiltrates; acute pulmonary edema pattern	Recovery may follow if drug stopped
Methothrexate	Fever, headache, malasie, dyspnea; peripheral eosinophilia 50%; skin rash 15%	Bibasilar infiltrates; pleural effusion rare	Recovery 1–6 weeks if drug stopped
Chlorambucil	Fever, anorexia, cough month to years after drug	Bibasilar interstitial infiltrates	Response to glucocorticoids variable; recovery may follow if drug stopped
Cytosine arabinoside	Noncardiogenic pulmonary edema within 4 weeks of taking drug or discontinuing it	Diffuse interstitial infiltrates	Fatal noncardiogenic pulmonary edema
Busulfan	Subacute onset of symptoms occurs during drug therapy	Diffuse pattern, intersitital or acinar; pleural effusion rare	Usually no recovery even if drug stopped
Azathioprine	Fever, dyspnea	Diffuse intersitital infiltrates	Recover may follow if drug stopped

be determined noninvasively; for example, serologic tests for fungi or *Dirofilaria* can help rule in infectious etiologies, and anti-native DNA, antinuclear antibody (ANA) titers, and the rheumatoid factor test can help point to a collagen-vascular disease.[17–20] The presence of a pleural effusion is of great importance for the diagnosis of collagen-vascular diseases and malignancy and to a lesser extent for pulmonary embolic disease or pulmonary drug reactions. Once again, rarely is a single finding pathognomonic; rather, all findings must be considered together in the proper clinical context, which goes far for determining a definitive diagnosis[1] (Table 11.4). The aphorisms for malignant disease, collagen-vascular disease, drug reactions, radiation pneumonitis, and miscellaneous conditions are presented below.

Neoplastic Pitfalls

1. Hilar enlargement is frequently associated with middle mediastinal adenopathy. The most common causes of unilateral hilar adenopathy are bronchogenic carcinomas, particularly squamous cell or small-cell anaplastic carcinomas, primary tuberculosis, fungal infections, lymphomas, and metastatic carcinomas.

2. A fine reticular pattern on chest film in association with hilar adenopathy never indicates an infectious process. The differential diagnosis includes sarcoidosis, lymphoma, leukemia, small-cell carcinoma, metastases, or silicosis.

3. Unilateral hilar adenopathy secondary to lymphoma is unusual. Involvement is usually asymmetric but bilateral with lymphomas.

4. Lymphangitic spread of a carcinoma may also rarely lead to bilateral hilar adenopathy.

5. Viruses may cause bilateral hilar adenopathy in children but not commonly in adults. Bilateral hilar adenopathy secondary to malignancy is more common in children.

6. Leukemias occasionally are associated with bilateral hilar adenopathy in concert with bronchopulmonary adenopathy. Pleural effusion and parenchymal lung involvement with leukemia occurs in 25% of patients.

7. Lymphoma is associated with hilar adenopathy where it is calcified following radiation therapy.

8. Bilateral hilar adenopathy in acquired immunodeficiency syndrome (AIDS) patients may be due to pneumonia or AIDS-related lymphomas.

9. With sarcoidosis hilar nodes decrease as the disease progresses; and with lymphoma the nodes increase as the disease progresses.

10. Pseudolymphoma involving the hilar nodes in the absence of a pulmonary infiltrate suggests phenytoin (Dilantin).

11. Ten percent of bronchogenic carcinomas cavitate. Cavitation is most common with squamous cell carcinomas and never occurs in small-cell anaplastic (oat cell) carcinomas.

TABLE 11.4. Pneumonia: eosinophilic pulmonary infiltrates.

Disorder	History of asthma	Signs and symptoms	Laboratory tests	Diagnosis
Drug-induced eosinophilic pneumonias		Dry cough, fever, chills, dyspnea	Chest film: patchy infiltrates, eosinophic pleural effusions in some Blood eosinophilia	Withdrawal of causative drug results in rapid improvement
Chronic eosinophilic pneumonia	±	High fevers, night sweats, chills, dyspnea, weight loss, sometimes coexisting bronchial asthma	Chest film: peripheral infiltrates Blood eosinophilia	Lung biopsy: eosinophils with mononuclear cell
Bronchopulmonary aspergillosis		Chronic asthmatics with brownish sputum, wheezing	Fleeting infiltrates on chest film Blood and sputum eosinophilia	↑ Serum *Aspergillus* precipitins; eosinophils and *A. fumigatus* in sputum
Loeffler syndrome	–	Low-grade fever, myalgias, dry cough, not "sick"	Chest film: peripheral densities or fleeting infiltrates Blood and tissue eosinophilia	Benign, acute, self-limiting; diagnosis of exclusion
Churg-Strauss allergic granulomatosis	+	Skin, renal, and CNS involvement with fever, wheezing; mimics CHF	Chest film: nodular densities Blood eosinophilia	Lung biopsy: granulomatous eosinophilia; vessels of different size involved (i.e., vasculitis)
Parasitic infestations	–	Dry cough, not "sick"	Migratory pulmonary infiltrates Blood eosinophilia	*Wuchereria* or *Toxocara* serologies; *Ascaris*, *Ancylostoma*, *Strongyloides* in stools
Hypereosinophilic syndrome	–	Fever, weight loss, hepatosplenomegaly, adenopathy	Migratory pulmonary infiltrates Blood and tissue eosinophilia	Bone marrow: eosinophilic preleukemia

12. Metastases cavitate less commonly than bronchogenic carcinomas and usually have thick-walled cavities. Thin-walled cavities in metastatic lesions suggest a primary cancer of the head or neck. A cavitating lesion with an air-fluid level suggests an abscess or a lymphoma.

13. Air-fluid levels may be found with lymphomas and *S. aureus*, *Klebsiella*, or *Proteus* oat cell lesions. A single thick-walled upper lobe cavity suggests *Klebsiella*.

14. Bronchial adenomas are most common in women 30–50 years of age; they are centrally located and may be associated with an obstructive pneumonia. Hemoptysis occurs in 50%. They have a predilection for the upper and middle lobes; and calcification and cavitation are rare. Twenty percent are solitary peripheral nodules, well circumscribed, and lobulated.

15. Linear stranding is characteristic of carcinoma extending from the lesion toward the pleura. Alveolar cell carcinoma tends to be peripheral and may be associated with an air bronchogram or bulging fissure sign, but cavitation rarely occurs.

16. Calcifications argue against the diagnosis of bronchogenic carcinoma except when carcinoma develops in a calcified scar. Which is usually an adenocarcinoma.

17. Hematogenous metastases are multiple in 75% of cases and solitary in 25%. Pulmonary metastatic lesions rarely cause clinical symptoms.

18. Calcification in a metastatic lesion occurs only with osteogenic sarcomas, mucinous adenocarcinomas, and bone-forming sarcomas.

19. Lymphomas rarely obstruct bronchi and may be associated with air bronchograms. Cavitation is rare. Most cases are associated with hilar or mediastinal adenopathy.

20. Metastatic calcifications due to secondary hyperparathyroidism or multiple myeloma occur predominatly in upper zone lung fields.

21. Solitary nodules that may calcify but are malignant include chondrosarcomas, mucinous adenocarcinomas of the colon or breast, papillary carcinoma of the thyroid, carcinoids, and cystadenomas of the ovary.

22. AVMs are well defined and usually lobulated. Calcification is rare. A feeder vessel is usually present.

23. Commonest metastases to the lungs are from breast, thyroid, kidney, gastrointestinal tract, and tests. In children one sees Wilms' tumor, Ewing's sarcoma, neuroblastoma, or osteogenic sarcoma.

24. Metastatic lesions tend to be peripheral on the lower lobe. Hilar adenopathy and effusions are uncommon. Ill-defined lesions suggest a primary lesion in the prostate, breast, stomach, or testes. Central nervous system (CNS) tumors rarely metastasize to the lungs.

25. A right pleural effusion is found 65% of the time and a left pleural effusion 10% of the time. Bilateral pleural effusion is seen 20% of the time with Meigs' tumor.

26. The mediastinum shifts away from the hilum if there is a pleural effusion; but if the effusion is due to bronchogenic carcinoma, the

mediastinum deviates toward the tumor. Bilateral effusions are never due to bronchogenic carcinoma.

27. Bilateral effusions are usually due to heart failure, nonbronchogenic carcinomas, metastatic carcinomas, lymphomas, and SLE.

28. Carcinomatous effusions are usually due to bronchogenic carcinomas when associated with cough or chest pain.

29. Malignant effusion is uncommon in individuals under age 40. Malignant pleural effusion is likely if there is splenomegaly, superior vena cava syndrome, hepatomegaly, pelvic mass, clubbing, tibial periostitis, or superclavicular adenopathy.

30. Pleural effusion associated with a fine or reticular parenchymal pattern does not suggest an infectious etiology. Other causes include congestive heart failure, rheumatoid nodules, lymphangitic spread, and leukemias and lymphomas.

31. Bloody pleural effusions suggest a malignant process, thromboembolism, or trauma. Red blood cells (RBCs) are needed to give pleural fluid a red color. More than 100,000 RBCs produce a grossly red pleural fluid.

32. Carcinomatous effusions are usually bloody with a lymphocytic predominance (2000–4000), a normal though slightly depressed glucose level, and pH over 7.3.

33. Among the malignant causes of pleural effusion, only mesotheliomas commonly produce pH less than 7.3. A clue to a mesothelioma is a bloody pleural effusion fluid that is highly viscous.

34. Rapidly occurring pleural effusion suggests hemorrhage or group A streptococcal pneumonia, whereas rapid recurrent accumulation of pleural fluid suggests malignancy.

35. The commonest malignancies with a pleural effusion are lymphomas and alveolar cell carcinoma.

36. Pleural effusion without hilar adenopathy suggests an occult retroperitoneal lymphoma.

37. Diffuse pulmonary nodules with pleural effusions and a normal heart size suggest metastatic carcinoma.

38. The only chest finding with carcinoma of the pancreas is isolated pleural effusion.

39. Pleural effusion with an otherwise normal chest film suggests peripheral carcinogenic carcinoma, metastases, mesothelioma, SLE, rheumatoid arthritis, or primary tuberculosis.

Collagen-Vascular Disease Pitfalls

1. Recurrent pleural effusion with subsequent pleural thickening suggests rheumatoid arthritis or tuberculosis.

2. Patients with sarcoidosis and a pleural effusion should be considered to have tuberculosis or metastatic carcinoma until proved otherwise.

3. Bilateral pleural effusion in SLE patients with cardiomegaly suggests pericardial effusion.

4. Pleural effusion may be a presenting sign of rheumatoid arthritis.

5. Bilateral hilar adenopathy associated with a pleural effusion suggests lymphoma or tuberculosis and argues against the diagnosis of sarcoidosis.

6. "Lobulated" bilateral hilar adenopathy suggests the diagnosis of sarcoidosis. A clear channel between the cardiac shadow and the hilum suggests sarcoidosis versus lymphoma. An enlarged azygos node also suggests sarcoidosis.

7. Five percent of patients with sarcoidosis have eggshell calcifications of the symmetric bilateral hilar adenopathy. Calcifications take more than 6 years to appear and are associated with advanced pulmonary disease.

8. Unilateral or bilateral paratracheal adenopathy suggests sarcoidosis with bilateral or hilar adenopathy.

9. Lymphomas, when associated with paratracheal lymphadenopathy, are usually asymmetric, in contrast to sarcoidosis.

10. The most common cause of bilateral hilar adenopathy is sarcoidosis, which may be mimicked by lymphoma or metastatic carcinoma.

11. Sarcoid presents as unilateral hilar adenopathy in fewer than 1–5% of cases.

12. Rheumatoid nodules may be thick- or thin-walled and have a smooth inner surface; they are most common in the lower lobes.

13. Rheumatoid nodules cavitate commonly but do not calcify. Caplan syndrome nodules occur in crops, and both calcification and cavitation occur.

14. Dressler syndrome usually occurs 1 week after cardiothoracic surgery. Pain is usually pleuritic and may involve the shoulder. Pain after myocardial infarction lasts 1 day only.

15. A miliary pattern on the chest film may be caused by tuberculosis, histoplasmosis, or coccidiodomycosis. There are many noninfectious diseases that may mimic these disorders as well, including eosinophilic granuloma, sarcoidosis, hypersensitivity pneumonitis, carcinoma with lymphangitis spread, lymphoma, or alveolar cell carcinoma.

16. The best way to diagnose miliary tuberculosis is by liver or bone marrow biopsy. The chest film is often negative in miliary tuberculosis patients.

17. In SLE patients recurrences with pleural effusions are the rule; and pleural effusions may be the only sign of lupus pneumonitis.

18. Lupus effusions are never bloody, never large, never full of PMNs; and they never have a low glucose level.

19. Only rheumatoid arthritis and SLE among the collagen-vascular diseases are commonly associated with pleural effusions.

20. Increased pleural fluid protein suggests tuberculosis or rheumatoid arthritis.

21. Rheumatoid arthritis may be associated with a negative chest film.

22. Rheumatoid arthritis is associated with chronic pleural effusions that vary in size, as do the subcutaneous nodules.

23. One-third of rheumatoid effusions are bilateral and are prone to empyema.

24. Rheumatoid effusions are characterized by "debris" and "tadpole-shaped" epithelial cells, as well as by extracellular material.

25. Undetectably low pleural fluid glucose suggests rheumatoid arthritis.

26. A low pleural fluid pH and low glucose level suggest rheumatoid arthritis or tuberculosis, rarely carcinoma.

27. Transudates are due to cirrhosis, congestive heart failure, or nephrosis. Transudates are occasionally seen with pulmonary emboli or sarcoidosis.

Miscellaneous Pitfalls

1. Acute pulmonary drug reactions are frequently associated with pleural effusions, whereas with chronic pulmonary drug reactions effusion is rare.

2. The pleural effusion from a pulmonary embolus takes a few days to develop. PMNs are characteristic, but they are present in low numbers.

3. Ten to fifteen percent of patients with cirrhosis have an effusion, more commonly on the right than on the left.

4. The "shaggy heart" sign may be found with asbestosis or pertussis.

5. Honeycomb lung, which is a generalized reticular nodular pattern, never appears with an infectious process.

6. Empyema can be distinguished from chylothorax by centrifugation, after which, if due to empyema, a clear supernatant results.

7. Abdominal hydatid cysts are multiseptate and usually calcified; calcification does not occur in lung lesions.

8. A regular inner surface of a right lower lobe cavity with pleural effusion suggests amebiasis. A thin-walled cavitary lesion with a "hump" on the inner surface suggests paragonamiasis.

9. Do not confuse pulmonary artery enlargement for unilateral hilar adenopathy. Pulmonary artery enlargement may be due to poststenotic dilatation on the left side, massive pulmonary embolus to one lung, or aortic aneurysm.

10. Silicosis is always symmetric, as is extrinsic allergic alveolitis and chronic berylliosis.

11. Calcification of the hilar lymph nodes is seen in about 5% of patients with silicosis. The anterior and posterior mediastinal, cervical, or intraperitoneal nodes may be calcified as well. Only 1% of patients with coalminers' pneumoconiosis have eggshell calcifications of the hilar nodes.

12. "Eggshell calcifications" of the hilar nodes should not be confused with aortic calcifications and the wall of a saccular aneurysm.

13. Be wary of fibromas and dermoid cysts of the anterior mediastinum with "rim calcifications" mimicking the eggshell calcifications of the hilar nodes.

14. Other causes of symmetric hilar adenopathy include the eosinophilic granuloma, idiopathic pulmonary hemosiderosis, Goodpasture syndrome, and drug-induced pulmonary reactions.

15. Air-fluid levels argue against the diagnosis of Wegener's granulomatosis. Multiple thick-walled cavities bilaterally with an irregular inner surface are characteristic, as the irregular inner surface is due to hemorrhage.

16. Cavitation in a pulmonary infarct suggests septic pulmonary emboli rather than bland pulmonary emboli, as cavitation of bland emboli in infarcts is unusual.

17. Pancreatitis usually produces a left-sided pleural effusion, but it may be on the right or bilateral.

18. "Yellow nail syndrome" is the association of pleural effusion with lymphedema and yellow nails. It is benign and requires no further workup.

19. A chylous pleural effusions is milky in appearance and usually accompanied by an elevated triglyceride level without cholesterol crystals.

20. Peripneumonic effusions may be differentiated from chylous effusions by the cholesterol crystals and normal triglyceride levels in the pleural fluid.

21. One-third of patients with nephrotic syndrome have associated thromboembolism.

22. Most transudates have WBC counts under 1500 cells/mm^3.

23. In the absence of a positive Gram stain, PMNs in low number in the pleural fluid suggest CHF or pulmonary embolism.

24. Pneumothorax may be associated with eosinophilic pleural fluid and

suggests pulmonary thromboembolism or asbestosis.

25. Transudates usually have a normal pH, few WBCs with a lymphocytic predominance, and a normal glucose level.

26. A pleural effusion with ascites suggests Meigs syndrome, nephrosis, cirrhosis, or CHF.

Tuberculosis Pitfalls

1. Pleural calcification indicates empyema, tuberculosis, hemothorax, talc, or asbestos exposure.

2. The only atypical pneumonia with a bloody pleural effusion is tularemia.

3. Pleural effusion argues against the diagnosis of viral pneumonia and is uncommon with *Mycoplasma* pneumonia.

4. Eosinophils argue against the diagnosis of tuberculous pleural effusion.

5. Pleural fluid in tuberculosis may be serosanguineous but is rarely grossly bloody.

6. The higher the lymphocyte count in the pleural fluid, the more likely is tuberculosis.

7. One-third of patients with tuberculosis eventually develop a tuberculous pleural effusion. Axillary pleural pain is a clue to tuberculous effusion.

8. Tuberculosis is not associated with clubbing, eosinophilia, or gross blood in the pleural fluid. A count of more than 3000 WBCs goes against the diagnosis of tuberculous pleural effusion.

9. Tuberculous pleural effusions characteristically have low glucose and elevated protein levels and are prone to spontaneous resolution.

10. Atypical tuberculosis produces smaller effusion than that caused by *M. tuberculosis*.

11. Sixty-five percent of idiopathic pleural effusions in PPD-positive individuals develop tuberculosis within 5 years. The protein in tuberculosis-related pleural effusions is characteristically more than 4 g/dl.

12. Nocardiosis and actinomycosis are associated with empyema and rib involvement. Thick-walled large solitary cavitary lesions, especially of the upper lobes, favor a diagnosis of actinomycosis or nocardiosis.

13. Tuberculosis and coccidioidomycosis may have air-fluid levels.

14. Primary tuberculosis is unilateral 60% of the time. Bilateral node enlargement is rare, and ipsilateral paratracheal node enlargement is present in 40% of cases. There is no hilar adenopathy with reactivation tuberculosis.

15. Tuberculous cavities have a predilection for the apical and posterior segments of the upper lobes and superior segment of the lower lobes.

16. Air-fluid levels argue against the diagnosis of tuberculosis, as does an irregular wall cavity because tuberculous cavities tend to have a smooth inner surface.

17. Pneumatoceles are found in children with staphylococcal pneumonia; less commonly they are seen in adults with PCP and group A streptococcus pneumonia in AIDS patients.

18. Cavitation argues against the diagnosis of *S. pneumoniae* and legionnaires' disease.

19. Most thick-walled cavities become thin-walled over time.

20. The larger the lung cavity, the more likely it is due to anaerobic bacteria.

21. Upper lobe cavitary lesions due to bacteria include chronic *Klebsiella* and *Proteus* lesions, of both which cause upper lobe abscesses. A clue to a *Klebsiella* lesion is the "shaggy border" within the thick-walled cavity.

22. Tropical eosinophilia is occasionally associated with bilateral node involvement when caused by filariasis.

23. Tularemia is characterized by unitaleral hilar node involvement, with "ovoid" parenchymal densities and bloody pleural effusion. Unilateral hilar adenopathy occurs in 25–50% of tularemic pneumonias.

24. Mediastinal widening and hemorrhagic mediastinitis associated with pleural effusion suggest anthrax.

25. Lymph node enlargement is rare in adults with *Mycoplasma* pneumonia but is not uncommon in children. Unilateral ill-defined lower lobe infiltrates are the rule with *Mycoplasma* pneumonia.

Fungal Pitfalls

1. Patients with leukopenia do not usually develop fungal pneumonias until after at least 2 weeks of profound leukopenia.

2. "Satellite calcifications" suggest tuberculosis or histoplasmosis.

3. Leukopenic compromised hosts, when infected with *Mucor*, do not get rhinocerebral mucormycosis; rather, pulmonary mucormycosis develops.

4. A cavitary lesion of the lower lobe is not blastomycosis or cryptococcosis. *Cryptococcus* is characteristically pleura-based, but effusions are uncommon.

5. Calcifications and cavitation are uncommon with coccidioidomycosis.

6. A large lower lobe peripheral lesion without rib involvement favors the diagnosis of cryptococcosis or carcinoma. Cavitation and hilar adenopathy are not features of cryptococcosis.

7. Unlike tuberculosis, coccidioidomycosis has a predilection for the anterior segment of the upper lobes.

8. Histoplasmosis may mimic tuberculosis by having a similar upper lobe location, and it may coexist as a coinfection in the same patient.

9. Hilar adenopathy is a common feature of all fungal pneumonias except blastomycosis.

10. Enlargement of the paratracheal lymph nodes in a patient with coccidioidomycosis may indicate imminent dissemination, as may the disappearance of erythema nodosum.

11. The presence of an ipsilateral paratracheal node in a fungal pneumonia with unilateral hilar adenopathy favors the diagnosis of coccidioidomycosis.

Summary

Noninfectious diseases mimicking the infectious pneumonias usually present with little or no fever. Their presentation is subacute or chronic, and there are associated extrapulmonary laboratory or physical findings. When obtaining the history, doing a physical examination, interpreting the chest film, and interpreting laboratory data, the physician should be on the lookout for clues to a noninfectious explanation for the pulmonary symptomatology or the roentgengraphic findings. Almost always it is possible, by combining various diagnostic parameters and using the aphoristic approach, to differentiate between infectious and noninfectious processes as well as to arrive at a working diagnosis within each of the broad diagnostic categories (e.g., malignancies, collagen-vascular diseases, drug hypersensitivy reactions). The definitive diagnosis usually requires an invasive diagnostic procedure in the case of malignancies, but the diagnosis may be made by noninvasive means for a variety of other disorders (e.g., angiotensin-converting enzyme in sarcoidosis, ANA and SLE, eggs or parasites in the stools of a patient with pulmonary infiltrates and eosinophilia).

References

1. Cunha BA, Strampfer MJ: Pearls and pitfalls. In Brandstetter RD (ed): Pulmonary Medicine. Oradell, NJ: Medical Economics, 1989.
2. Wilson JD, Braunwald E, Isselbacher KJ, et al: (eds): Harrison's Principles of Internal Medicine, 12th ed. New York: McGraw-Hill, 1991.
3. Gorbach SL, Bartlett JG, Blacklow NR (eds): Infectious Diseases. Philadelphia, Saunders, 1992.
4. Mandell GL, Gordon-Douglas R Jr, Bennett JE (eds): Principles and Practice of
Infectious Diseases, 3rd ed. New York: Churchill Livingstone, 1985.
5. Brandstetter RD, Hausen HS, Desvarieux H: Noninfectious pulmonary disorders radiographically mimicking infection. Infect Dis Pract 1991;15:1–8.
6. Leatherman JW (ed): Noninfectious pulmonary infiltrates. Semin Respir Infect 1988;3(3):179–274.
7. Sapira JD: The Art and Science of Bedside Diagnosis. Baltimore: Urban & Schwarzenberg, 1990.
8. Reed, JC: Chest Radiology, 3rd ed. St. Louis: Mosby-Year Book, 1991.
9. Lippington GA, Jamplis RW: A Diagnostic Approach to Chest Diseases, 2nd ed. Baltimore: Williams & Wilkins, 1977.
10. Chapman S, Nakielny R: Aids to Radiological Differential Diagnosis, 2nd ed. London: Baillière, Tindall, 1990.
11. Burgener FA, Kormano M: Differential Diagnosis in Conventional Radiology, 2nd ed. New York: Thieme, 1991.
12. Cunha BA: Pneumonias acquired from others. Postgrad Med 1987;82:126–156.
13. Wollschlager CM, Khan FA, Khan A: Utility of radiography and clinical features in the diagnosis of community acquired pneumonia. Clin Chest Med 1987;3:393.
14. Levison ME (ed). The Pneumonias. Boston: John Wright-PSG, 1984.
15. Pennington JE (ed): Respiratory Infections: Diagnosis and Management. New York: Raven Press, 1983.
16. White DA, Cooper JAD Jr: Drug-induced lung disease. In Brandstetter RD (ed): Pulmonary Medicine. Oradell, NJ: Medical Economics, 1989.

17. Matthay RA (ed): Clinics in Chest Medicine: Pulmonary Manifestations of Systemic Disease, Vol. 10. Philadelphia: Saunders, 1989, pp. 469–818.
18. Hunnighake GW, Fauci AS: Pulmonary involvement in collagen vascular diseases. Am Rev Respir Dis 1979;119:471.
19. Sarosi GA, Davies SF (eds): Fungal Diseases of the Lung. Orlando, FL: Grune & Stratton, 1986.
20. Davis SF: Fungal disease. Semin Respir Infect 1990;5(2):91–154.

12
Discharge Strategies for the Patient with Pneumonia

ROBERT D. BRANDSTETTER and ANDREW PUGLIESE

Pneumonia is a significant cause of morbidity and death in the United States, affecting more than 3 million people each year and necessitating the hospitalization of more than 500,000 annually.[1] Although most patients with pneumonia are not admitted to hospital, those who are have a mortality rate of 10–25%.[2] Accordingly, the decision to admit patients with pneumonia is predicated on the fact that they are more ill and likely to have complications of their disease. Furthermore, they represent a group of patients who probably have coexisting chronic disease.

When a patient is admitted with pneumonia, many institutions with utilization review committees immediately inspect the chart and place a sticker in it to remind the physician of the number of hospital days allotted for the pneumonia. Although many variables exist that affect this number, several facts are clear. The cost of hospitalization for a patient with pneumonia is extraordinary. Indeed, some of the newer antibiotics are particularly expensive, coupled with the intravenous fluids administered. Patients with pneumonia may be debilitated, adding another burden to the cost of the admission. Additional ancillary services and subspecialty consultants further contribute to the final charges ultimately generated by the time of discharge.

The purpose of this chapter is to offer some guidelines that may result in the earlier discharge of a patient hospitalized with pneumonia. No published data are available, so what are offered are suggestions and common sense thoughts. Of primary concern is to not allow a situation where premature discharge from the hospital results in the compromise of a patient and ultimate readmission.

At the time of the decision to admit a patient with pneumonia, the physician should plan the likely length of hospitalization. Although it is easier said than done, the reason for admission frequently dictates the duration of hospitalization. For example, patients who have single or multiple lobe involvement on chest roentgenogram, and have nausea or vomiting or are clinically dehydrated, may do surprisingly well with the institution of intravenous antibiotics and hydration. On the other hand, patients with known cardiopulmonary disease or diabetes mellitus who have the simplest pneumonia may require weeks of supportive therapy before successful discharge. This chapter focuses therefore on that gray area between the short hospital stay in the non-intensive-care unit (non-ICU) and the long hospitalization (ICU care).

At the time of admission it seems appropriate to consider all avenues that can speed up the effectiveness of antibiotic therapy and to keep in mind that the compromise of extrapulmonary organs should be minimized or avoided. Finally, at the time of admission, ancillary services such as discharge planning, social services, and home care planning should be contacted so a prompt, nondelayed discharge can be expected. The institution of a flow sheet is not unreasonable to allow the physician to affirm the presence and activity of these important health care professionals. (Fig. 12.1).

The effectiveness of antibiotic therapy must initially be related to the correct diagnosis and selection of the most appropriate antibiotic. Other chapters in this book deal with this point in detail, but suffice it to say a wrong diagnosis resulting in inappropriate antibiotic treatment at the very least results in a longer hospitalization. Once specific or empiric antibiotics are chosen, the route, dose, and interval of administration must be decided. As routine as this process may be, delay in resolution of the pneumonia and prolongation of hospitalization may be anticipated if these aspects are not correctly addressed at the time of admission. There is nothing in the literature stating that everyone admitted with pneumonia must receive parenteral antibiotics. The severity of the pneumonia and the nature of the extrapulmonary manifestations, coupled to the realization that a sense of security is established with parenteral antibiotics, however, makes such therapy preferred. It should be mentioned, though, that most oral antibiotics are not only well tolerated but well absorbed by the intestinal mucosa.

Intravenous routes are employed most often, and it is at this point that intravenous access should always be guaranteed by the physician. Should any question exist on admission as to poor venous access, a central venous line should be considered so antibiotic delivery is guaranteed during the course of hospitalization. Little hesitation should be given to this mode of administering antibiotics, as the morbidity is low, and its benefits are clear.

The dose of antibiotic and interval of administration are variable. It is good practice to consult the hospital pharmacist, the *Physician's Desk Reference*, or other reliable source when a question arises, so the right amount of antibiotic is given over a safe period. Coexisting heart, liver, or renal disease may be present, affecting dosage. The metabolism and excretion of antibiotics must thus be taken into account if the physician is to use correct dosages and intervals. Promptness of clinical improvement is also miximized.

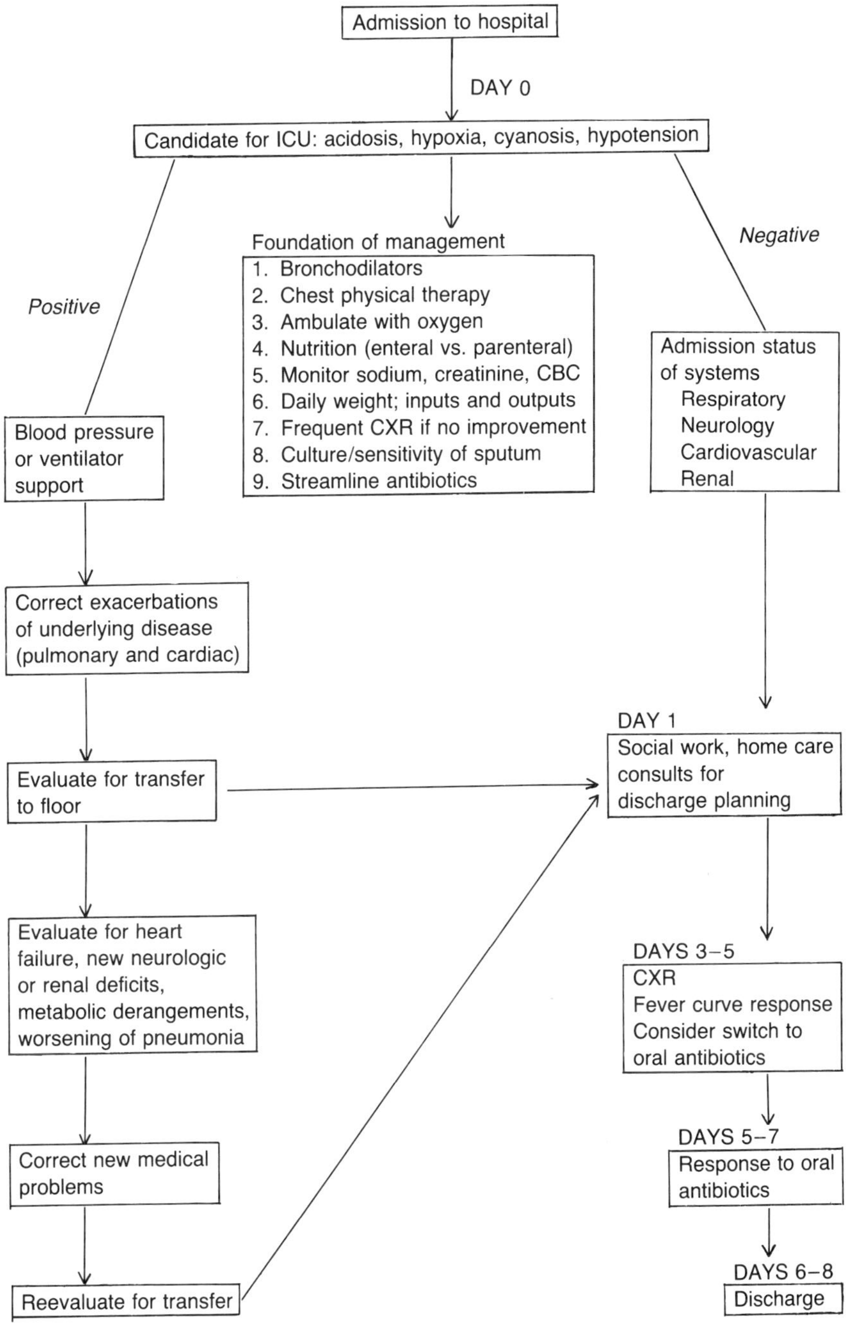

FIGURE 12.1. Discharge planning strategy for pneumonia.

Pulmonary function should be fully addressed at the time of admission and during the course of the hospitalization. Patients who have bilobar infiltrates, cyanosis, or a respiratory rate greater than 30 breaths/minute should have an arterial blood gas assay to determine the degree of hypoxia, the presence of acidemia, and the amount of supplemental oxygen to be administered. Correcting hypoxia can be expected to improve tissue oxygenation and possibly avoid other organ dysfunction.

If there is a problem with giving oxygen to hospitalized patients, it is that it tends to keep them bedridden. Portable oxygen should therefore be considered so the patient can ambulate. Most pneumonias do not dictated "bed rest" and in fact can be harmful if deep vein thromboses occur. Furthermore, ambulation encourages improved pulmonary function by enhancing diaphragmatic excursion and respiratory inspiratory muscle movement. Getting out of bed is also associated with a sense of well-being and in older patients allows early identification of mobility problems. Indeed, in this group of patients intervention by physical therapists is essential, especially early during the course of hospitalization.

It makes sense to utilize methods to enhance pulmonary secretions and to make them less viscid upon expectoration. The use of pharmacologic agents that enhance cilial function in the tracheobronchial tree has been described. These medicines, used principally by the inhalation route, are employed under most circumstances for their bronchodilatory effect. Accordingly, the patient may particularly benefit by the opening of closed lung units and the movement of mucus up and out of the tracheobronchial tree. The use of chest physical therapy early during the course of pneumonia may also be employed to promote drainage of copious and thick secretions.

After consideration of the respiratory system requirements, the physician should then embark on a trouble-shooting scheme to maintain other organ systems in preadmission shape. This point is of particular concern in the elderly, who often display a "domino-like effect" when they are hospitalized: synchronous failure of otherwise stable organs in the setting of a serious illness. Neurologic, cardiac, and renal function are the systems the physician should monitor. Problems can thus be minimized by early identification and a lengthy hospitalization avoided.

There is no question that neurologic dysfunction hampers resolution of pneumonia and thus prolongs hospitalization. Altered mental function, swallowing disorders, and ineffective cough contribute to mobidity associated with pneumonia. Those patients identified with decreased awareness should be discouraged from taking oral feedings for fear of aspiration. Although nasogastric feeding tubes do not guarantee the absence of aspiration (and indeed they may increase aspiration by compromising the seal of the gastroesophageal sphincter), adequate nutrition can be maintained. Avoiding malnutrition, preventing colonization of the gastrointestinal tract with gram-negative organisms, and reducing gastrointestinal bleeding can be expected by giving gastric nutrition. Those patients who cannot have such nasogastric feedings require peripheral administration to ensure nutrition.

The group of patients with swallowing abnormalities would be benefited by consultation with a speech and swallowing specialist. Not infrequently such patients can be "instructed" how to swallow so aspiration does not occur.

Patients who do not have an effective cough should not receive sedatives and should be actively encouraged to cough. Although the cough reflex is spontaneous, it can be enhanced voluntarily. Such patients should also benefit from mucokinetic agents (bronchodilators that enhance cilial function). Furthermore, these patients may also derive improvement in the cough reflex by talking more to other patients, where airflow mechanics may trigger a cough if mucus is present. Getting together with other patients again should foster a better sense of well-being, hopefully resulting in earlier discharge.

During the course of hospitalization an effort should be made to identify new neurologic deficits early in their presentation, so management and intervention can be initiated. Transient ischemic attacks and metabolic encephalopathy may indeed compromise swallowing, leading to aspiration, or result in a depressed cough reflex.

Patients who have Parkinson's disease, or those who pool secretions in the oropharynx should have frequent oral suctioning. The use of anticholinergics to dry up secretions may seem appropriate; however, the overall effect may result in inspirated pulmonary secretions. Accordingly, patients may experience additional difficulty in mobilizing mucus from the lower airways.

In addition to recognizing preexisting and new neurologic deficits, it is important to maintain a good cardiovascular system during the course of managing someone with pneumonia. It is an all too frequent scenario, in particular with the elderly, that respriatory infection exacerbates heart disease. The cardiac response to fever and hypoxia is tachycardia. Additionally, there are potent vasoactive substances, as well as a myocardial depressant factor, that alters myocardial contractility during serious infection. Ischemic episodes or more unstable rhythms, such as supraventricular tachycardia and multifocal atrial tachycardia, may then occur. The early identification and correction of these rhythm disturbances should result in a more stable cardiovascular system during the treatment of pneumonia.

Another common cardiac problem exacerbated by respiratory tract infection is left heart failure. The reason for it may be the aggravating tachycardia and ischemia as well as changes in total body water in the circulating vascular compartment. In patients with preexisting lung disease or pneumonia alone, antidiuretic hormone (ADH) may be released, resulting in increased water and hyponatremia. It has also been shown that volume and pressure changes on the right side of the heart can result in release of an atrial peptide, which in turn can affect renal function—once again by elaboration of ADH. Finally, an increase in water volume may occur as a result of intravenous fluids delivered with the antibiotic.

Addressing these water disturbances is important, as symptoms of heart failure may be indistinguishable from those of pneumonia with preexisting lung disease. Certainly "cardiac asthma" is not uncommon. Daily weights, strict fluid inputs and outputs, prompt mobilization of the patient, cautious use of diuretics, and the early discontinuation of intravenous fluids should result in not only the early recognition of water problems but also prompter discharge from the hospital.

The final organ system not infrequently compromised during the course of pneumonia is the renal system. In addition to responding to ADH release and maintaining the delicate balance between water, sodium, and other electrolytes, renal insufficiency can result from associated hypotension or the use of antibiotics. Frequent monitoring of the blood pressure may allow early recognition of a hypotensive trend, thereby avoiding renal failure. Unfortunately, an acute fall in blood pressure may not be promptly identified, with renal tubular acidosis resulting. Finally, antibiotics such as the aminoglycosides should have appropriate dosages and intervals of administration to prevent renal failure. In addition, peak-and-trough blood levels should be routinely monitored for any change in excretion of the drug that may result in renal toxicity.

Conclusion

The material presented is the basis of good overall medical management of patients with pneumonia. Even though it is principally anecdotal, adhering to these suggestions should result in early discharge from the hospital. It seems unlikely that longer hospitalizations would occur. Figure 12.1 is a practical flow sheet that serves as a reminder of these important factors to the physician when a patients is admitted with pneumonia. If there is any final recommendation, it is that discharge from the hospital. It seems unlikely that longer hospitalizations would occur. Figure 12.1 is a practical flow sheet that serves as a reminder of these important factors to the physician when a patient is admitted with pneumonia. If there is any final recommendation, it is that discharge planning strategies should commence on the day of admission—and not a day later.

References

1. Wollschlager CM, Khan FA, Khan A: Utility of radiography and clinical features in the diagnosis of community-acquired pneumonia. Clin Chest Med 1987;8:393–404.
2. McKellar PP: Treatment of community-acquired pneumonias. Am J Med 1985;79(Suppl 2A):25–30.

INDEX

Q

R